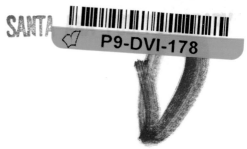

Falls in Older People

Prevention & Management

FOURTH EDITION

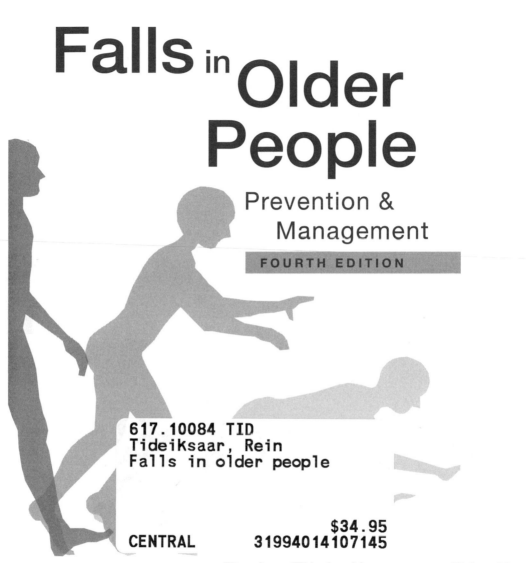

Falls in Older People

Prevention & Management

FOURTH EDITION

Rein Tideiksaar, Ph.D.

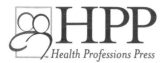

HPP
Health Professions Press

Baltimore • London • Sydney

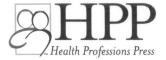

Health Professions Press, Inc.
Post Office Box 10624
Baltimore, MD 21285-0624
www.healthpropress.com

Typeset by Barton Matheson Willse & Worthington, Baltimore, Maryland.
Manufactured in the United States of America by Sheridan Books, Ann Arbor, Michigan.

Illustrations by Juanita Wassenaar-Beggs.
Interior and cover designs by Erin Geoghegan.

The publisher and the author have made every effort to ensure that all of the information and instructions given in this book are accurate and safe, but they cannot accept liability for any resulting injury, damage, or loss to either person or property, whether direct or consequential and however it occurs.

All of the case studies in this book are composites of the author's actual experiences. In all instances, names have been changed; in some instances, identifying details have been altered to protect confidentiality.

Library of Congress Cataloging-in-Publication Data

Tideiksaar, Rein.
    Falls in older people : prevention and management / Rein Tideiksaar.—4th ed.
        p. cm.
    Includes bibliographical references and index.
    ISBN 978-1-932529-44-9 (pbk.)
    1. Falls (Accidents) in old age.   2. Falls (Accidents) in old age—Prevention.   3. Older people—Hospital care.   4. Older people—Nursing home care.   I. Title.
    [DNLM: 1. Accidental Falls—prevention & control. 2. Aged. 3. Risk Factors. WA 288 T558f 2010]
    RC952.5.T53 2010
    617.10084'6—dc22

                                                                   2010002242

British Library Cataloguing in Publication data are available from the British Library.

Contents

About the Author

Rein Tideiksaar, Ph.D., is President of FallPrevent, LLC, a company that provides educational, legal, and marketing services in connection with preventing falls in older adults. Dr. Tideiksaar has been active in the area of fall prevention for more than 25 years. He has directed numerous research projects on falls and has developed fall prevention programs in the community, assisted living, home care, acute care hospital, and nursing facility settings. Dr. Tideiksaar has written numerous articles and book chapters on falls and related topics. In addition to three previous editions of this professional resource, he is the author of *Falling in Old Age: Its Prevention and Treatment, 2nd edition* (Springer Publishing Company, 1997) and the *Essential Falls Management Series* (Health Professions Press), which includes:

- Assessment & Training Tools (2004)

- Guide to Bed Safety (2006)

- Guide to Exit Alarms (2006)

- Managing Falls in Adult Day Services (2006)

- Managing Falls in Assisted Living (2006)

- After the Fall (2007)

- Guide to Hip Protectors (2007)

- Falls and People with Intellectual & Developmental Disabilities (2007).

From 2000 to 2003, Dr. Tideiksaar was the Senior Vice President of Fall Prevention and Injury Reduction Systems, ElderCare Companies, Inc., Point Pleasant Beach, NJ. Prior to 2000, he was Director of Geriatric Educational and Clinical Programs and Director of the Falls and Immobility Program, Department of Geriatrics, Southwest Medical Associates, Inc., Las Vegas, NV; Director of Geriatric Care Coordination, Sierra Health Services, Inc., Las Vegas, NV; and Director of the Falls and Immobility Program, Department of Geriatrics and Adult Development, Mount Sinai Medical Center, New York, NY.

Dr. Tideiksaar obtained a doctorate from Columbia Pacific University and physician assistant certification from the State University of New York at Stony Brook. He completed his geriatric training at the Parker Jewish Geriatric Institute, New Hyde Park, NY.

Preface to the Fourth Edition

Since *Falls in Older People* was first published in 1993, falls have been and continue to be a common problem for hospital patients and nursing facility residents. In fact, falls consistently make up the largest single category of reported incidents and, in some organizations, falls account for up to 70% of adverse events. More important, falls are associated with a host of negative outcomes, including serious injury and even death. In addition to potentially devastating patient and resident outcomes associated with falls, there are also troubling economic outcomes. As of October 2008, the Centers for Medicare and Medicaid Services (CMS) announced that Medicare will no longer pay the extra costs of treating preventable errors or injuries resulting from falls in acute care hospitals. Fall-related injury (or death) is not covered in the list of "Never Events" published by CMS, which are defined as "errors in medical care that are clearly identifiable, preventable, and serious in their consequences." As a result, hospitals will be responsible for the treatment of impacted patients. Most significantly, a facility will be burdened by being responsible for 100% of the cost of such treatment. Many other insurance carriers and secondary payers may soon follow CMS's lead. Medicaid, which covers reimbursement for nursing facilities, may also eventually implement the Never Events policy. As a consequence, it is important that hospitals and nursing facilities seriously and effectively address the problem of falls, especially injurious falls.

Since the early 2000s, acute care hospitals and nursing facilities have devoted a great deal of effort to developing fall prevention programs, especially with Never Events on the front burner. However, despite the existence of solid hospital- and nursing facility-based fall research, which has focused on identifying patients and residents at risk of falls and identifying and addressing individual risk factors, there is a scarcity of concrete evidence of successful preventive efforts in hospitals and nursing facilities.

In my role as a fall prevention expert over many years, I have had the privilege of shadowing or walking in the shoes of a number of caregivers in hospitals and nursing facilities across the United States. I have walked alongside nurses and physicians, nursing assistants, physical therapists, occupational therapists, and administrators. I have learned much from these experiences, and have witnessed tremendous interest and extraordinary efforts by hospitals and nursing facilities to try to prevent falls. And yet patients and residents keep falling. Why?

Despite the best efforts of caregivers, and short of gluing all patients and residents to their beds, we will never be able to completely prevent falls. Nevertheless, there is a great deal that can be done to reduce the likelihood of falls. The ability to prevent falls is largely dependent on caregivers adhering to a clinical process or practice of fall prevention, which identifies factors contributing to falls as well as solutions to reduce the risk of falls. While this is a necessary step, it is insufficient in completely getting the job done. The effectiveness of any fall prevention program is reliant not only on having in place a process of care, but also administrative support, which is crucial in enabling and facilitating a care process. Some of these support activities include promoting a culture of safety (i.e., an atmosphere of "no shame, no blame," in which caregivers are not blamed for falls, but rather falls are looked at as an opportunity to do things better); ongoing caregiver education regarding fall prevention to increase caregiver confidence, knowledge, skills, and ability to identify patients and residents at risk of falls and to select appropriate interventions for the prevention of falls; and appointing a caregiver who can support, coordinate, and champion prevention initiatives. Having in place an organized clinical approach or process as well as administrative leadership are the foundation of a successful fall prevention effort.

The aim of this fourth edition of *Falls in Older People* remains the same—to educate caregivers in hospitals and nursing facilities about falls and what can be done to prevent them. It continues to be my firm belief that if organizations and caregivers are knowledgeable about what causes falls and how to prevent them, then the risk of falls can be greatly minimized. Many years ago when I was a student and learning about falls, one of my professors told me something that remains with me today: "Without a base of knowledge of how things are (and why), you can't really have a reasonable idea about how things ought to be." In writing this edition, I have kept those words in the back of my mind.

In addition to updating the chapters, bibliography, and case study exercises, I have included chapters on key process steps and interventions, organizational requirements and evidence-based practice, and new guidelines and forms for helping hospital and nursing facility professionals develop their fall prevention programs. (All guidelines and forms from Section Three are also available as electronic PDF files on the CD-ROM *Falls in Older People: Assessment and Training Tools*.)

As in previous editions, my hope is that this book will be read from cover to cover until its pages are worn thin through repeated readings. Hopefully this will mean that I have been successful in making the problem of falls understandable and played a part in helping to reduce the risk of falls.

Content of the Book

The book is divided into three sections. Section One, Understanding Falls and Fall Management, gives an overview of and specific suggestions for helping the reader understand the underlying causes of falls and how to develop and maintain an effective fall management program. Chapter One examines the outcome of falls with respect to their consequences for patients and residents, their families, and the institution. Chapter Two reviews the multiple age-related physiological changes, pathological conditions, medications, and environmental and institutional factors associated with falls and fall risk. The clinical approach to the assessment of both falls and fall risk is examined in Chapter Three. Chapter Four explores a number of medical, rehabilitative, and environmental strategies that reduce fall risk. Common environmental causes of falling (e.g., lighting conditions, ground surfaces, furnishings) and their modifications are covered in Chapter Five. Chapter Six is devoted to a discussion of the issues surrounding mechanical and chemical restraints in the management of falls, including a framework for reducing physical restraints.

Section Two, Fall Prevention Practice, which is entirely new to this edition, is designed to support, reinforce, and, in some instances, expand on the information in Section One. Chapter Seven examines key clinical process steps and interventions that are crucial to achieving effective fall prevention. Chapter Eight explores a number of organizational requirements that are important in implementing and maintaining fall prevention programs. Chapter Nine presents a summary of evidence-based practices related to fall prevention.

Section Three, Resources, is divided into three parts: Fall Prevention Guidelines, Home Safety Guidelines, and Forms. Fall Prevention Guidelines discusses a "best clinical practice" approach to the management of falls and fall risk in acute care hospitals and nursing facilities, how best to utilize common safety technologies (e.g., hip protectors, fall alarms, low beds), how to implement effective safety technology solutions, designing monitoring strategies for high-risk patients and residents, and the specific role of nurses and certified nursing assistants in fall prevention. Guidelines are also provided to help readers understand the structure and process of fall prevention and restraint-avoidance programs (i.e., what is needed and what has to happen to achieve success). Home Safety Guidelines is a handout that can be used to educate patients and residents as well as their family members on how to avoid falls when leaving the facility and returning home. Forms, which are photocopiable and referenced throughout the book, includes the comprehensive Performance-Oriented Environmental Mobility Screen (POEMS), a restraint and non-restraint assessment and care planning tool, a wheelchair problems and modifications checklist, discharge teaching sheets that can be given to families when a patient or resident leaves a facility to ensure the optimum safety of the individual at risk of falling at home, high-fall risk room setup, steps to reduce bedside falls, components of a successful fall prevention program, a checklist to audit care plans, safety walk rounds, and a safety culture checklist.

The Appendix includes a number of case study exercises and a problem-solving questions and answers section, which can be used by staff to assist in their fall prevention activities.

While going through *Falls in Older People, Fourth Edition*, the reader will notice some redundancy or repetition of certain materials. This is intentional and with a purpose in mind. It is often said that we remember only about 10% of what we read; therefore, to fully appreciate and understand the topic of fall prevention, some of the subject matter needs to be presented several times in different ways. (In essence, learning is best achieved through repetition!) I'm hopeful that this approach will not only increase the reader's knowledge base, but also will be useful for those who wish to prepare policies, guidelines, procedures, training materials, and other related clinical and/or teaching materials.

Introduction

One of the most common and often critical problems faced by institutionally based health care providers is that of falls among older adults. Hospital falls represent a leading cause of adverse events, accounting for 25%–89% of all reported inpatient incidents.[1] According to hospital fall statistics, the overall risk of a patient falling in the acute care setting is approximately 1.9% to 3% of all hospitalizations.[2] Inpatient fall rates range from 1.7 to 25 falls per 1,000 patient days, depending on the care area, with geropsychiatric patients having the highest risk.[3] To a large extent, this wide range is attributable to differences in various institutional policies (i.e., how falls are defined and reported) and the specific site or location of fall occurrence (e.g., rehabilitation, psychiatric, critical care, orthopedic, medical, surgical). For instance, in subacute or rehabilitation settings up to 46% of patients fall,[4, 5] and in psychiatric hospitals up to 36% of patients experience one or more falls.[6] In the psychiatric or behavioral health setting, fall rates range from 4.5 to 25 falls per 1,000 patient days.[7] In addition, more than 50% of falls in hospitals are not witnessed,[8] which is another factor responsible for inexact knowledge of fall frequencies.

Regardless of exactly how many people fall, people age 65 and older experience the majority of these falls. Studies that compare the age distribution of people with falls show that older people are overrepresented,[9, 10] averaging about 1.5 falls per bed annually.[11] As many as 50% of these older inpatients fall repeatedly.[12] In the nursing facility, a setting to which older people are often admitted for safety reasons, falling is equally problematic. Up to 75% of all nursing facility patients fall each year and greater than 40% experience recurrent episodes. Approximately 50% of those who fall once will have at least one additional fall.[13, 14, 15, 16] An average nursing home with 100 beds will experience anywhere from 100 to 200 falls annually, with the typical nursing home patient experiencing a fall 2.6 times per year.[16] The probability of falling, in both hospitals and nursing facilities, increases with advancing age; the highest incidence of falling occurs in the 80- to 89-year-old age group.[17, 18] This high incidence is more a reflection of the increasing illness and frailty that accompanies aging than it is of old age itself. Falls, particularly repeated falls, are a major cause of physical and psychological trauma. Falls that occur repeatedly are likely to produce a cumulative adverse effect on the individual's capacity for mobility, causing periods of immobility and, as an outcome of complications, premature death (see Figure I-1).

In an effort to prevent falls, health care professionals have tried to protect patients by limiting their mobility, often resorting to the use of mechanical or chemical restraints. However, mobility restrictions and restraint use have

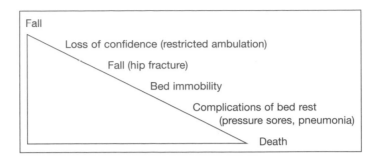

Fall
　　Loss of confidence (restricted ambulation)
　　　　Fall (hip fracture)
　　　　　　Bed immobility
　　　　　　　　Complications of bed rest
　　　　　　　　(pressure sores, pneumonia)
　　　　　　　　　　Death

Figure I-1.　The downward-spiraling effects of falls.

proven to be ineffective in reducing falls and are associated with a host of negative outcomes for older people. Moreover, federal and state governing bodies responsible for regulating hospitals and nursing facilities are focusing their attention on the problem of mechanical and chemical restraints and the methods employed to reduce them. In particular, they have stated strongly that mechanical restraints have a very limited role in the prevention of falls and are asking institutions to implement restraint-reduction programs. A better understanding of the phenomenon of falls will help health care professionals to prevent falls without resorting to traditional methods of restraint use.

Historically, the blame for falling has, for the most part, been borne by the host, the person who falls. Popular mythology holds that falls are attributable to either individual carelessness or the process of aging. Falls are considered to be either a "normal" phenomenon of aging—a manifestation of a general decline that is bound to occur—or, in people with multiple disorders, one aspect of a "hopeless" state in which one disorder after another leads inevitably to a negative conclusion. Many health care providers have dealt with falls and their adverse consequences for so long that they have become hardened; they no longer identify them as problems with solutions, other than to restrict the individuals' mobility. Moreover, providers may be reluctant to consider the possibility of better solutions.

Contrary to popular myth, falls, to a large degree, rarely "just happen"—they are neither accidental nor random events. They are predictable occurrences, the outcome of a multitude of host-related and environmental factors that occur either alone or in conjunction with one another. Many of the factors that contribute to falls are potentially amenable to interventions. By minimizing or eliminating these risk factors, falls can be reduced or prevented altogether.

In order to implement preventive measures, health care providers must first understand the conditions under which falls occur and the factors that are associated with fall risk. With an increased knowledge of why older people fall and what factors are associated with fall risk, providers will be able to more easily identify patients at risk and explore appropriate solutions aimed at reducing fall risk. Many of the factors responsible for falls are quite easy to fix, particularly for someone with a practiced eye, a different perspective, and different expertise. The second step health care providers must take is to mount an organized approach to the clinical assessment of fall risk and falls and put in place intervention strategies for both.

Table I-1.   Characteristics of hospitals and nursing facilities

Characteristic	Hospitals	Nursing facilities
Goal	Diagnose and treat acute disease	Manage chronic disease
Population	Patients are medically unstable (i.e., are experiencing acute illness and/or exacerbations of chronic disease) Institutional stay is temporary	Residents are medically stable but require ongoing medical or personal assistance In general, institutional stay is long term
Staff	Acute care orientation Daily physician presence Higher nursing staff–patient ratio	Chronic care orientation Irregular physician presence Lower nursing staff–patient ratio
Environment	Designed to facilitate acute medical care services	Designed to accommodate residents' levels of function

Although hospitals and nursing facilities more or less differ in their goals, distribution and orientation of staff, population of individuals cared for, and environmental design principles (see Table I-1), the factors associated with falls as well as intervention strategies within each institution are similar in many respects. An apple-to-apple comparison between the two institutional settings may not always be possible (e.g., what works for hospitals with respect to preventing falls may not work for nursing facilities and vice versa); so when it becomes necessary to consider the specificity of each institution, it is noted and differences appropriate to each are set forth.

Falls by hospital patients and nursing home residents are a complex problem. Acquiring a base of knowledge is an important start. An awareness of falls (e.g., their extent, complications, risk factors, and causes) and strategies and approaches aimed toward their prevention can lead to a greater understanding of how to solve the puzzle. Although it is unrealistic and unreasonable to assume that all falls are preventable, there is much that can be done to reduce falls in hospitals and nursing homes. The possibility that we as health professionals can identify people at risk—and do something about a condition that may not be inevitable (i.e., falling) after all—is what fall prevention is about. Therefore, although it may not always be possible to prevent a fall from occurring, anticipating a fall is possible. By using a multidisciplinary team approach in which all staff members participate in the creation of fall prevention activities and understand the reasons behind certain required actions, institutions can significantly reduce the risk of falls.

I have been involved in fall prevention for more than 20 years. In closing, I would like to leave the reader with my wisdom or lessons learned over the years, which I hope can be put to good use.

- An important starting point in redesigning a fall prevention program and its components is recognition that the existing program and activities are not working. Remember, every system or fall prevention program is perfectly designed to achieve the results it gets.

- There is no quick fix for preventing falls; getting all the gears in place, working in harmony or unison takes time. Fall prevention programs that

are pushed or rushed into place often do not succeed. Rather, it is important to start slow.

- Fall prevention takes organizational commitment; without buy-in and involvement from top management, effective fall prevention is not possible.

- Although nurses in many ways are the foundation of fall prevention, their involvement is simply not enough; fall prevention requires a multidisciplinary team approach.

- Fall prevention, like politics, is local. Hospitals and nursing homes vary greatly; what works in one may not work in another.

- In redesigning a fall prevention program, it is important to rethink, refocus, and retool rather than simply repuff (i.e., change the name but do the same thing over and over again).

- Designate a fall expert. With so many safety issues and safety regulations being put forward, it is easy for hospitals and nursing homes to go into crisis mode and lose their focus on fall prevention. An outside fall expert can be instrumental in helping organizations refocus, provide valuable feedback on program shortcomings, and support redesign efforts.

- Education, education, education! In order for change to take hold, the importance of staff education and training cannot be overemphasized.

ENDNOTES

1. Kerzman, H., Chetrit, A., Brin, L., & Toren, O. (2004). Characteristics of falls in hospitalized patients. *Journal of Advanced Nursing, 47,* 223–229.
2. Vassalo, M., Sharma, J.C., Allen, S.C. (2002, May/June). Characteristics of single fallers and recurrent fallers among hospital in-patients. *Gerontology, 48,* 147–150.
3. Halfon, P., Eggli, Y., Van Melle, G., et al. (2001). Risk of falls for hospitalized patients: A predictive model based on routinely available data. *Journal of Clinical Epidemiology, 54*(12):1258–1266.
4. Tutuarima, J., van der Meulen, J., de Haan, R., van Straten, A., & Limberg, M. (1997). Risk factors for falls of hospitalized stroke patients. *Stroke, 28,* 297–301.
5. Teasell, R., McRae, M., Foley, N., et al. (2002). The incidence and consequences of falls in stroke patients during inpatient rehabilitation: Factors associated with high risk. *Archives of Physical Medicine and Rehabilitation, 83*(3):329–333.
6. Tay, S.C., Quek, C., Pariyasami, S., Ong, B.S., Wee, B.M., Yeo, J., & Yeo, S. (2000). Fall incidence in a state psychiatric hospital in Singapore. *Journal of Psychosocial Nursing, 38,* 11–16.
7. Draper, B., Busetto, G., & Cullen, B. (2004). Risk factors for and prediction of falls in an acute aged care psychiatry unit. *Australasian Journal on Ageing, 23*(1): 48–51.
8. Nyberg, L., & Gustafson, Y. (1995). Patient falls in stroke rehabilitation: A challenge in rehabilitation strategies. *Stroke, 26,* 838–842.
9. Goodwin, M.B., & Westbrook, J.I. (1993). An analysis of patient accidents in hospital. *Australian Clinical Review, 13*(3), 141–149.
10. Rigby, K., Clark, R., & Runciman, W. (1999). Adverse events in health care: Setting priorities based on economic evaluation. *Journal of Quality Clinical Practice, 19,* 7–12.
11. Rubenstein, L.Z., Robbins, A.S., Schulman, B.L., Rosado, J., Osterweil, D., & Josephson, K.R. (1988). Falls and instability in the elderly. *Journal of the American Geriatrics Society, 36,* 278–288.

12. Krauss, M.J., Nguyen, S.L., Dunagan, W.C., Birge, S., Costantinou, E., Johnson, S., et al. (2007). Circumstances of patient falls and injuries in 9 hospitals in a midwestern healthcare system. *Infection Control and Hospital Epidemiology*, *28*(5), 544–550.
13. Nygaard, H. (1998). Falls and psychotropic drug consumption in long-term care residents: Is there an obvious association? *Gerontology*, *44*, 46–50.
14. Kiely, D., Kiel, D., Burrows, A., & Lipsitz, L. (1998). Identifying nursing home residents at risk for falling. *Journal of American Geriatrics Society*, *46*, 551–555.
15. Thapa, P.B., Brockman, K.G., Gideon, P., et al. (1996). Injurious falls in non-ambulatory nursing home residents: A comparative study of circumstances, incidence, and risk factors. *Journal of the American Geriatrics Society*, *44*(3):273–278.
16. Vu, M.Q., Weintraub, N., Rubenstein, L.Z. Falls in the nursing home: Are they preventable? (2004, November/December). *Journal of the American Medical Directors Association*, *5*(6):401–406.
17. Luukinen, H., Koski, L., Hiltunen, L., & Kivela, S.L. (1994). Incidence rate of falls in an aged population in northern Finland. *Journal of Clinical Epidemiology*, *47*, 843–850.
18. Rubenstein, L.Z., Robbins, A.S., Josephson, K.R., Schulman, B.L., & Osterweil, D. (1990). The value of assessing falls in an elderly population: A randomized clinical trial. *Annals of Internal Medicine*, *113*, 308–316.

Understanding Falls and Falls Management

Chapter One

Consequences of Falls

Falls are a major cause of death and disability in older people and pose a serious threat to their health and well being. The consequences of falls are not confined to older people. They place a burden on family members, make excessive demands on health care professionals, and strain the resources of institutions.

MORTALITY

Falls and their consequences are a leading cause of death in people 65 years old and older.[1] About 10,000 older adults die each year as a result of falls.[2, 3] The risk of dying from a fall increases as people age. Fall-related death rates among people 65 years old and older are 10–150 times higher than those in younger age groups. Of all deaths due to falls, 66% involve people age 75 or older; these people have a mortality rate eight times higher than that for people 65–74 years of age.[3] More than two thirds of injury-reported deaths after age 85 are related to falls.[4] Of people admitted to the hospital after a fall, only about 50% will be alive 1 year later. In the hospital setting, fall-related deaths are a rare occurrence. Although less than 1% of inpatient falls result in death, this translates to approximately 11,000 fatal falls in the hospital environment per year nationwide. In nursing facilities, approximately 1,800 fatal falls occur annually.[4] For people age 85 and older, it is estimated that one in every five falls results in death.[5] A clustering of falls (i.e., multiple falls occurring over a short period of time) is associated with increased mortality.[6] (For the definition of this term and others used throughout this chapter, see the Terminology sidebar on page 4.)

Fall-related mortality appears to be the direct result of the fall (e.g., from injuries sustained) and current comorbidity (e.g., pneumonia, heart failure, pulmonary disease). Older people have decreased body reserves or lower thresholds, and once injured from a fall they have a much higher likelihood of dying than do younger people. The use of mechanical restraints to guard against the risk of falls also has been implicated as a cause of death. Most commonly, with the restraint device in place, a person falls or climbs out of bed, slides off a chair, or slips downward in a raised hospital bed. He or she becomes entangled and suspended in the restraint—which is usually pressed tightly against the chest or throat—and dies of asphyxia.[7]

Terminology

Clustering of falls	Multiple falling events occurring over a short period of time
Colles fracture	Distal forearm fracture (or fracture of the wrist)
Comorbidity	Presence of additional diseases or illnesses
Contraction (of joint)	Shortening or tightening of a muscle that causes decreased joint motion
Femoral neck	Head of the long bone of the thigh
Orthostatic hypotension	Lowered blood pressure that occurs on rising to an erect position
Osteoporosis	Decrease in bone strength
Protective reflex	Extension of the arms outward and/or a shift of the feet to maintain balance and avoid a fall
Pulmonary embolism	Blockage of pulmonary artery or one of its branches
Soft-tissue injury	Injury to nonbony tissues, for example, sprains and strains
Subdural hematoma	Accumulation of blood resulting from injury to the brain
Venous stasis	Blood trapped in an extremity (e.g., arm, leg) by compression of veins
Vestibular function	Mechanism within the inner ear involved in balance control

MORBIDITY

The consequences of falls are numerous, from physical injury to immobility, to psychosocial trauma, to a morbid fear of falling again.

Physical Injury

In hospitals, injuries occur in approximately 6%–44% of falls. Moreover, half of all hospitalizations resulting from injurious falls are experienced by people older than age 65, and people hospitalized for fall-related trauma are discharged to nursing facilities more often than are people without falls. In the institutional setting, between 9% and 15% of falls result in physical injury; approximately 4% result in fractures, and approximately 12% result in other serious injuries such as head injuries, soft-tissue injuries, musculoskeletal sprains, and lacerations.[5] The most common fractures are those of the distal forearm and hip. Distal forearm, or Colles, fractures occur when an older person loses balance and attempts to break a fall in progress by extending the arms outward. After age 70, there is a decrease in the incidence of forearm fractures, at which time there is a steep increase in the incidence of hip fractures and head injuries. Older adults' decreased ability to exhibit the protective reflex is believed to be the cause of the decline in distal forearm fractures.

Some hypothesize that a decline in the protective reflex may be attributed to age-related changes in central nervous system function (e.g., decreased reaction and response times), concomitant diseases (e.g., stroke, Parkinson's disease, arthritis), and certain drugs (e.g., psychotropics, hypnotics).[8] Consequently, older people who fall are at great risk for head trauma, spinal cord trauma, and hip fracture.

Falls are a leading cause of head injury in older people. Aside from bruises and lacerations, subdural hematomas are the most significant head injuries. They tend to occur more often than other injuries because of certain age-related changes in the older brain, such as decreased cerebral reserve. As a result, older people are less able than younger people to withstand even minor trauma, such as might occur from bumping into a wall, a bedside rail, or a headboard. Any time a person exhibits mental confusion after a fall, a neurological evaluation should be conducted to rule out a subdural hematoma. Any lingering subdural hematoma that has not healed within a short period of time can lead to permanent cognitive dysfunction.

Approximately 2.9% of falls result in hip fracture.[9] Although the incidence of hip fractures is low, the subsequent mortality and morbidity are substantial. Of all patients with hip fracture, 4% die in the hospital,[10] and within 1 year after their injury, up to 23% are dead;[11] people 75 years old and older have the highest mortality rates.[1] A high incidence of coexisting chronic diseases in people with hip fracture contributes to this increased mortality rate. After a hip fracture, many older people never regain their premorbid level of ambulation. Approximately 60% of people with hip fracture have decreased mobility; another 25% become functionally dependent in walking and need mechanical assistance (e.g., the use of a cane or walker) or the assistance of another person.[1] Of all hip fracture survivors, 14% remain in the nursing facility 1 year after injury.[12]

The risk of sustaining a hip fracture from a fall depends on a number of interacting factors, including the height of the fall, the impact surface, protective reflexes, "shock absorbers," and bone strength.

Height of the Fall and Impact Surface

In order to build sufficient momentum to produce injury (e.g., bone fracture), a person must fall a considerable distance. For example, an unexpected fall from a standing height (e.g., from a slip or a loss of consciousness) or a fall from an elevated bed height (e.g., over bedside rails) is more likely to result in injury because of the increased force of impact than a fall from a low height, such as from a chair or toilet. Falls on hard, nonabsorptive floor surfaces such as linoleum tile, concrete, and wood are more likely to result in injury than falls onto absorptive surfaces such as carpeting.

Protective Reflexes

The onset of a fall elicits several protective reflexes, including extending the arms outward and initiating quick shifting movements of the feet in order to regain balance. Both may avert a fall or minimize the force of impact. Conversely, a loss of protective reflexes stemming from neuromuscular dysfunction that affects the extremities or from sedation induced by medication may increase the impact of falling and the risk of injury.

"Shock Absorbers"

Fat and muscle bulk surrounding vulnerable areas, such as the hip, is capable of absorbing the impact of a fall, decreasing the risk of fracture. Fractures are more likely to occur in people whose muscles have atrophied or who have less fat padding (i.e., thin people).

Bone Strength

A loss of bone strength attributable to osteoporosis at the femoral neck may result in fractures. These fractures may be either "spontaneous" hip fractures that occur during weight-bearing episodes or fractures that occur even with minimal ground impact against the bone. Bone loss is a particular problem in older women: By age 80, women may have lost up to 50% of their bone strength, compared with 15% in men.

Immobility

In the absence of physical injury, falls are often associated with a restriction of activities—either self- or staff-imposed—and immobility. As a consequence, people are at risk for a host of morbid complications that increase with the duration of immobility (Table 1-1). In turn, any concomitant loss of functional status places people at additional risk for falls (Figure 1-1).

Psychosocial Trauma

Falls, particularly those that recur, are associated with a number of traumatic psychosocial consequences. Threats of impending falls can alter self-image and create feelings of increasing frailty and incompetence. Often, people experience increased anxiety while performing activities of daily living (ADLs; e.g., getting out of bed, transferring from the toilet) because they are uncertain as to whether they can perform the ADLs safely. Such people become increasingly apprehensive, and their sense of vulnerability to falling and self-injury is heightened. These people may become depressed, especially if their mobility or freedom to move about independently is diminished and they become functionally dependent on staff for assistance. Any limitations in mobility have broad lifestyle implications for these older adults. For example, they may remain in their rooms or sit alone in the unit, which decreases their sociability and participation in leisure activities. Often, compromised mobility that becomes permanent necessitates placement in a long-term care facil-

Table 1-1. Physiological and psychological consequences of immobility

System	Consequences
Musculoskeletal	Joint contractions, causing decreased range of motion
	Muscle weakness/atrophy
	Osteoporosis
Integumentary	Pressure sores
Respiratory	Pneumonia, causing decreased ventilation
	Pulmonary embolism
Cardiovascular	Orthostatic hypotension
	Venous stasis
Urinary	Urinary infections
	Incontinence
Gastrointestinal	Constipation
Neurological	Vestibular dysfunction/loss of balance
Psychological	Social isolation
	Decreased self-image
	Depression
	Anxiety
	Confusion

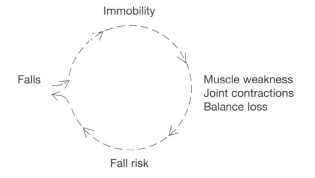

Figure 1-1. Falls that are associated with immobility and subsequent functional decline can increase the risk of additional falls.

ity. Falls and immobility account for up to one third of all admissions to nursing facilities,[13] thus constituting one of the leading causes of nursing facility placement.

Patients and residents with falls may voice a number of other worries or fears, which include the following:

- Being belted or restrained, experiencing a loss of autonomy

- Having their relatives informed of the episode, which may cause further embarrassment for the patient or resident

- Being transferred to "dependent" units for their care, thus experiencing a loss of independence

- Fearing that nursing staff will not be available or come to their aid in time to prevent another fall

- Being forced to use a cane or walker, thus losing self-esteem

- Becoming a burden to family and staff members

- Dreading that the next fall will result in a hip fracture or other injury.

Fear of Falling

Falls can lead to patients or residents losing confidence in their ability to function because of a fear of falling. Conservative estimates indicate that up to 50% of people who fall avoid ADLs because they fear additional falls and injury.[14] Such fear may be protective, or it may be harmful. To a certain degree, it may be protective if it motivates people to avoid activities they can no longer perform safely, to recognize their limitations, and to become more cautious. However, a fear of falling also can be detrimental, adversely affecting mobility and independence. As a response to their fear, some people alter their walking patterns; typically, their steps become hesitant and irregular.

Ambulation is accompanied by a great deal of anxiety and often is accomplished by the person clutching or grabbing onto furnishings for support, a strategy that may increase the risk of falls. Subsequently, many people experience multiple near falls, which can heighten their fear of falling and may lead to a curtailment of all physical activity. Many older people reject devices that assist in safe mobility because they are reluctant to project an image of frailty and thus endure social rejection from their peers, or they may feel that their cane or walker provides insufficient support. Other people who are fearful of falling may eventually become chairbound or bedridden, reluctant to attempt independent activities, and in need of human assistance to accomplish ADLs. Many patients and residents in this category develop a fear of being dropped by staff members during transfer activities and may be hesitant to leave their beds or chairs.

Fear of falling may lead to a number of morbid outcomes. Older hospital patients may delay or eventually avoid discharge to the community, particularly if they live alone. Stalling can affect these patients adversely because many times it ultimately leads to placement in a nursing facility. Similarly, many nursing facility residents with a fear of falling become socially isolated and functionally dependent. Thus, the risk of complications associated with immobility increases.

FAMILY CONCERNS

Family members of people with falls in hospitals and nursing facilities also experience the consequences of falls. They may feel guilty about the fall, blaming themselves for not being there to prevent the event, or they may blame the nursing staff for allowing the fall to happen, sometimes even accusing the staff of neglect. Concerned for the safety of their relative, family members may insist on restricting activities and may inquire about the use of mechanical restraints and bedside rails to safeguard the patient or resident. These restrictions are especially likely to occur if the older person experiences multiple falls or a fall that results in injury. Although many family members become dismayed at the sight of restraints, they reluctantly accept their use for safety reasons. However, other families may insist on restraint removal, even if it places their loved ones at risk for falls. Most families do not seek a guarantee that no harm will come to their relative; rather, they simply want assurance that the staff will assess the problem or the risk for subsequent falls and take appropriate measures to guard against falls. When alternatives to the use of mechanical restraints are discussed with family members, they often feel comfortable with the prospect of reducing or eliminating restraints.

In the hospital setting, many families question staff about whether their loved ones can safely return home, particularly if they live alone. Families seek alternatives such as altered living arrangements (e.g., moving the relative with falls in with them) or placement in a group home or assisted living facility. If these options are not feasible, families may resort to nursing facility placement.

INSTITUTIONAL EFFECTS

The consequences of falls are challenging for institutions as well as families and the patients or residents themselves. The complications include increased health care costs and effects on staff.

Health Care Costs

Falls and their complications often result in increased costs from potential liability risks and health care needs. The institution and its employees are responsible for the safety of their patients or residents for the length of their stay in the institution and may be held responsible if older adults fall and sustain injuries. Thus, both institution and staff are at risk for legal liability and increased costs associated with legal fees and settlement awards. Falls are the largest category of incident reports submitted to risk management for review because of potential liability.[15] The risk of legal action is highest in patients and residents whose falls are associated with serious injury, such as a fracture. Family members, rather than the patients and residents themselves, are likely to file a complaint against the institution, perhaps partly because of guilt about their relative's poor outcome.

Falls and injuries generate other expenses as well, including the following:

- *Labor costs:* Nursing, physician, and rehabilitative services accrued as a result of the time spent evaluating fall events, completing documentation (e.g., filling out occurrence reports, charting), providing postfall care (e.g., treating injury and immobility complications, restorative care), and monitoring patients and residents at fall risk (e.g., hourly nursing rounds, in-room sitters).[16]

- *Equipment costs:* Mobility devices (e.g., canes, walkers, wheelchairs), bed rails, fall alarm systems, and durable medical equipment (e.g., grab bars, toileting devices, restraints, restraint-alternative devices).

- *Utilization costs:* Prolonged hospitalization (e.g., increased length of stay, increased bed-days) and permanent placement,[17] in the case of nursing facilities; recurrent falls and their complications are common causes of rehospitalization and readmission to nursing facilities.[18, 19]

Many times, institutions must bear the brunt of these expenses. Hospital reimbursement systems may not pay for the necessary services or extended days due to complications that stem from falls and injuries. In nursing facilities with reimbursement capitation, the necessary care that results from fall-related complications may exceed coverage. In general, hospitals and nursing facilities that hold capitation contracts with managed care organizations are responsible for any expenses accrued, and managed care plans that enroll residents of nursing facilities are responsible for covering fall-related costs.

Effects on Staff

Nursing staff caring for patients and residents with recurrent falls may find the responsibility of constantly deciding between the individuals' desires for autonomy and the families' requests for safety and protection against the risk of falls emotionally demanding. Staff easily can become disheartened when patients and residents continue to fall, despite all their attempts to prevent falls. Often, staff may experience stress, guilt, and self-doubt about their ability to deliver safe care.

ENDNOTES

1. Davis, A.E. (1995). Hip fractures in the elderly: Surveillance methods and injury control. *Journal of Nursing Trauma, 2*(1), 15–21.
2. Centers for Disease Control and Prevention. (1995). *Injury mortality, 1986–1992.* Atlanta: Author.
3. Stevens, J.A., Ryan, G., & Kresnow, M. (2006). Fatalities and injuries from falls among older adults—United States, 1993–2003 and 2001–2005. *Morbidity and Mortality Weekly Report, 55,* 1221–1224.
4. Baker, S.P., O'Neill, B., Ginsburg, M.J., & Guohua, L. (1992). *The injury fact book* (2nd ed.). New York: Oxford University Press.
5. Hook, M.L., & Winchel, S. (2006). Fall-related injuries in acute care: reducing the risk of harm. *MEDSURG Nursing, 15,* 370–377, 381. Peel, N.M., Kassulke, D.J., & McClure, R.J. (2002). Population based study of hospitalised fall related injuries in older people. *Injury Prevention, 8*(4), 280–284. Fischer, I.D., Krauss, M.J., Dunagan, W.C., Birge, S., Hitcho, E., Johnson, S., Costantinou, E., & Fraser, V.J. (2005). Patterns and predictors of inpatient falls and fall-related injuries in a large academic hospital. *Infection Control and Hospital Epidemiology, 26,* 822–827.
6. Wolinsky, F.D., Johnson, R.J., & Fitzgerald, J.F. (1992). Falling, health status, and use of health services by older adults. *Medical Care, 30,* 587–597.
7. Miles, S.H., & Irvine, P.I. (1992). Deaths caused by physical restraints. *Gerontologist, 32,* 762–766.
8. Melton, L.J., Chao, E.Y.S., & Lane, J. (1988). Biomechanical aspects of fractures. In B.L. Briggs & L.J. Melton (Eds.), *Osteoporosis: Etiology, diagnosis, and management* (pp. 111–131). New York: Raven.
9. Nadkarni, J.B., Iyengar, K.P., Dussa, C., Watwe, S., & Vishwanath, K. (2005). Orthopaedic injuries following falls by hospital in-patients. *Gerontology, 51,* 329–333.

10. U.S. Department of Health and Human Services, Public Health Service, National Center for Health Statistics. (1992). (Unpublished data from the 1988 and 1991 National Hospital Discharge Survey.)

11. Fisher, E.S., Baron, J., Malenka, D.I., Barrett, J.A., Kniffin, W.D., Whaley, F.S., et al. (1991). Hip fracture mortality in New England. *Epidemiology, 2*(2), 116–122.

12. Kennedy, E.M. (1994). *Hip fracture outcomes in people age fifty and over.* Background paper OTA-BP-H-120. Washington, DC: U.S. Government Printing Office.

13. Tinetti, M.E., & Speechley, M. (1989). Prevention of falls among the elderly. *New England Journal of Medicine, 320,* 1055–1059.

14. Franzoni, S., Ronzzini, R., Boffelli, S., Frisoni, E.B., & Trabucchi, M. (1994). Fear of falling in nursing home patients. *Gerontology, 40,* 38–44.

15. Quinlan, W.C. (1994). The liability risk of patients who fall. *Journal of Healthcare Risk Management, 14,* 29–33.

16. Titler, M., Dochterman, J., Picone, D.M., Everett, L., Xie, X-J, Kanak, M., & Fei, Q. (2005). Cost of hospital care for elderly at risk of falling. *Nursing Economics, 23*(6), 290–306.

17. Bates, D.W., Pruess, K., Souney, P., & Platt, R. (1995). Serious falls in hospitalized patients: Correlates and resource utilization. *American Journal of Medicine, 99*(2), 137.

18. Hill, K.D., Vu, M., & Walsh, W. (2007). Falls in the acute hospital setting—impact on resource utilization. *Australian Health Review, 31,* 471–477.

19. Greene, E., Cunningham, C.J., Eustace, A., Kidd, N., Clare, A.W., & Lawlor, B.A. (2001). Recurrent falls are associated with increased length of stay in elderly psychiatric inpatients. *International Journal of Geriatric Psychiatry, 16,* 965–968.

Chapter Two

Causes of Falling and Fall Risk

A fall can be defined as any event in which a person inadvertently or intentionally comes to rest on the ground or another low level such as a chair, toilet, or bed. As an initial step in designing any intervention to reduce falls, it is essential to know why falls occur and under what circumstances they take place. The risk of falling occurs when a person engages in an activity that results in a loss of balance, a displacement of the body beyond its base of support. Loss of balance may occur while one is carrying out everyday activities such as walking; transferring on or off chairs, wheelchairs, beds, and toilets; and reaching up or bending to retrieve or place objects. A fall is likely to follow an episode of balance loss if the neuromuscular systems responsible for balance stability fail to recognize and correct the displacement of the body in time to avert a fall.

Falls in older people are often precipitated by a number of factors. These factors include intrinsic factors (e.g., age-related physiological changes, disease states, medications) and extrinsic factors (e.g., hazardous environmental conditions, faulty devices, footwear). In addition, several situational circumstances, such as length of stay in institutional settings, time of day when falls take place, and staff characteristics, influence the occurrence of falls.

Falling should be viewed as a nonspecific sign or symptom of an underlying problem that can be attributed to either intrinsic or extrinsic factors. In the past, falls have been assigned to a single cause and ascribed to a medical event or accidental environmental encounter. As researchers are beginning to understand, in general, falls in older people are not the result of a single intrinsic or extrinsic factor occurring in isolation; rather, falls are complex events caused by a combination of both types of factors (Figure 2-1). However, for ease of understanding the etiology, or causes, of falls, it is useful to divide falls into strict intrinsic and extrinsic categories.

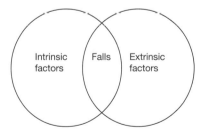

Figure 2-1. Falls are caused by the interaction of intrinsic and extrinsic factors.

INTRINSIC FACTORS

A number of intrinsic factors play an important role in fall causation. These factors consist of age-related changes (e.g., changes in vision, changes in

balance, changes in gait, changes in the musculoskeletal system, changes in
the cardiovascular system), pathological conditions (e.g., acute diseases,
chronic diseases), and medications.

Age-Related Changes

Mobility, the ability to maintain upright posture and to ambulate and transfer effectively, depends on the operation and integrity of many systems, primarily the visual, neurological, musculoskeletal, and cardiovascular systems.
With advancing age, these systems decline gradually in function; they affect
gait and balance and influence the risk of falling (Table 2-1).

Changes in Vision

The ability of the eyes to adjust to varying levels of light and darkness diminishes as people age. As a result, the eyes of older people need more time
to adjust to changes in environmental lighting. Dark adaptation is especially

Table 2-1. Aging changes to consider in safety planning

System	Age-related changes	Clinical consequences
Genitourinary	Reduced bladder capacity	Frequency of urination and toileting
	Weakness of bladder muscles	Urine leakage, inadequate bladder emptying, and risk of incontinence
	Nocturia	Frequency of nighttime urination and toileting
	Enlarged prostate gland in men	Increased frequency of urination, dribbling, obstruction, and retention; increased risk of urinary infections
Nervous	Deterioration of nerves	Slow reflexes and coordination; decreased reaction time and balance
	Reduced flexibility of the lens in the eye	Visual impairment
	Decreased nerves and blood supply to the ears	Hearing loss
	Decreased blood flow to the brain	Risk of mental confusion and memory loss
Musculoskeletal	Reduced muscle mass	Decreased strength; risk of impairment; decreased endurance and tone; increased reaction time
	Brittle bones (osteoporosis)	Risk of fractures
	Loss of back muscle strength, reduced flexibility of spine	Poor posture (including leaning or slumping) and balance impairment
	Degenerative joint changes	Increased joint stiffness and pain; decreased mobility, gait and balance impairment
Integumentary	Loss of elasticity, fragile blood vessels, reduced subcutaneous fat	Increased risk of bruising and skin tears, slow healing
Cardiovascular	Slow heart rate, sluggish blood flow	Risk of low blood pressure during postural changes

affected by aging and may compromise a person's visual capacity, particularly under conditions of low illumination (e.g., when walking about or toileting at night). When moving from a dimly lit room into bright lighting and vice versa, people often experience temporary blindness until the eyes adjust to the dramatic change in illumination.

A greater sensitivity of the aging eye to glare can lead to visual dysfunction. Common sources of glare include sunlight shining through windows and reflecting off waxed floors or glossy tabletops and bright light from un-shielded light fixtures directed toward the eye. Glare from floor surfaces is particularly troublesome because it can mask potential ground hazards. Also, glare can create visual distortions in older people that may result in their perceiving floor surfaces as excessively slippery. As a consequence, older people sometimes alter their gait to compensate. They walk more slowly and more flat-footed and use a wider base of support, a pattern reminiscent of that which people adopt to walk on ice. However, this gait change may not be safe and can lead to unsteadiness and falls. At other times, people cope with the glare emanating from floors by avoiding the surface altogether. Some view excessive floor glare, especially if it restricts a person's mobility, as a passive form of restraint. (For a definition of *glare* and other terms, see the Terminology sidebar on pages 16–17.)

Restriction of a person's visual field leads to an inability to see objects in the pathway that lie outside the person's view, increasing the likelihood of slips and trips. A loss of visual acuity and contrast sensitivity can make perception of objects in the environment more difficult. In particular, the inability to detect low-contrast objects can lead to unsafe ambulation and transfers. If not visualized clearly, objects such as extended chair and table legs, door thresholds, and carpet edges can cause people to trip. Furnishing surfaces (e.g., chair and toilet seats, bed mattress edges) that are not visually distinguishable can interfere with the achievement of stable seating positions, which increases the likelihood of falls while transferring. The loss of visual acuity and contrast sensitivity or decreased functional vision are more evident under conditions of low illumination (e.g., walking to the bathroom at night).

A decline in depth perception can cause certain ground surfaces (e.g., patterned or checkered linoleum, carpet designs) to appear to be elevations or depressions on the ground, surfaces that older people prefer to step around or avoid walking on entirely. In addition, a loss of depth perception makes it difficult to perceive objects that lie in areas of shadows, low illumination, or excessive brightness.

Changes in Balance

The body's ability to maintain balance depends on the central nervous and musculoskeletal systems, requiring adequate vision, proprioceptive feedback, vestibular input, muscle strength, and joint flexibility to detect and correct balance displacement. Combined, these systems culminate in postural sway, a process of antero-posterior and lateral motion of the standing or seated body that controls stability and protects against the forces of gravity (i.e., loss of balance and falls).

Terminology

Agnosia	Neurological disorder that leads to disturbances in the recognition or perception of familiar sensory information
Apraxia	Loss of the ability to execute previously learned motor skills
Ataxia	Impairment of coordination of muscular activity
Cardiac arrhythmia	Any deviation from the normal pace of the heart
Cardio-acceleration	An increase in the pulse rate
Cervical spondylosis	Breakdown of cervical vertebrae
Chronic obstructive pulmonary disease	General term for disease involving airway obstruction (e.g., chronic bronchitis, emphysema, asthma)
Congestive heart failure	Chronic inability of the heart to maintain an adequate output of blood, resulting in an inadequate blood supply to the body
Contrast sensitivity	The ability to perceive spatial detail and object contrast
Dark adaptation	The ability of the eyes to adjust to low levels of illumination
Dorsiflexion	Bending or flexing
Dysarthria	Difficulty in articulating single sounds in speech
Dysphasia	Disturbance in speech evidenced by lack of coordination and failure to express words in proper order
Electrolyte disorders	Disorder in compounds that play an essential role in function of the body
Extracellular volume regulation	Homeostatic mechanisms that regulate against volume depletion
Extrinsic	External to the system
Gait cycle	The manner of progression in walking or style of walking
Glare	A dazzling effect associated with a source of intense illumination
Hemianopsia	Blindness in half of the visual field
Hemiplegia	Paralysis involving one side of the body, generally an arm or leg
Hypotension	Low blood pressure
Hypovolemia	Low fluid states in the body

or the greater the precision and speed needed to accomplish the movement, the greater the importance of vision. When visual input is diminished by age-related changes, balance becomes difficult to maintain. This concept is demonstrated when an older person stands with his or her eyes closed or walks into a dark room; in both cases, balance is unsteady.

The vestibular system works in conjunction with the visual and proprioceptive systems to achieve balance; it helps to maintain stable visual perception and body orientation as a person moves about the environment. During periods of displacement of balance, the vestibular receptors detect movement and prompt antigravity extensor muscles to execute compensatory head, trunk, and limb movements, which oppose postural sway. In other words, the system located in the inner ear that regulates balance senses that the body has been placed out of balance and signals the neuromuscular system to activate one or more movements to ensure that a fall does not take place. This body-orienting response, known as the righting reflex, diminishes with age. Consequently, when an older person slips, trips, or loses balance while transferring, his or her chance of regaining stability and avoiding a fall declines.

Usually, some redundancy occurs in the sensory information necessary to maintain balance, and the failure of one source of input such as vision can be counteracted with feedback from intact proprioceptive and vestibular systems. However, deprivation in more than one system is likely to lower the balance threshold and increase fall risk. This risk becomes evident when older people who have fallen are compared with older people who have not fallen. Older people who fall have greater postural sway or unsteadiness than people without falls, and people with multiple falls demonstrate appreciably more sway or unsteady balance than those with single falls.[1]

Changes in Gait

The gait cycle consists of two phases: stance and swing. The stance phase occurs when one leg is in contact with the ground, and the swing phase occurs when the other leg is advanced forward to take the next step (Figure 2-5).

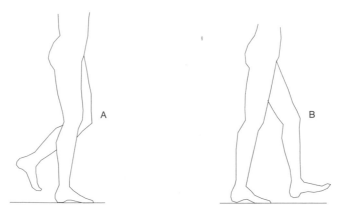

Figure 2-5.   (A) The stance phase and (B) the swing phase of the gait cycle.

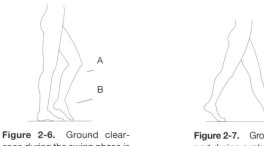

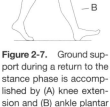

Figure 2-6. Ground clearance during the swing phase is accomplished by (A) knee flexion and (B) ankle dorsiflexion.

Figure 2-7. Ground support during a return to the stance phase is accomplished by (A) knee extension and (B) ankle plantar flexion.

Ambulation is accomplished via a series of reciprocal leg movements that alternate between stance and swing—pushing off on the leg in stance phase while swinging the other leg forward. To allow adequate ground clearance during the swing phase, the leg is flexed at the knee and dorsiflexed at the foot (Figure 2-6). When the heel of the swing leg strikes the ground, the return to the stance phase, the knee is extended and the foot is plantar flexed to provide support to the body (Figure 2-7).

As compared with younger people, older people experience a number of changes in the gait cycle. The speed of walking, step length, and steppage height decline (Figure 2-8). Changes in gait are also specific to each gender, although they are not well understood. Women tend to develop a narrow standing and walking base, often take small steps, and exhibit a pelvic waddle during ambulation. The pelvic waddle has been attributed in part to a loss of muscular control in the lower extremities. Conversely, older men tend to adopt a wide standing and walking base and assume a more shuffling gait.

Whether age-related changes in gait are compensatory and serve to maintain balance or are hazardous and thus influence fall risk remains speculative. However, changes in gait are more evident in people with a history of falls, and this influences fall susceptibility to a certain degree. When the swing phase is interrupted (Figure 2-9), either the foot fails to adequately clear the ground or it encounters an irregularity on the surface of the floor, such as curled-up carpeting or a raised tile edge, which results in tripping. When a bare foot or shoe bottom either encounters a surface of low frictional resistance (e.g., a wet or highly polished floor surface) or approaches the ground with a change in stride length during a return to the stance phase, a slip can occur (Figure 2-10). Whether a trip or slip results in a fall depends on the person's ability to initiate and execute maneuvers that correct his or her balance.

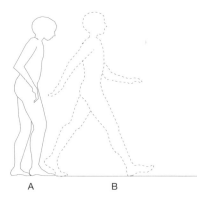

Figure 2-8. The gait of (A) an older person is compared with that of (B) a younger person, demonstrating a decrease in step length and steppage height.

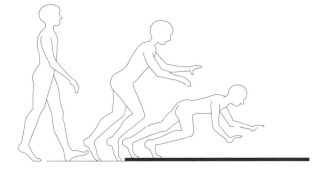

Figure 2-9. The movement of the right foot is interrupted during the swing phase. A trip and fall forward occurs as a result.

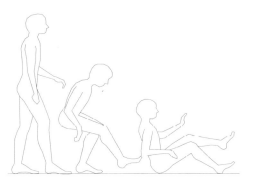

Figure 2-10. The movement of the right foot during a return to the stance phase encounters a surface of low frictional resistance. A slip and fall backward occurs as a result.

Changes in the Musculoskeletal System

The capacity to maintain balance while walking and transferring, and thus accomplish these activities safely, is affected by a number of age-related changes in the musculoskeletal system. Such changes include muscle atrophy, calcification of tendons and ligaments, and increased curvature of the spine due to osteoporosis, which results in kyphosis. In response, older people develop a stooped posture (Figure 2-11) and have difficulty extending their hips and knees fully when walking, which can affect their ability to maintain stability and to correct any displacements of balance that occur. A severe forward-leaning posture may change the body's balance threshold: The center of gravity is shifted forward, past the base of support (i.e., the critical point of stability), making it more difficult for older people to thrust the foot forward quickly enough to preserve balance. Poor ankle muscle strength complicates the execution, and older people find it difficult to adjust their center of gravity in line with the base of support rapidly enough to prevent a fall. In fact, with age, general muscular strength declines, particularly in the proximal muscles.

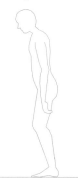

Figure 2-11. Age-related musculoskeletal changes can lead to a stooped posture.

The deterioration of articular cartilage in the hips and knees becomes prominent in older adults. In concert, these changes can impair transfer activity (e.g., sitting down and rising from chairs, toilets, and beds). An inability to flex the knees and hips sufficiently and the loss of lower extremity strength may impair the capacity of the legs to exert maximum push or force during the attempt to transfer. Similarly, a decrease in shoulder and upper extremity flexibility and strength may cause the body to fail to provide optimal upper extremity leverage during transfers.

Changes in the Cardiovascular System

Aging is associated with several physiological changes that impair homeostasis or regulation of blood pressure, which can predispose older adults to falls. The baroreceptor reflex, which consists of stretch receptors located in large arteries, is sensitive to sudden changes in blood pressure and serves as a regulatory mechanism that helps to maintain sufficient blood flow to the brain. This reflex occurs despite changes in posture, such as suddenly standing up after remaining seated or in a prone position for some time. As people age, they experience a progressive decline in baroreflex stimulation, caused by arteriosclerosis. This arterial hardening may cause transient episodes of hypotension, which becomes evident in the presence of hypotensive stimuli such as hypovolemia (e.g., dehydration, blood loss) or medication side effects. Therefore, the aged heart is less able than a younger heart to cardioaccelerate to compensate for any hypotensive effects. Also, older people have impaired extracellular volume regulation, and as a result, sodium conservation declines. Diminished sodium conservation can lead to sodium imbalance and dehydration, which can influence blood pressure regulation and subsequently lead to hypotension.

Pathological Conditions

Diseases and their associated impairments, superimposed on age-related physiological changes, play a more decisive role in falls than do physiological changes occurring by themselves. Older people have reserve capacity beyond what they may need for ordinary mobility tasks. Therefore, aging per se and age-related physiological changes are less likely to cause falls in the absence of associated disease. Often, falls are markers for an underlying acute disease or diseases. Indeed, evidence indicates that, in general, people with repeated falls have more medical comorbidity than do people without falls.[2]

Acute Diseases

A fall may be the initial sign or an early indication of an underlying acute illness, representing the onset of a new disease or an unstable existing disease, as in the following case example:

B.R. is an 89-year-old man with severe Parkinson's disease who experienced five falls during a 2-week period. The falls were ascribed to poor mobility resulting from his neurological disease. However, subsequent investigation revealed the presence of a gastrointestinal bleed (i.e., blood in the stool with anemia), which was caused by a stomach ulcer. After treatment of the ulcer, his falls ceased.

Falling episodes that precede an episode of illness are called prodromal falls. Illnesses most often identified as causative of falls are those present at the time of the fall that interfere with postural stability; such illnesses include syncope, hypotension, cardiac arrhythmias, electrolyte disorders, seizures, stroke, febrile conditions (e.g., urinary tract infections, pneumonia), and acute exacerbations of underlying chronic diseases (e.g., congestive heart failure, chronic obstructive pulmonary disease, kidney failure). Approximately 10% of falls in older people are attributed to acute illness.

Chronic Diseases

A fall often heralds a deterioration in health that is attributable to a chronic disease. Disease processes that predispose to falls include any persistent physical condition that interferes with mobility (e.g., the ability to walk about the environment; safe transfer on and off chairs, beds, and toilets). The most common disease processes originate in the visual, neurological, and musculoskeletal systems. Degenerative cognitive disorders compound the effects of falls and increase the risk for them.

Visual Disorders   Diseases of the eye such as cataracts, macular degeneration, glaucoma, and hemianopsia interfere with visual fields and decrease visual perception, visual acuity, and dark adaptation. Cataracts result in an overall blurring of vision, causing images to appear hazy or cloudy, and cause increased sensitivity to glare. Macular degeneration affects only central vision; peripheral vision remains intact. Glaucoma results in the loss of peripheral vision, and hemianopsia causes loss of vision in half of the visual field. When combined with poor illumination, visual disorders can result in poor recognition of environmental hazards and predispose people to trips and slips. Visual impairment is most likely to interfere with safe mobility at night.

Neurological Disorders   Dementia, especially of the Alzheimer's type, is associated with neurological disorders: ataxia, proprioceptive loss, apraxia, visuospatial dysfunction in object recognition, and agnosia. These changes lead to misinterpretation of environmental conditions, resulting in trips and slips, balance loss, and a reduced ability to correct imbalance and falls.

Neuropathy—the result of conditions such as diabetes mellitus, vitamin B_{12} deficiency, and cervical spondylosis—is associated with lower extremity weakness and altered proprioception, which can lead to poor balance and abnormal gait. Lower extremity hemiplegia or paresis resulting from stroke can result in a narrow, unstable standing and walking base of support, which is maintained typically on the unaffected foot, and increases the risk of loss of balance. A decrease in ankle dorsiflexion of the affected limb results in a diminished ability to initiate quick postural responses, and reduced foot–ground clearance during ambulation precipitates tripping. Parkinsonism affects postural control; it institutes a loss of autonomic postural reflexes, propulsion, retropulsion, and certain gait changes (e.g., short-stepping and shuffling, barely clearing the ground; poor initiation; freezing or sudden halting of gait) that can lead to a displaced center of gravity, loss of balance, and fall risk.

Musculoskeletal Disorders   Proximal muscle weakness, concomitant with conditions such as thyroid disease, polymyalgia rheumatica, osteomalacia, or deconditioning, can lead to unstable, waddling gaits and problems with transferring. Osteoarthritis of the knees and hips, with limited joint flexibility, may result in similar problems. Disorders of the foot (e.g., toe deformities, calluses, bunions) lead to mechanical problems during ambulation and to unsteady gaits.

Cognitive Disorders   Changes in thought processes resulting from dementia or depression are associated with falls. Older adults may misperceive environmental dangers, err in judgment, or fail to discriminate between safe and dangerous environmental conditions or activities. Consequently, they may place themselves in hazardous situations and take chances that people who are cognitively intact would avoid. People with dementia who wander, especially those with mobility problems, can be at particular risk, and they may lack the ability to communicate their needs. Conversely, despite their functional frailty, some people who are cognitively intact insist on maintaining a risky level of autonomy, particularly if they are accustomed to being active and independent. Their stubbornness can increase the risk of falls.

Language Disorders   Impaired communication attributable to conditions such as dysarthria and dysphagia may seriously compromise an older adult's safety. An inability to make one's wishes known (e.g., needing help with bed transfers, wanting to walk to the bathroom) or an inability to understand safety risks causes people to attempt activities that may be inadvisable or risky. In addition, any frustration or anxiety resulting from a failure to communicate can increase the risk of falls. Avoiding a fall is probably not the primary concern of people who are frustrated or anxious. Rather, they become consumed emotionally by an immediate problem, such as toileting. As a result, they may be less alert to surrounding environmental hazards.

The care of patients and residents with communication deficits consists of identifying the language problems and any specific precautions needed to ensure their safety. In general, older adults need to be informed about hazardous activities and environmental conditions and about ways to call for help when it is needed, despite the difficulty in communicating. The use of pictures, pantomime, notebooks, communication boards, and cards that have pictures of familiar objects should be encouraged. A speech-language pathologist can help to identify other communication-enhancing techniques.

Medications

Physiologic responses to medications change as people age.[3-5] A number of pharmacokinetic and pharmacodynamic changes take place, affecting how the body handles a drug and the specific action of the drug on the body. Major pharmacokinetic changes in the distribution, metabolism, and excretion of medications occur with aging. An increase in total body fat and decrease in lean muscle mass cause changes in the effects of lipophilic, or fat-soluble, medications. For example, clearance of benzodiazepines and psychotropic medications from the body is delayed, prolonging the half-life of these drugs. A decrease in total body water and albumin levels may lead to high serum levels of medications or accumulation of water-soluble and protein-binding drugs. The capacity of the liver to metabolize medications is also impaired, and the effect is acute with benzodiazepines. A reduction in hepatic blood flow can decrease the clearance of drugs traveling through the liver, thus increasing their half-lives. Psychotropics appear to be affected the most by the aging metabolism. A reduction in renal blood flow and glomerular filtration rate in the kidney leads to a decreased excretion of drugs that are eliminated renally.

Pharmacodynamic changes, which influence the onset, duration, and intensity of drug action or the response to a given dosage, are attributed to changes occurring at organ system receptor sites. The central nervous system and cardiovascular system receptor sites are affected the most profoundly with regard to postural stability. Drug action for most medications, particularly psychoactive drugs, is increased in the central nervous system because of degenerative changes in brain matter and neurotransmitters. An increase in body sway or unsteadiness has been demonstrated to occur shortly after the administration of psychotropic medications. In the cardiovascular system, a decline in baroreflex activity increases the body's sensitivity to antihypertensive agents and contributes to the risk of postural hypotension.

Taken together, pharmacokinetic and pharmacodynamic changes make older people susceptible to drug interactions and side effects that increase the risk of falls and injury. The classes of medications associated most commonly with falls include diuretics, hypnotics and sedatives, antidepressants, psychotropics, and antihypertensives. Any of these drugs can interfere with postural control, motor and sensory coordination, or cognitive function, which may adversely influence gait and balance and induce a fall. Other medications, such as nonsteroidal anti-inflammatory drugs and laxatives, have been implicated as a cause of falls. Their action is not direct but contributory, adding to the effects of underlying arthritis or a mobility dysfunction. Thus, older people may exceed their capabilities—for example, when rushing to the bathroom—and fall.

The risk of falling is greatest when a person is taking drugs with extended half-lives (greater than 24 hours) and increases with the number of medications the person consumes. In principle, the risk of falls and injury should always be taken into consideration when medications are prescribed. Particular care must be taken with drugs that have the potential for adverse effects on cognitive function or gait and balance. Although these medications may be acceptable for treating the underlying problem, their side effects can increase the risk of falls and injury (Figure 2-12).

EXTRINSIC FACTORS

A number of extrinsic factors play an important role in fall causation. These factors consist of the physical environment, the design of furnishings, the condition of ground surfaces, and illumination. In addition, several devices used to promote mobility (e.g., walkers, wheelchairs) or guard against falls (e.g., mechanical restraints, bedside rails) have been implicated in causing falls. Also, the type and condition of footwear worn by patients and residents can play a primary role in fall causation.

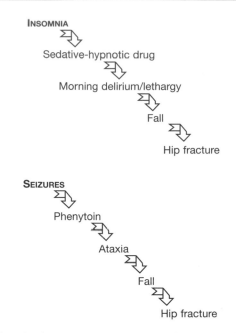

Figure 2-12. Example of medications prescribed for the treatment of medical problems such as insomnia and seizures and the potential side effects leading to falls and injury.

Physical Environment

Most institutional falls experienced by older patients and residents occur in the bedroom, bathroom, and dining areas, reflecting the amount of time people spend in these areas.[6] In conjunction with patient- or resident-initiated activities, several environmental obstacles and design features are associated with falls: transferring from inappropriately low or high beds or climbing over bedside rails; sitting on and rising from low-seated, unstable, armless chairs and low-seated toilets lacking grab bar support; walking in poorly illuminated areas and tripping over low-lying objects or floor coverings, such as thick-pile carpeting or upended linoleum or tile flooring; and slipping on highly polished or wet ground surfaces and sliding rugs. The probability of the physical environment contributing to falls is highest for people with mobility problems (e.g., altered gait and balance, impaired transfers), wherein the physical demands of activities or tasks may exceed the person's competence.

Relocation—moving from home to hospital or nursing facility, from one facility to another, from hospital to nursing facility and vice versa, or from one hospital unit to another—can increase the risk of falls. New environments can affect frail older people adversely, particularly those with mobility problems. Also, people with dementia may not tolerate change well, increasing their confusion and their risk of falls. Relocation to a new environment, which includes unfamiliar surroundings; new roommates, social situations, and nursing and other staff; and changes in daily activities, can be stressful and potentially disorienting for people with dementia.

Devices

Devices such as mechanical restraints and, more often, side rails are used for people who are at risk for falls in an attempt to protect them. It is ironic that these devices may actually increase fall risk in some instances. When patients or residents exit the bed by climbing over elevated bedside rails, perhaps catching their arms or legs in the rails, transferring becomes dangerous and increases fall risk (Figure

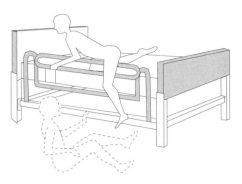

Figure 2-13. Transfers over elevated bedside rails can increase fall risk.

2-13). Also, people are more susceptible to injury, such as a fracture, when a fall from a great height occurs. In addition, bedside rails are associated with a host of other injuries, such as soft-tissue bruises, contusions, lacerations, and fractures. These injuries result when people become entrapped in bedside rails, bump into rails, or fall between the mattress and bedside rail while attempting to get out of bed. Bedside rails have been known to break or become unhitched from bed frames during transfers. Most bedside rail injuries are associated with full-length rails. However, this statement does not imply that half side rails are benign (i.e., in some instances, half side rails are not sturdy enough to support safe bed transfers).

The use of mechanical restraints can contribute to falls. Older adults can untie or slip out of restraints when they are applied improperly. As a result, older adults can fall from chairs and wheelchairs or out of bed. Patients and residents also may become entangled in restraints while attempting to get out of bed. Using restraints may increase older adults' risk of falls because of the effects of immobilization caused by restraint devices (e.g., deconditioning, muscle weakness, loss of joint flexibility, vasomotor instability). In addition, restraints can lead to increased anxiety, anger, agitation, and confusion, which heighten risk for falls. Moreover, the effectiveness of mechanical restraints in preventing falls and related injuries is doubtful. Restrained patients and residents experience more falls and serious fall-related injuries than do unrestrained people. Institutions that have limited their use of mechanical restraints have experienced either no increase in falls or only a slight increase. However, any increase in falls that may have resulted from eliminating restraints has not been accompanied by an increase in serious fall-related injuries.

Canes and walkers, devices prescribed to support mobility, can contribute to unsafe mobility if they are the wrong size, are used improperly, or are in a poor state of repair (e.g., worn rubber tips, structural breakdown). Patients and residents with inappropriate or malfunctioning walking devices may abandon or use their ambulation aids sparingly, which increases the risk of falls. Wheelchairs contribute to falls when a poor transfer technique (i.e., not locking wheel brakes, feet not clearing the footplates) is used. Wheelchairs may roll away or tip over during transfers. At other times, poor wheelchair design (e.g., inaccessibility of wheelchair brakes, short handles, improper footrest placement) and the condition of the chair itself (e.g., broken equipment, worn brakes and footrests) can be responsible for falls. In addition, falls from wheelchairs sometimes occur when patients or residents reach for objects or lean too far forward in their chairs, leading to wheelchair instability. People with cognitive impairments and lower extremity problems are at special risk for wheelchair falls; for example, they do not remember to lock wheelchair brakes, or they fail to clear the footplates when exiting the chair. Some people in wheelchairs who are agitated may rock their chairs to the point of tipping them over.

Footwear

Improper footwear can change gait and balance and lead to falls.[7] High-heeled shoes narrow the standing and walking base of support, decrease stride length, and place people in a forward-leaning posture, causing their balance to become precarious and making them susceptible to falls. Poorly fitting shoes, loose shoes in particular, can affect ambulation adversely. In an effort to keep their shoes on, people may shuffle when they walk, then trip. Leather-soled shoes promote slipping, as does wearing socks without shoes. Rubber crepe soles, although slip resistant, may stick to linoleum floor surfaces. Such sticking can halt gait precipitously, causing forward balance loss and falls, particularly in older adults with decreased foot-ground clearance. Thick-soled footwear such as running shoes or sneakers may decrease the proprioceptive feedback that is derived from the foot striking the ground during ambulation and cause a loss of balance.

Situational Circumstances

Situational circumstances also are responsible for predisposing older adults to falls and for contributing to falls. The circumstances examined here are length of stay in the health care facility, time at which the fall occurs, and specific characteristics of the facility staff.

Length of Stay

Commonly, older adults fall during the first week and after the third week of institutional stay. Various explanations have been offered. Incidents during the first week may be attributable to lack of familiarity with the environment or the presence of acute (i.e., altered homeostasis) or chronic diseases (i.e., altered mobility). Hospital patients who are perceived by both themselves and the staff as ready for discharge after the third week may be more likely to fall because they have been allowed full mobility. Residents of nursing facilities with functional limitations necessitating staff assistance at the time of admission can improve their functional status with restorative care and thus may be allowed independent movement. However, they may not have recovered their mobility fully, placing them at greater fall risk, which may account for falls after the third week. In acute care hospitals, increased length of stay is positively correlated with an increase in falls, presumably because of a greater chance of iatrogenic (i.e., induced inadvertently by a physician or by medical or surgical treatment, such as anesthetic effects) factors contributing to the risk.

Time of Fall

Most falls occur at night (i.e., 11 P.M.–7 A.M.) and certain daylight hours (i.e., 6 A.M.–10 A.M., 4 P.M.–8 P.M.). The primary explanation for nocturnal falls has been that older people get up to toilet, despite the fact that their ability to transfer safely out of bed is diminished, and that they travel to the bathroom under poor illumination. Also contributing to fall risk is the fact that there is less staff available at night and on weekends to assist patients and residents. The hours of peak frequency of falls during daylight hours correspond with peak waking activity levels.

Staff Characteristics

Staffing patterns, the number of nurses and nursing assistants available on any one shift, may also influence fall occurrence.[8] Most research shows an inverse correlation between falls and the number of staff available: Falls increase as staff is decreased, and as the number of staff increases, the frequency of falls declines. Sometimes the correlation is reversed; that is, falls increase with the addition of staff members. The reason for this reversed correlation is not entirely clear and may not relate strictly to the absolute number of nurses or to the ratio of staff to patients or residents but rather to their availability and their attitudes toward assisting people with impaired mobility. In other words, positive staff attitudes with respect to caring for older people may decrease the occurrence of falls, and negative attitudes may lead to acts of omission (e.g., failure to assess for risk and implement preventive strategies) and thus increased falls. Some speculate that the presence of agency nurses may increase risk of falls on weekends (i.e., agency nurses may not be familiar with patients and residents under their care and may lack appropriate attitudes toward patient and resident safety). Therefore, falls may not be related to the number of staff or ratio of staff to patients or residents but instead to the availability of staff at the time of the fall and the attitudes of the staff. Other complicating factors include the location of the rooms of people who fall, particularly if patients or residents reside a long distance from the nurses' station and time-consuming trips by staff are needed, and the number of staff present on different nursing shifts, weekends, and holidays.

RISK FACTORS FOR FALLS AND INJURY

Although a number of intrinsic and extrinsic factors predispose older people to falls and injuries, designing effective preventive measures entails identifying the specific risk factors involved. Several host-related or intrinsic factors have been found repeatedly to be strongly associated with the risk of institutional falls:

- History of falling

- Decreased vision (e.g., cataracts, macular degeneration, glaucoma, hemianopsia)

- Lower extremity dysfunction (e.g., arthritis, muscle weakness, peripheral neuropathy, foot disorders)

- Gait or balance disorders (e.g., Parkinson's disease, stroke, cane or walker use)

- Cardiovascular disorders (e.g., orthostatic hypotension, arrhythmia, syncope)

- Bladder dysfunction (e.g., nocturia, incontinence, frequency of urination)

- Special toileting needs (e.g., functional incontinence)

- Cognitive or emotional dysfunction (e.g., dementia, depression, anxiety, fear of falling, denial of physical and functional limitations, refusal to use necessary assistive devices)

- Communication disorders (e.g., dysarthria, dysphasia)

- Medications (e.g., diuretics, antihypertensives, sedatives, psychotropics, nonsteroidal anti-inflammatory drugs, number of drugs or polypharmacy).

These factors, in isolation or in combination, contribute to altered mobility, the ability to achieve and maintain safe ambulation, transferring activities (e.g., on or off beds, chairs, toilets, wheelchairs), and bending and reaching activities (e.g., obtaining objects from or placing objects onto nightstands, reaching into closets, cabinets, or dressers) or the ability to ask for assistance with mobility tasks.

Diseases associated with lower extremity dysfunction contribute greatly to gait and balance problems. These diseases impair ambulation and the speed and reliability of postural reflexes to correct balance displacements. In addition, loss of lower extremity strength is significantly associated with transfer difficulties that arise when one is sitting on or rising from chairs, beds, and toilets. Visual disorders can impair the detection of ground surfaces or low-lying objects and can interfere with the physiological compensation that corrects balance instability. Cognitive disturbances influence how a person perceives and adapts to the environment and to activity demands. As a risk factor, urinary dysfunction is complex. Toileting requires people to rise from a bed or chair, ambulate to the bathroom, adjust their clothing, position themselves on the toilet, maintain their balance on the toilet, stand up, leave the bathroom, and return to the point of origin. A fall may occur at any time. In addition, there is a risk that on the way to the bathroom a person will become incontinent and slip in his or her urine. The synergistic effects of medications at inappropriate dosages and the overzealous use of hypnotic-anxiolytic agents contribute to gait and postural instability. The risk of falling increases with the number of intrinsic risk factors present; multiple risk factors are more likely to be present in people with recurrent falls than in people without recurrent falls. Furthermore, the risk of falls is greatly increased in patients and residents with a history of falls during the past 3 months or recurrent falls (i.e., multiple episodes occurring over a short period of time, days to weeks).

When these intrinsic risk factors are combined with undesirable environmental conditions or extrinsic factors, the risk of falling is increased further. For example, unsuitable environments such as low-seated furnishings and toilets, reduced illumination, and hazardous ground surfaces may be negotiated easily by people who are functionally healthy. However, in people with altered mobility, the condition of the environment can be a major obstacle, increasing fall risk. The risk of injury after a fall is heightened by the presence of the following factors:

- *History of falls:* People with prior falls have a greater likelihood of falling again.

- *Advanced age:* Older women with osteoporosis are at particular risk.

- *Lower extremity weakness, loss of joint flexibility, or gait disturbances:* Greater risk of balance loss and inability to recover balance.

- *Ambulation with a cane or walker:* Increased likelihood of gait or balance disorder and fall risk.

- *Poor vision:* Inability to detect ground surface hazards, which can lead to trips and slips.

- *Confusion and dementia:* Errors in judgment between safe and hazardous tasks or the environment; reduced ability to correct imbalance.

- *Immobility:* Increased probability of lower extremity weakness and joint inflexibility, resulting in balance loss and poor balance recovery.

The risk of falls and injury occurs in three phases. Phase 1 is the initiating event that displaces the person's base of support and balance when walking. For patients and residents, these initiating events may be the result of lower extremity dysfunction such as muscle weakness, unstable joints, and diminished postural reflexes; or environmental hazards such as a slippery floor. Phase 2 occurs when the person's systems for maintaining upright posture or balance stability fail to recognize and correct the balance displacement in time to avoid a fall. Older people who fail to recover balance during falls may be experiencing a loss of sensory and motor functions, which may be the result of neurological and musculoskeletal disorders. Phase 3 of the fall, commonly called the impact phase, occurs when the person hits the floor or other surface. It is during this phase that the forces of the impact are transmitted to the body, possibly resulting in an injury. Efforts to prevent falls and injury must begin at Phase 1; the cause of falls must be evaluated and fall risk must be assessed, and subsequently, an attempt must be made to modify the risk factors discovered in an effort to prevent the occurrence of Phases 2 and 3. This approach is examined in the chapters that follow.

ENDNOTES

1. Salgado, R.I., Lord, S.R., Ehrlich, F., Janji, N., & Rahman, A. (2004). Predictors of falling in elderly hospital patients. *Archives of Gerontolology and Geriatrics, 38,* 213–219. Walker, P.C., Alrawi, A., Mitchell, J.F., Regal, R.F., & Khanderia, U. (2005). Medication use as a risk factor for falls among hospitalized elderly patients. *American Journal of Health-System Pharmacy, 62,* 2495–2499.
2. Myers, A.H., Baker, S.P., Van Natta, M.L., Abby, H., & Robinson, E.G. (1991). Risk factors associated with falls and injuries among elderly institutionalized persons. *American Journal of Epidemiology, 133,* 1179–1190.

3. Campbell, A.J. (1991). Drug treatment as a cause of falls in old age: A review of the offending agents. *Drugs and Aging, 1,* 289–302.
4. Hartikainen, S., Lonnroos, E., & Louhivuori, K. (2007). Medication as a risk factor for falls: Critical systematic review. *Journal of Gerontology: Medical Sciences, 62A*(10), 1172–1181.
5. Keller, R.B., & Slattum, P.W. (2003). Strategies for prevention of medication-related falls in the elderly. *Consultant Pharmacist, 47,* 223–229.
6. Hignett, S., & Masud, T. (2006). A review of environmental hazards associated with in-patient falls. *Ergonomics, 49,* 605–616. Tzeng, H.M., & Yin, C.Y. (2008). The extrinsic risk factors for inpatient falls in hospital patient rooms. *Journal of Nursing Care Quality, 23,* 233–241.
7. Koepsell, T.D., Wolf, M.E., Buchner, D.M., Kukull, W.A., LaCroix, A.Z., Tencer, A.F., Frankenfeld, C.L., Tautvydas, M., & Larson, E.B. (2004). Footwear style and risk of falls in older adults. *Journal of the American Geriatrics Society, 52,* 1495–1501.
8. Dunton, N., Gajewski, B., Taunton, R.L., & Moore, J. (2004). Nurse staffing and patient falls on acute care hospital units. *Nursing Outlook, 52*(1), 53–59.

Chapter Three

Clinical Assessment and Evaluation

The accumulated effects of multiple diseases, medications, and resulting disabilities, combined with extrinsic factors (i.e., environmental settings that are hazardous or unsuitable for safe mobility), predispose many older patients in hospitals and nursing facility residents to falls and subsequently cause them. However, the degree of individual fall risk and the etiology, or causes, of falls among older people vary widely. Because of interindividual variability (e.g., differences in coexisting medical problems and their number and severity; the number, types, and dosages of medications used; the level of cognitive function and mobility; design and structure of institutional environments), some people are at greater fall risk than others, and thus the etiology of falls is different. Consequently, both the prediction of individual fall risk and the determination of fall etiology are difficult without a comprehensive systematic approach.

The primary aim of the clinical assessment is to identify people who are at risk for falls and to discover the causative factors. Once these factors have been identified, a clinical evaluation is performed in order to design preventive or interventional strategies to reduce fall risk. The steps involved in the fall and fall risk assessment are outlined in Figure 3-1.

FALL ASSESSMENT

A falling episode should be followed by an evaluation and treatment of any physical injury or life-threatening medical conditions that precipitated or followed the falling event. Any time a fall occurs, the patient or resident should not be moved or assisted in getting up from the floor until the possibility of injury has been eliminated. Also, any symptoms or signs of acute medical problems must be referred for medical attention immediately. An injury and medical emergency checklist that nurses can use as a referral tool is provided in Section Three.

Once the patient or resident is medically stable, a history of the circumstances surrounding the fall should be taken to help determine the differential diagnosis. Taking a history is analogous to inquiring about any other medical symptoms such as abdominal pain or chest pain. To discover the etiology, a history of the circumstances should be obtained, as should descriptive information on the duration, severity, and location of the discomfort.

Step 1
    Patient or resident has fallen: Proceed to Step 2. If patient or resident has not fallen: Proceed to Step 4.

Step 2
    Evaluate for physical injury and/or acute medical problems. Provide treatment as indicated.

Step 3
    Obtain fall history, circumstances of incident.

Step 4
    Review fall risk factors (medical, psychological, and functional histories).

Step 5
    Obtain Peformance-Oriented Environmental Mobility Screen (POEMS).

Step 6
    Perform physical examination.

Step 7
    Obtain laboratory and diagnostic studies as indicated.

Step 8
    List differential diagnosis of fall(s) and/or identified fall risk factors.

Step 9
    Implement interventions to reduce fall risk.

Step 10
    Monitor/follow-up to determine success of interventions.

Step 11
    Repeat assessment if patient or resident continues to fall or experiences new falls. If no falls, proceed to Step 12.

Step 12
    Repeat fall risk assessment on a regular basis.

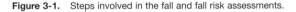

Figure 3-1. Steps involved in the fall and fall risk assessments.

Taking a fall history consists of asking the person about any symptoms experienced at the time of the fall or those occurring before the fall (e.g., dizziness, heart palpitations, loss of consciousness or balance, legs giving away, trips or slips) and for a description of the activity the person was engaged in at the time of the fall. Because older adults may have poor recollection of these events because of cognitive impairment, reports from nurses, other staff members, and family members who witnessed the fall can be helpful. In addition, the location, time (hour of the day) of the fall, and any injuries sustained should be documented.

Asking patients and residents to recount the circumstances of their falls provides valuable clues to the etiologies. For example, falls associated with rising from a bed or chair and experiencing symptoms of dizziness may point to orthostatic hypotension (for a definition of this and other terms related to the chapter, see the Terminology sidebar). An absence of symptoms may implicate the design, height, or stability of the bed or chair as a causative factor. If a person complains of tripping or slipping, the environment (e.g., hazardous ground surface camouflaged by poor lighting, wet floors, upended carpet edges or linoleum tiles) may be the precipitating cause, either by itself or in combination with an underlying gait disorder.

Terminology

Differential diagnosis	Distinguishing between two or more diseases with similar symptoms by systematically comparing their signs and symptoms
Hypoglycemia	Low blood sugar
Orthostatic hypotension	Lowered blood pressure that occurs on rising to an erect position
Proprioception	Muscle and joint sensations of body's position in space
Syncope	Fainting; temporary unconsciousness

In addition, the history should include inquiry about previous falls and their circumstances. This inquiry helps to determine whether there is a pattern to the falls. The majority of people who fall repeatedly do so under similar circumstances. If not available from the patient or resident, this information may be gathered from a review of past incident reports or medical records. It is equally important to solicit information about near falls. Near falls are events in which a person loses balance but manages to avert a fall to the ground by grabbing onto an object such as the back of a chair, a headboard, or a table edge for support. (If the object had not been available for support, the person probably would have suffered a fall to the ground.) Observational studies of older people residing in institutions have demonstrated that in the course of their daily activities, many frail adults have a high frequency of near falls, which increases the risk of falling.[1]

Other questions that should be asked about previous falls include whether the person has experienced any physical injury or loss of self-confidence in performing activities, or, subsequently, has restricted his or her mobility in any way. A positive response to the latter may indicate a fear of subsequent falls.

A thorough history aimed at identifying the circumstances associated with falling represents the foundation of determining fall etiology because all subsequent evaluations are based, in part, on the information obtained. As such, the fall history (Figure 3-2) can be incorporated into existing hospital and nursing facility incident reports and thus becomes a standard part of any investigation of falls.

Symptoms experienced at time of fall(s)

Previous number of falls or near falls

Location of fall(s)

Activity engaged in at time of fall(s)

Time (hour of day) of fall(s)

Trauma (physical, psychological) associated with fall(s)

Figure 3-2. Fall history to be gathered on an individual, using the acronym SPLATT.

FALL RISK ASSESSMENT

The assessment of fall risk in older adults in hospitals and nursing facilities begins with the identification of individual risk factors from the thorough history.[2]

Identification of Individual Risk Factors

A thorough history can detect most people who are at high risk for falling. The person taking the history should inquire about the occurrence of falls during the previous 3 months and the circumstances surrounding the fall(s) and review the medical history for conditions and medications that place patients or residents at risk. Individual fall risk factors include

- Visual impairment

- Postural hypotension

- Reduced lower extremity strength

- Impaired gait and balance

- Impaired mobility

- Use of ambulation assistive devices

- Bladder dysfunction

- Altered cognition

- Polypharmacy (taking four or more medications)

- Sedatives, psychotropics, hypnotics, and antihypertensive drugs.

These factors, particularly when they occur simultaneously, have been associated repeatedly with fall risk; attempts to ascertain their presence should be included in the risk assessment of patients and residents. Although these factors by themselves increase susceptibility to falls, their relationship as a true measure of fall risk is more accurately reflected in their effects on a person's ability to ambulate and transfer safely and independently in the living environment. Any impairment in gait and balance that results from these factors is a strong predictor of fall risk. Therefore, a performance-oriented environmental mobility screen (POEMS), which evaluates how competently patients and residents execute a number of positional changes and movements during their daily activities, should be obtained. (A blank, photocopiable master form is included in Section Three.)

Performance-Oriented Environmental Mobility Screen

POEMS is the second step of the assessment of fall risk and is beneficial in identifying host-related situations and environmental conditions that cause dysmobility in people at fall risk. POEMS assesses the following performance items: balance maintained in sitting and rising from a chair, bed, and toilet; standing balance; ability to bend down from a standing position; and ability to ambulate in the bedroom and bathroom. Transfer and ambulation maneuvers are tested with or without assistive devices as applicable. Testing the person's capacity to ambulate in different locations takes into account that the space limitations, ground surfaces, and illumination of the space are dissimilar and represent different risks. The person is scored on each task as being either normal (i.e., independent mobility) or impaired (i.e., person is unsteady during performance or unable to accomplish the task or perform the task safely). Any impaired execution indicates that the person is at fall risk.

Depending on the patient's or resident's state of health, the sequence of POEMS maneuvers may be altered to accommodate individual needs. In patients and residents who are ill, the length of the POEMS is determined by the person's ability to continue performing the maneuver safely. The following list suggests sequences for people who are ill and for people who are well.

Illness

- Transfer off bed

- Stand after rising from bed (eyes open)

- Stand with eyes closed

- Stand in place (sternal nudge)

- Bend down, pick up object

- Walk around bedroom or bed

- Walk to and around bathroom

- Sit down and rise from toilet

- Walk up and down hallway

- Transfer onto bed.

Wellness

- Sit down and rise from chair

- Stand after rising from chair (eyes open)

- Stand with eyes closed

- Stand in place (sternal nudge)

- Bend down, pick up object

- Transfer onto and off bed

- Walk around bedroom or bathroom

- Sit down on and rise from toilet

- Walk up and down hallway.

POEMS is initiated in the older person's bedroom. The person is asked to sit down and rise from a chair. The person doing the screening should observe the person's ability to complete the activity in a smooth and controlled movement, without loss of balance or the use of armrests. The chair should not tip

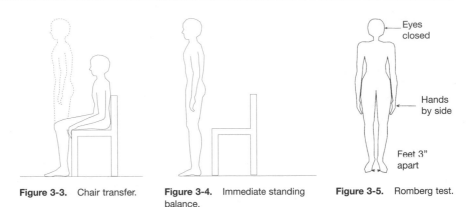

Figure 3-3. Chair transfer.   **Figure 3-4.** Immediate standing balance.   **Figure 3-5.** Romberg test.

or slide away, and the person's feet should not slide but rest flat on the floor (Figure 3-3). Next, the person should be instructed to rise from the chair and remain standing in place for approximately 30 seconds. The person doing the screening should observe whether the person is able to stand without loss of balance or support from the chair to maintain balance (Figure 3-4). The person should be asked to perform the Romberg test, which assesses proprioceptive function: He or she should remain standing with eyes closed, arms placed at his or her sides, and feet planted approximately 3 inches apart. Inability to maintain balance, as demonstrated by increased postural sway or grabbing furnishings for support, indicates an abnormality (Figure 3-5).

The examiner should perform a sternal push test with the person standing still with his or her eyes open. The push test consists of nudging the person's sternum lightly with the fingers, applying enough force to induce balance displacement (Figure 3-6). This maneuver tests postural competence in response to loss of balance. The normal reaction is to stretch the arms forward, away from the body, and to take one or two steps backward (Figure 3-7). Both movements represent the body's ability to compensate for sudden balance shifts. The inability to maintain balance (e.g., a fall backward) signifies an abnormality (Figure 3-8). During these postural tests, another staff member should be positioned behind the person to intervene in the event of a fall. In extremely frail people or in those who, from appearances, would obviously have difficulty recovering from imbalances, the sternal push test may be omitted for safety reasons.

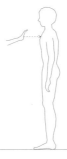

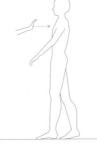

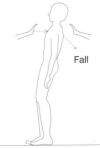

Figure 3-6. Sternal push test.   **Figure 3-7.** A normal reaction to body displacement.   **Figure 3-8.** An abnormal reaction to body displacement.

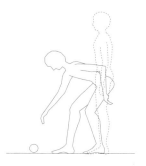

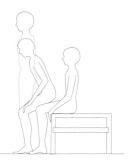

Figure 3-9. Bending-down performance.

Figure 3-10. Bed transfer.

After the body displacement tests, the person should be asked to bend from a normal standing position as if to retrieve an object from the floor. The examiner should observe whether the person is steady and able to maintain balance without holding onto furnishings for support (Figure 3-9). The person's reaching activities, such as obtaining clothing from closets and other storage areas, can be assessed in a similar fashion.

Next, the person should be asked to transfer onto and off of the bed. The person's ability to perform this maneuver in a smooth, controlled manner without loss of balance or need for arm support to maintain sitting balance on the mattress should be observed and rated. Also, the bed should remain steady, without moving or sliding away. The older person's feet should rest flat on the floor in the seated position (Figure 3-10).

The next performance item tests ambulation ability. The person should be asked to walk about and turn around, first in the bedroom and then in the bathroom, using the ambulation device if applicable. The examiner should observe the person's gait and balance, whether the person's gait is continuous and whether it occurs without hesitation or excessive deviation from side to side; whether both feet clear the surface of the floor; whether the person staggers, loses balance, or grabs environmental surfaces (e.g., bed, chair backs, sink edge, walls) for support; and whether the ambulation device is used safely and fits into spaces (e.g., both sides of the bed, in the bathroom) (Figure 3-11).

Toilet transfer is the next area to be tested in POEMS. The person should be asked to transfer onto and off the toilet. As with other tests, the

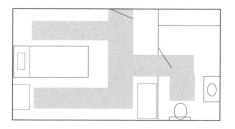

Figure 3-11. Common environmental walking routes are reflected by the shaded areas. A person should be able to use his or her ambulation device safely in all areas.

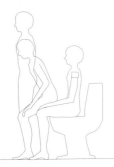

Figure 3-12. Toilet transfer.

person should be observed for his or her ability to perform this activity in a smooth, controlled movement, without loss of balance or the need to hold onto the sink edge or grab bars for support (Figure 3-12). Finally, the person should walk from the bedroom and down the hallway to the nurses' station and other locations, such as the dining room. The person should be observed for his or her ability to walk without gait and balance difficulties or fatigue.

If the person's POEMS results are normal (i.e., the patient or resident is able to perform the maneuvers independently), the person is at low fall risk. However, any impairment in execution of a task indicates the presence of underlying intrinsic or extrinsic factors (Table 3-1) that place the person at fall risk.

Advantages of POEMS

POEMS has several advantages: It is easy to understand and administer by nurses and nursing assistants in both hospital and nursing facility settings. In general, it takes no longer than 10 minutes to complete, even with the frailest people. In addition to detecting mobility dysfunction, POEMS can be used to help design rehabilitative and environmental interventions and to monitor clinical changes or outcomes (e.g., the effects of medical conditions, medications, environmental influences) over time.

Table 3-1. POEMS differential diagnoses

Impaired maneuver	Intrinsic factors	Extrinsic factors
Chair, bed, and toilet transfers	Parkinsonism Arthritis Deconditioning Adverse drug effects	Poor chair, bed, or toilet design
Standing balance	Postural hypotension Vestibular dysfunction Adverse drug effects	
Romberg test	Proprioceptive dysfunction Adverse drug effect	Poor illumination Overly absorptive footwear, carpeting, or both
Sternal push	Parkinsonism Normal pressure hydrocephalus Adverse drug effects	
Bending down	Central nervous system dysfunction Adverse drug effects	
Walking/turning	Foot disorders Parkinsonism Hemiparesis Sensory dysfunction Adverse drug effects	Improper footwear Improper size/use of ambulation device Hazardous ground surfaces

Administering POEMS

Optimally, the fall risk assessment should be completed when people are first admitted to the hospital or nursing facility because the risk of falling is greatest during the first few days of institutional stay. However, completing the assessment may not always be feasible or practical, particularly in an acute care hospital. On admission to an acute care facility, patients may be injured (e.g., hip fracture) or severely ill. Often, people with rapidly fluctuating medical conditions are maintained by bed rest. In these instances, risk assessment is best administered after any acute problem or condition is treated and stabilized or at a time when the patient is permitted to assume an independent level of function. In both hospitals and nursing facilities, risk should be reassessed whenever the person's medical condition, medication regimen (e.g., the addition or subtraction of drugs, dosage modifications), or functional status changes.

In nursing facilities and certain hospital units such as psychiatric wards, where people reside for prolonged periods of time, risk assessment, particularly POEMS, should be repeated at established intervals, approximately every 3–6 months. This should be done so as to identify people with gradually deteriorating health conditions because any decline in mobility can be an early sign of disease and fall risk.

POEMS can be incorporated into the Minimum Data Set 2.0 (MDS 2.0; Long-Term Care Facility Resident Assessment Instrument) in nursing facilities as follows:

MDS Full Assessment Form
Section G: Physical Functioning and Structural Problems

Bed mobility

Transfer

Walk in room

Walk in corridor

Locomotion on unit

Toilet use

Test for balance

Modes of locomotion

Modes of transfer

Change in ability to perform activities of daily living (ADLs)

MDS Quarterly Assessment Form
Section G1: ADL Performance

Bed mobility

Walk in room

Walk in corridor

Toilet use

Modes of transfer

Resident Assessment Protocols

Failure to thrive

ADLs

Functional rehabilitation potential

Falls

Psychotropic drug-related side effects (unsteady gait or balance)

Physical Restraints (risk of falls)

A fall risk checklist is presented in Section Three that can be used to help identify and record individual risk factors. In addition, the checklist can be incorporated into existing institutional examination forms, medical and nursing records, and incident reports. Once a patient or resident is identified as being at fall risk, all staff must be alerted. A number of measures have been used by nursing staff to recognize people at risk: application of brightly colored stickers placed on the medical and nursing charts, bedroom door, and bedside; and distinctively colored wrist identification bands or slippers to be worn by the person at risk.

Several hospitals and nursing facilities have developed standard fall risk assessment tools that predict a person's susceptibility to falls (see Bibliography). The sources of data used to develop these risk profiles vary greatly (e.g., incident report data, literature reviews of risk factors, staff experiences). A number of potential problems with these risk assessment tools have been identified. Staff members have varying definitions of a fall they report; some institutions may require only falls resulting in physical injury to be reported; profiles developed from the literature are often skewed toward characteristics of a particular institution, hospital, or nursing facility; and within each institution, specific factors derived from specialized units (e.g., oncology, orthopedic, surgery, psychiatric, rehabilitation, neurology, stroke, dementia-specific care) may not apply to different institutions or settings.

Staffing patterns and environmental designs also may affect fall risk; indeed, in some instances they may be a greater determinant of risk than the characteristics of patients or residents by themselves. The most effective procedure is to examine the risk assessment tools available and choose several that seem to reflect the particular population of the facility. Each procedure should be used in a pilot program within hospital units and nursing facility floors that have a high incidence of falls. Their success is measured by assessing a group of people who have experienced falls and comparing them with a group of people without falls. Using the tool in this way should determine whether it is sensitive enough to differentiate fall risk. Questions that should be answered while using the tool include the following: Does the tool work? Does it accurately identify patients and residents at risk for falling? Is the tool practical? Do nurses find the instrument convenient for routine use? Being able to accurately identify patients and residents at risk on a regular basis enables resources (e.g., nursing and rehabilitative staff, safety equipment, assistive devices) to be targeted toward prevention.

CLINICAL EVALUATION

Once the fall and fall risk assessments have been completed, multiple fall etiologies and risk factors may be identified via clinical evaluation. The primary aim of the clinical evaluation is twofold: First, in people with falls, it isolates a specific cause; in people with identifiable risk factors, it uncovers the presence of remediable or modifiable factors. Second, the clinical evaluation determines in both groups the existence of any new risk factors that were not detected previously. Although in general the clinical evaluation is the province of physicians, allied health professionals (e.g., physicians' assistants, nurse practitioners, clinicians) are equally adept in assessment techniques. The services of these professionals are useful, particularly in the nursing facility, where the presence of physicians is rare.

The clinical evaluation of patients and residents with falls begins with a review of the medical records, current medical problems, and medications. This review may provide important clues to the factors contributing to falls. For example, if a person experiences dizziness before a fall and records indicate the recent addition of a diuretic to the person's medicines, the association of the two factors may indicate that the fall was caused by an adverse medication effect. Similarly, if a person has arthritis in the knees and falls while transferring from a chair, the arthritis may be partially responsible for the fall.

Once the person's historical information is compiled, a POEMS should be obtained. As in people at fall risk, the value of POEMS for people who have fallen lies in isolating organ systems and environmental problems that may provide insight into the possible etiology of the fall. The next step is to perform a physical examination that includes comprehensive cognitive, neurological, musculoskeletal, and cardiac evaluations. Information gathered from the fall and fall risk assessments and POEMS can serve as a focus for the physical examination. For example, if the fall history reveals that a fall occurred in association with dizziness and changes in position and POEMS demonstrates a loss of balance, unsteadiness, or the complaint of dizziness on immediate standing, postural changes in blood pressure must be assessed to rule out or confirm orthostatic hypotension. Similarly, if the person demonstrates difficulty with chair or bed transferring during POEMS, the physical examination should concentrate on evaluating the musculoskeletal system for reduced muscle strength. Not only will any abnormality discovered during the physical examination help to identify the cause of falls and modifiable risk factors, but other findings may be detected that are not directly related but may increase the risk of subsequent falls.

Once the physical examination has been completed, the next step is to perform laboratory and diagnostic studies. The extent of testing is dictated by the information gathered from all previous evaluations. For example, if the physical examination confirms the presence of orthostatic hypotension, blood and stool testing for volume-depleted states such as dehydration, blood loss, and anemia must be ordered. If the person is diabetic and the history suggests falls resulting from hypoglycemia, a blood glucose test should be obtained. If the fall is associated with a syncopal episode and the physical examination reveals an irregular pulse rate, an electrocardiogram and possibly a Holter monitoring study should be considered. A history of bladder dysfunction

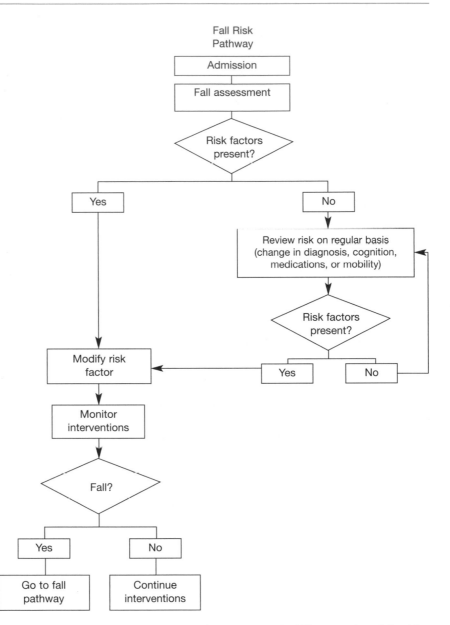

Figure 3-13. The fall risk assessment pathway. This assessment should be repeated regularly to identify new or changing risk factors.

demands urine and blood tests and urodynamic studies to search for underlying causes. Similarly, manifestations of lower extremity weakness on physical examination indicate the need for tests that may explain the etiology.

After all evaluations are complete, a list of intrinsic and extrinsic factors responsible for fall risk or falls can be compiled. From the list, interventions to reduce the risk of subsequent falls should follow (see Chapter 4). Follow-up ensures that the intervention strategies used are effective. Repeat the fall risk

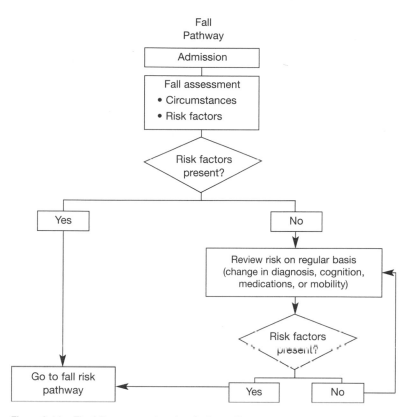

Figure 3-14. The fall assessment and evaluation pathway.

assessment by using flowcharts or pathways, as shown in Figures 3-13 and 3-14, on a regular basis to identify new or changing risk factors (Figure 3-13). If the person continues to fall, repeat the fall assessment and evaluation (Figure 3-14). Some factor may have been missed or overlooked from previous evaluations, or the person may have developed an additional condition that causes falls. It is important to remember that falls and fall risk are not fixed or static processes but rather are dynamic events, and the causes can change as often as do the person's medical conditions and environmental surroundings.

ENDNOTES

1. Connell, B.R., & Wolf, S.L. (1993). Patterns of naturally occurring falls among frail nursing home residents. *Gerontologist, 33*(Special Issue), 58.
2. Rutledge, D.N., Donaldson, N.E., & Pravikoff, D.S. (2003). Update 2003: Fall risk assessment and prevention in hospitalized patients. *Journal of Clinical Innovation, 6*(5), 1–55.

Chapter Four

Preventive Strategies to Reduce Fall Risk

The goal of fall prevention strategies is to design interventions that minimize fall risk by ameliorating or eliminating contributing factors while maintaining or improving patients' and residents' mobility. Potential preventive strategies are based on known risk factors and postulated causes of falls and can be classified as medical, rehabilitative, and environmental. In most cases, fall prevention includes components in each category. Although little direct evidence exists on the effectiveness of any of these particular approaches in preventing falls, common sense suggests that they are promising and should be attempted. A description of these measures designed to prevent or reduce the incidence of falls, which can be used by hospital and nursing facility staff, along with an elaboration of fall prevention programs developed in institutional settings, follows.

MEDICAL STRATEGIES

The importance of identifying patients and residents at fall risk and those with falls and following up with a clinical evaluation of each to identify modifiable factors cannot be overemphasized. Each factor may represent a sign or symptom of an underlying disease or medication effect that warrants a clinician's attention in order to rule out reversible acute problems, identify chronic medical conditions that may contribute, and treat each appropriately. Of equal importance is the assessment of medications. All drugs should be reviewed carefully in terms of their risks and benefits. Dosages should be examined with an eye toward reduction when possible. Any combination of drugs should be monitored on a regular basis for potential drug interactions. In particular, drugs that affect mobility or increase fall risk such as sedatives, hypnotics, and psychoactives should be scrutinized routinely.

As a general rule, medications in older people should be initiated at their lowest effective dose, increased slowly with monitoring for side effects and clinical efficacy, maintained at the lowest possible dose, and discontinued when no longer effective. For patients and residents with osteoporosis who are at risk for injurious falls, consideration of drug treatment (e.g., calcium supplements and medications that reduce bone loss) to modify the risk of hip and other fractures is advised.

REHABILITATIVE STRATEGIES

Patients and residents who do not respond or improve with medical treatment and continue to remain at fall risk, particularly those with chronic neuromuscular disorders, may respond to a number of rehabilitative strategies. These strategies include engaging in exercise therapy, wearing proper footwear, using hip-protective pads, and using appropriate ambulation devices to assist with mobility.

Exercise

People with impaired muscular strength and altered gait and balance—the consequences of underlying medical conditions, deconditioning, or both—may benefit from low-intensity leg strengthening and weight-bearing exercises as well as gait, balance, and transfer training generally provided by physiatrists and physical therapists. These kinds of exercise and training programs are designed to restore and maintain muscle strength and coordination, bone mass, joint flexibility and movement, vestibular and proprioceptive function, and postural control reflexes and to teach people effective bed, chair, and toilet transfer techniques. In addition, there are a variety of exercise programs that nurses and nursing assistants can easily perform on their own to help maintain patient and resident mobility (Table 4-1). Figure 4-1 illustrates a set of simple exercises designed to maintain or improve mobility. These exercises can be performed by staff either at the person's bedside or in a group setting, depending on the institution. These exercises should be started gradually and be done twice daily. The facilitator should work at the

Table 4-1.   Types of ambulation programs

Daily Floor Ambulation Program

Ambulatory patients or residents are encouraged to walk at least three times daily, or 30–45 minutes a day as tolerated, to the dining room, planned activities, and so forth. Assistance with ambulation is provided for individuals with poor gait and balance and/or fear of falling. The use of wheelchairs is discouraged.

"Walkers Group"

Ambulatory patients or residents are encouraged to walk daily from bed to bathroom, from bedroom to nurses' station, from bedroom to the end of the hallway, from one end of the hallway to the other end, and so forth, with set goals determined by physical condition. Rewards are given for achieving each goal.

Wheelchair Walking Program

Patients or residents are encouraged to "walk" with their chairs—to move their wheelchairs along by using their legs. This exercise helps them to maintain effective and safe transfers and improves lower extremity function. Removing the footrests discourages their use.

Mobility Program

Patients or residents are encouraged to ambulate and/or stand at least three times daily and to walk to the activity room for group exercises and meals daily. Patients, residents, and/or their caregivers are taught active and passive range-of-motion exercises, weight-bearing exercises, and resistive and aerobic exercises.

patient's or resident's own pace and level of stability. (Strength building can be intensified by adding 1- to 2-pound weights when performing Exercises 2 and 3.) For most patients and residents, these exercise therapy programs pose a minimal risk of adverse effects (i.e., injury), and they may be effective in combating impaired mobility and decreasing the risk of falls and injury.

A growing body of evidence suggests that older people respond to exercise therapy, even those who are very old and frail. Exercise can enhance the functioning of other organ systems involved in mobility endurance, such as

Exercise 1: Chair Rise/Sit (improves lower extremity strength and joint motion)

Ask the patient or resident to stand up from a stable chair and then sit down. If necessary, the patient or resident should use the armrest of the chair for support. 8–10 reps, as tolerated.

Exercise 2: Modified Sit-Up (improves lower extremity strength and joint motion)

Ask the patient or resident to lift each leg from the knee. 6–8 reps, as tolerated.

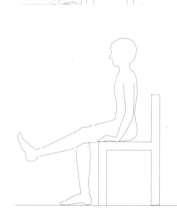

Exercise 3: Standing Knee Bend (improves lower extremity strength and balance)

Ask the patient or resident to lift leg, bend, and straighten at knee. Alternate right and left legs. 10 reps, as tolerated.

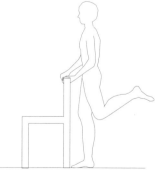

Figure 4-1. Flexibility and balance exercise program.

(continued)

Figure 4-1. *(continued)*

Exercise 4: Shoulder Shrug (improves upper extremity range of motion)

Ask the patient or resident to sit up or stand up straight, shrug the shoulders up high, and release. 10 reps, as tolerated.

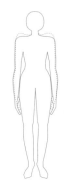

Exercise 5: Arm Circles (improves upper extremity range of motion)

Ask the patient or resident to sit up or stand up straight. With each arm make a circle, which gradually increases to become as large as possible. Begin the exercise with the arms 6 inches from sides and circle arms upward and down again. Each circle, 20 seconds; 2 reps, as tolerated.

Exercise 6: Ankle Pumps (improves ankle strength and balance)

Ask the patient or resident to lift up body on tiptoes and lower body back down while holding on to the back of a stable chair. This exercise may be done in a chair if the patient or resident has poor balance: Ask the individual to lift up heels on tiptoes and lower the heels back down again. 15 reps, as tolerated.

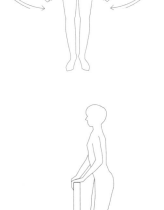

Figure 4-1.   Flexibility and balance exercise program.

cardiovascular and pulmonary performance. In addition, because they build patients' and residents' self-confidence in performing activities, fear of falling or instability may be reduced. Because these people may be susceptible to falls and injury, caution is advised; a renewed sense of confidence and ability to execute mobility tasks may lead these people to attempt activities that exceed their capabilities. This possibility should not dissuade staff from encouraging patient and resident independence in mobility, however. Instead, patients and residents should receive assistance at the beginning of such a program, and the assistance should continue until the person can participate in the activities safely and independently.

For people who fall, mobility should be encouraged as soon as possible in order to avoid the consequences of immobility. If patients or residents need assistance with walking, nursing staff can use a gait belt (Figure 4-2). The belt serves as a ready "handle" to grasp in the event that the older person begins to fall. Staff should hold on to the belt handles or the tail strap with one hand and, with the other hand, hold on to the person's shoulder, which helps to control balance if the older person falls forward or backward. If the patient or resident does lose balance, the staff member should maintain normal posture (i.e., should not bend over): The knees should be bent, with the feet spaced 12 inches apart. The person should be pulled gently toward the staff member, or his or her descent to the ground should be

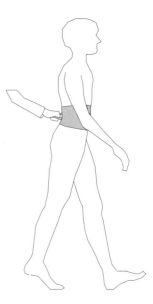

Figure 4-2. Assisted ambulation using a gait belt.

controlled gently. Some staff and even the older person may find that a gait belt provides added security. To assist a person walking without a cane, the staff member should position himself or herself in back and slightly to the side of the person. If the person uses a cane or hemiwalker, the staff member should stand on the opposite side of the device. To ensure safety, the patient or resident should never be pushed beyond safe limits; the activity should be stopped if the person complains of fatigue or if gait and balance become unsafe. It is also a good idea to consult with a physical therapist on proper techniques for assisted walking.

Footwear

All shoes and slippers worn by patients and residents should fit properly and have slip-resistant soles. If foot problems such as hammertoes, bunions, calluses, and nail disorders prohibit the wearing of proper-sized shoes, the person should be referred for podiatric care. To accommodate foot problems, special therapeutic footwear (i.e., "Frankenstein" shoes) may be prescribed. Some frail older people may experience difficulty walking in this type of shoe, which can increase fall risk. The shoes are somewhat heavy to wear, and therefore the person may shuffle when walking, which can lead to tripping. Cutting out the toe box of the shoes may be a good alternative to therapeutic footwear, which interferes with safe walking.

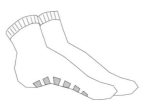

Shoes and slippers with rubber or crepe soles provide adequate slip resistance on linoleum floors. Socks with nonskid tread on the soles (Figure 4-3) are a good choice, particularly for people who make nocturnal bathroom trips. However, for

Figure 4-3. Socks with non-skid tread soles.

some people, such as those with a shuffling gait or poor steppage height (i.e., inability to pick up the feet an adequate distance from the floor), slip-resistant soles may interfere with safe ambulation because the soles adhere to ground surfaces. In particular, disposable foam "hospital slippers" and sneakers or running shoes with thick rubber soles can adhere to the ground surface when a person is walking in them. For such people, footwear with leather-type soles that promote gliding on linoleum and carpeted floor surfaces may be a better choice in institutional settings having a mixture of floor surfaces (i.e., both linoleum and carpeting); however, caution in the selection of soles is warranted. For some older people, footwear with smooth soles (lack of traction) can facilitate walking on carpeted surfaces but promotes slipping when walking on linoleum-covered surfaces.

Footwear with thick, soft soles may interfere with proprioceptive feedback (i.e., it may cause an inability to feel the ground while walking), resulting in a loss of balance. Wearing thin, hard rubber-soled shoes (e.g., boat shoes, Topsiders) can help a person preserve his or her balance. The best way to evaluate the adequacy of the sole surface of footwear is to observe patients and residents as they walk on different floor surfaces in their environment to see whether their footwear interferes with safe ambulation.

High-heeled shoes should be avoided because they narrow a person's standing and walking base of support, which can lead to a loss of balance.

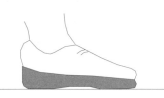

Figure 4-4. Shoes with wedge heels.

Footwear with low, broad heels is a better choice and should be encouraged. These shoes are better suited for safe walking and balance. However, if the patient or resident insists on wearing high heels—either out of vanity or because of a real need—she should be cautioned that high heels worn over a long period of time cause a shortening of the Achilles tendon, which then necessitates their use. Staff should then encourage the wearing of shoes with wedge heels (Figure 4-4). Wedge heels provide a better base of support than ordinary high-heeled shoes, and they are less likely to catch on an elevated floor surface, such as upended carpet, linoleum tile edges, or door thresholds.

Hip Protectors

More than 90% of hip fractures in older people are related to direct trauma against a hard ground surface after a fall. Hip protectors (Figure 4-5) are designed to act as shock absorbers around the hip (i.e., providing a cushion between the hip bone and impact surface), diverting the direct impact of a fall away from the bone, which helps to reduce the risk of a hip fracture. Three different types of hip protectors are available:

- *Hard shell pads:* Thin, elliptical plastic shields either sewn into specially designed undergarments or placed into pockets inside an ordinary pair of underwear; the shields are positioned to cover the hip bone.

- *Soft adsorbing pads:* Two shock-absorbent foam pads inserted into a lightweight wraparound garment that is worn under outer clothing and over underwear; Velcro closures are used to allow easy application and removal of the system.

- *Dual-mechanism hard and absorbing pads:* These can offer the best features of both types, with an absorbing component and a dispersing component.

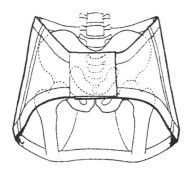

Figure 4-5. Example of a hip padding system (Hip-Guard). (Illustration reproduced with the permission of Prevent-Wise, Inc.)

Hip protectors can prevent hip fractures and have demonstrated benefits for both nursing facility residents and hospital patients.[1, 2] However, questions remain as to who should wear hip pads, how to convince people to wear them, and what kinds of hip pads are the most effective (see Fall Prevention Guidelines in Section Three, Part A).

Approximately 50%–80% of older people comply with hip protectors, wearing them regularly. Compliance is higher in people who are cognitively intact and in people who have recently experienced an injurious fall. A fear of falling improves a person's initial acceptance of hip protectors, perhaps because they offer the person peace of mind. Therefore, hip protectors may be most helpful as a preventive strategy against hip fractures in select groups of patients and residents such as those at risk for further hip fracture and those with a fear of falling or injury.[3]

Patients benefiting from a hip protector include those who have frequent falls and health related conditions associated with hip fracture:

- Osteoporosis
- Diabetes
- Stroke
- Arthritis
- Parkinson's disease
- Functional and balance impairment
- Cognitive impairment or dementia
- Diminished visual abilities
- Use of benzodiazepines or anticonvulsants.

Other conditions that may warrant the use of a hip protector include the following:

- Any sudden change of health conditions associated with dizziness or loss of balance
- Starting a medication associated with side effects of dizziness, orthostatic hypotension, or loss of balance
- Falls associated with dizziness or balance loss
- Low staff:patient ratios.

Noncompliance with wearing hip pads takes two forms: initial rejection (the person does not want to wear hip pads) or later rejection (the person initially accepts wearing hip pads but subsequently refuses to wear them). Several factors are associated with noncompliance,[4] including altered cognitive status and wearability (see Fall Prevention Guidelines in Section Three, Part A).

Altered Cognitive Status

Patients and residents with dementia may lack the capacity to comprehend or recognize the need for hip protectors, or they may become agitated while wearing the pads, forcing their removal. It is important to remember that not all people with dementia think about or respond to situations similarly; thus, some people reject hip pads or become disturbed by their presence, whereas other people accept and use hip protectors without complaint. In general, people with severe dementia are more tolerant of hip pads than are people with mild to moderate dementia. Because people with dementia are at significant risk for falling (e.g., from participating in hazardous activities, not asking for assistance with activities, or developing small-stepped gaits) and fracturing their hips, attempts to provide hip protectors to people with mild to moderate dementia should not be abandoned. Some patients and residents, especially those with dementia, may need to have the purpose of the hip protector explained to them each time it is applied in order to prevent agitation.

Wearability

Some older people complain that hip protectors are uncomfortable to wear, that they are too bulky for sitting in chairs or sleeping in bed, that they are too hot or tight to wear under clothing, and that they are too difficult to remove in readiness for toileting (this is especially the case for people with urinary incontinence and frequency). Staff members sometimes complain that hip protectors are difficult to care for, particularly when worn by people who are incontinent, or are too difficult to remove when assisting incontinent people with scheduled toileting regimens. Alternatives that increase compliance include the following:

- Selecting times when hip protectors are worn (e.g., days when people feel more unsteady) or not worn (e.g., during sleep, although nocturia, or excessive urination at night, is a risk factor for falls)

- Asking people to wear pants and dresses that are a few sizes larger than usual (to accommodate hip pads)

- Providing soft-seated chairs, which may be more comfortable for people to sit in.

Studies assessing the effectiveness of the different hip protectors in reducing hip fractures and increasing wearability are inconclusive. Therefore, it is too early to recommend any one hip protector over another with certainty. However, because sometimes the point of impact in a fall is not directly on the hip but on the buttock, the soft absorbing pad protector, which wraps around the pelvis, may offer more protection than the plastic or hard shell system. The soft absorbing pad protector may protect against hip fracture in frail people with osteoporosis and poor balance who are constantly bumping against hard surfaces, such as walls and table edges. In addition, staff may find the soft absorbing pad protector easier to use for people who are incontinent because it can be used in conjunction with adult incontinence pads. Because hip protectors used by themselves cannot preclude the possibility of sustaining a hip fracture, hip protectors alone cannot be relied on in the prevention of fractures but must be used in conjunction with other preventive efforts.

Ambulation Devices

Ambulation devices, such as canes and walkers, are designed to improve gait and balance and to decrease the risk of falls. They work by creating greater stability, which increases a person's standing and walking base of support because they provide an additional point or points of ground contact (Figure 4-6). Ambulation devices furnish proprioceptive feedback through the handles and reduce the load on weight-bearing joints, such as hips and knees. Also, devices provide visual physical support, which instills confidence during ambulation, helping to reduce the person's fear of instability and falls.

The choice of a cane, whether single- or multistemmed, or a walker, whether pick-up or wheeled type, should be determined by each person's needs (see Table 4-2 for a list of types of assistive ambulation devices). In some ways, ambulation devices should be treated as medications: They should be "prescribed" to correct a specific underlying gait and balance problem and, as a consequence, tailored to fit both the person and the environment. Also, people must be instructed in the proper use of the device in walking and transferring in order to prevent adverse effects, such as falls and subsequent injury; this is best accomplished by referring patients and residents to a physiatrist or physical therapist.

Despite best efforts to prescribe the correct device and instruct people in using an assistive device properly, many patients and residents use ill-fitting devices or use them inappropriately, which increases the risk of falls. Nurses and other hospital and facility staff are in a position to detect errors at an early stage and to decrease fall risk through corrective intervention. Corrective intervention can be accomplished by ensuring that canes and walkers are the

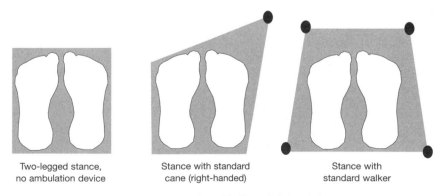

Two-legged stance,   Stance with standard   Stance with
no ambulation device   cane (right-handed)   standard walker

Figure 4-6. Base of support (shaded areas) provided by ambulation devices.

Table 4-2.   Types of assistive ambulation devices

Standard Cane

The standard cane is the most commonly used ambulation device. It is shaped like a candy cane and is usually made of wood or adjustable aluminum. The crook handle of the standard cane decreases grip strength, particularly in individuals with arthritis. The point of support is in the front of the hand, which makes this cane slightly unsteady. The cane should be held in the hand opposite to the disability (e.g., if pain is in right knee, cane is held in left hand). For balance support, however, the cane may be held in either hand.

Ortho Cane

The ortho cane is made of aluminum and is adjustable. It is similar to the standard cane. The shaft of the cane is offset, thereby placing the point of support directly below the handle. This design offers more stability than does the standard cane. The handle is molded, which provides a more comfortable grip than the standard cane.

Quad Cane

The quad cane has four legs and is used by individuals with impairment or weakness in one leg but who possess adequate balance control. This cane is more stable than the standard cane. It comes in a variety of base sizes. Base size is important because the wider the base, the greater the stability. Individuals with dementia may experience difficulty with quad canes. If the handle is not held facing the proper direction, the cane becomes very unstable, leading to loss of balance. Also, people with impaired vision may easily trip over the legs of the cane.

Hemi-Walker

The hemi-walker is a one-arm walker with four legs. This walker offers more support than the quad cane due to its broadly based legs. It is designed for individuals who are unable to use a standard walker (e.g., a hemiplegic with only one functioning upper extremity). Use of the hemi-walker requires good balance control and upper arm strength to move the walker.

Standard Walker

The standard walker consists of four adjustable legs equipped with rubber tips. The walker is designed for individuals with poor balance and lower extremity weakness or impairment. Walkers may be either nonfolding or folding. Nonfolding walkers offer greater stability and may be more appropriate than folding walkers for people living in long-term care facilities.

The device itself has several limitations: The individual using the walker must pick up the walker while walking, which results in a loss of balance when all four legs of the walker are off the floor. Individuals with poor balance and/or upper extremity weakness may push the device along the floor, causing the walker to suddenly halt and tip over, a particular problem on carpeted floor coverings. Applying metal furniture tips to the legs can overcome this problem, although the walker may slide away from some individuals.

Rolling Walker

The rolling walker is similar in design to the standard walker; however, it is equipped with either two front wheels or wheels attached to all four legs. The rolling walker does not require lifting and, therefore, is suited for individuals with poor balance and limited upper extremity strength. The two-wheeled walker is difficult to move on carpeted floor coverings because the rear legs drag along the floor; applying metal furniture tips to the rear legs overcomes this problem. The four-wheel walker is easier to move along, but may roll too far forward, causing users to lose their balance.

Rolling walkers equipped with weight-activated brakes are safer to use; the walker automatically stops when the user pushes down on the rear legs of the device. Some four-wheel walkers are equipped with baskets and seats that allow individuals to carry objects and sit down when tired, although sitting down requires good transfer technique and sitting balance.

Table 4-3.   Ambulation device inspection summary

Inspect	Examine canes and walkers for defects (e.g., worn rubber tips, defective wheels, structural problems). Replace device as indicated and/or refer all problems to physical therapy.
Inquire	Ask patients and residents about their device: Are they using their cane or walker? If not, why? Are they experiencing any problems with their cane or walker? If yes, what are the problems? Does the device improve or interfere with ambulation? Refer all problems to physical therapy.
Observe	Ask patients and residents to perform walking and transferring maneuvers with their device. Observe whether they are performing tasks correctly and safely. Is the person able to use the device properly in tight places (e.g., bathroom, bedroom) without interference? Refer all problems to physical therapy.

appropriate size (for an explanation of measurement techniques, see Fall Prevention Guidelines in Section Three, Part A), and ensuring that patients and residents are using their devices properly during activities (see Fall Prevention Guidelines in Section Three, Part A, for suggestions on how to help people use devices when walking, standing, turning, or sitting). In addition, ambulation devices should be inspected routinely for defects (Table 4-3). Inspection is of particular importance in nursing facilities, where the mobility status and device needs of residents are likely to change over time.

Wheelchairs

Wheelchairs are designed for patients and residents with limited ability to walk or who are totally dependent in walking. Wheelchairs come in a variety of sizes, designs, and materials, all of which are determined by the needs of the patient or resident. It is essential for nursing and other staff to work with physical and occupational therapists to ensure proper chair selection, fit, and use. The problems most commonly causing wheelchair falls and suggestions on how to correct them are described in Section Three.

ENVIRONMENTAL STRATEGIES

When older people enter a hospital or nursing facility, they are exposed to new environmental conditions such as the design of furnishings, illumination, and ground surfaces. If these conditions exceed a person's mobility capacity, he or she is at risk for falls. Patients and residents with functional disabilities are especially vulnerable. These people have a narrower adaptive range to help them cope with the increased demands of the environment (e.g., elevated bed heights, diminished lighting, glare-producing floor surfaces). In this context, the goal of environmental interventions to reduce fall risk is twofold: to identify and subsequently eliminate conditions that may interfere with mobility and to simplify or optimize individual mobility tasks by modifying the physical environment and the surrounding areas (see Chapter 5).

The most important environmental items to be assessed follow. To ensure that safe conditions are maintained, a complete and comprehensive assessment should be performed on a regular basis.

Illumination

- Are lights bright enough to compensate for reduced vision?

- Are lights glare-free?

- Are light switch plates, lamp pull cords, and switches in the bedroom and bathroom both visually and physically accessible?

- Are light switches available by the entryways of bedrooms and bathrooms (to avoid ambulating in the dark)?

- Are night-lights available in the bedroom and bathroom?

Floor surfaces

- Are floor surfaces slip resistant and glare-free?

- Are carpeted edges secured to the floor?

- Are throw rugs slip-resistant?

- Are frequently traveled pathways in the bedroom and ward area free of low-lying (i.e., difficult to visualize) objects?

Furnishings

- Are beds low enough and stable enough to support safe, independent transfers?

- Are chairs equipped with armrests, and are they stable enough (i.e., non-tippable) to support safe, independent transfers?

- Are bedside and dining room tables stable enough to support balance when leaned on?

Bathroom

- Are toilet grab bars available and securely fastened to the toilet or mounted on the wall?

FALL PREVENTION PROGRAMS

Fall prevention programs have been developed by several hospitals and nursing facilities.[5–10] These programs have met with varying degrees of success in fall reduction and have the following in common:

- A multidisciplinary safety committee to develop and implement an institution-wide fall prevention program.

- An in-service nursing and medical staff education program for all professionals involved in patient and resident care. Nursing education extends to staff on all three shifts.

- A mechanism to identify patients and residents at fall risk immediately on admission and, for each nursing shift, whenever a change of condition occurs.

- A mechanism (e.g., colored wrist identification bands, colored adhesive stickers near the bedroom door and bedside and on medical and nursing charts) for identifying patients or residents at fall risk.

- Assessment of patients and residents immediately after a fall.

- A formal program and policy for reporting and investigating incident reports. (The essential components of such policies and reports are described in Tables 4-4 and 4-5.)

- Implementation of strategies to prevent falls and follow-up to review whether the designed interventions have decreased falls on a regular basis. (These preventive strategies are presented in Table 4-6. This list is not

Table 4-4. Components of policy for incident reporting

The policy clearly defines what events constitute a reportable fall (e.g., an unanticipated event, usually of sudden onset, in which the patient or resident engages in an activity that results in balance loss and a subsequent fall).

The policy clearly describes what actions to take in the event of injury and/or acute medical conditions.

The policy clearly describes fall precaution measures to follow in order to prevent recurrence.

The policy clearly outlines a step-by-step procedure to follow for completing the incident report.

The policy clearly describes a step-by-step process to follow after the incident report is completed (e.g., documenting the incident in the patient's or resident's chart; forwarding a copy of the incident report for administrative review to the medical and nursing director, safety committee, or quality assurance committee).

The policy describes a process to inform all staff involved in patient or resident care of the current policy (e.g., during orientation, during in-service education).

The policy describes a time period in which statements are updated to reflect institutional attempts to practice reasonable standards of care related to fall prevention.

Table 4-5. Components of incident report

- Time and place of the fall
- Injuries and/or medical conditions present at the time and results of the medical examination
- Circumstance of the fall (patient/resident description of the event and/or eyewitness reports)
- Fall risk factors, both intrinsic and extrinsic, present at the time of the fall
- Preventive measures in place at the time of the fall, especially if the individual was at risk
- Immediate preventive strategies put in place to prevent additional falls
- Recommendations for treatment (i.e., intervention strategies) to prevent fall recurrence

meant to be all-inclusive, nor does it suggest that these strategies are effective. It represents the recommendations most commonly found in the literature.)

- An educational program for patients, residents, and family members that teaches the causes and prevention of falls during a stay in the hospital or nursing facility (Table 4-7).

- A discharge teaching program for patients, residents, and family members that teaches the prevention of risks of readmission (Table 4-8).

- The consistent recognition of staff (i.e., regular encouragement and praise).

- Informing staff that their efforts have led to a reduction of falls and an enhanced level of care.

Although further research is needed, ample evidence suggests that incorporating these components into existing or newly developed fall prevention programs is beneficial in reducing fall risk.

Table 4-6.   Strategies for fall prevention

Assessment

Identify fall risk on admission.

After admission, reassess risk level at regular intervals (e.g., daily, every shift, changes in medical and/or functional conditions).

Observe patient or resident mobility on a daily basis.

Monitor high-risk medications (side effects), polypharmacy.

Conduct environmental safety rounds on a regular basis (e.g., check wheelchair brakes/footrests, bed wheel brakes, bedside rail attachments, nonslip strips along the side of the bed, safety of assistive ambulation devices, condition of floor coverings, position of furnishings in bedroom, safety of bedside commodes, clutter in hallways, night-lights in bedroom, safety of footwear).

Nursing Care

Maintain regular toileting schedules (elimination rounds).

Use bedside commodes during hours of sleep.

Provide properly fitting, nonslip footwear.

Place confused patients or residents close to nurses' station for close observation.

Establish frequent nursing rounds on high-risk patients or residents.

Provide assistive ambulation.

Encourage daily exercise.

Increase nursing staff.

Environmental

Keep bed in a low position.

Keep the bed wheels locked.

Use bed half side rails to assist with safe bed transfers.

Place the call light and other objects within easy patient or resident reach.

Use bed/chair alarm systems to monitor unsafe activity.

Maintain adequate illumination in bedrooms and bathrooms.

Maintain nonslip floor surfaces.

Keep hallways clear.

Provide grab bars and toilet risers in the bathroom.

Table 4-7. Educational program for patients, residents, and family members

To reduce the risk of falls during a stay in the hospital or nursing facility:

Orient patients or residents to bedroom, unit, activities, and routines.

Orient patients or residents to staff members.

Instruct patients or residents on the proper use of equipment (e.g., electric beds, call lights, ambulation devices, wheelchairs, bathroom grab bars, bed half side rails, bedside commodes). Do not assume that individuals can figure out these things by themselves.

Teach patients or residents safe transfer techniques from bed, chairs, toilet, and wheelchair.

Instruct high-risk patients or residents to call for assistance when getting out of bed, ambulating, and toileting.

Educate family members about safety measures and fall prevention; provide instruction on how to identify risk and environmental hazards.

Provide a safety brochure that addresses important issues such as the need to wear nonslip footwear and use assistive devices whenever out of bed, the importance of calling for assistance during periods of increased risk, important side effects of medications, what to do if a fall occurs, and so forth. Material should be printed in large type for easier reading and reinforced verbally with patients or residents and family members at the time of admission.

Table 4-8. Discharge teaching program

To reduce the risk of falls and related injury at home:

Prevent the risk of down time (i.e., person is unable to arise unassisted from the floor following a fall). Provide patient or resident with a personal emergency response system (PERS). This is a button device worn by the individual as a pendant or wrist band and includes a radio transmitter connected to the person's home telephone. When the device is activated, the emergency signal goes out to a 24-hour monitoring center, which sends appropriate help (e.g., family member, neighbor, police, ambulance). The PERS can be purchased, leased, or rented. As an alternative, individuals can be taught how to rise from the floor by themselves (i.e., move themselves to a side-sitting position). They can then kneel with the support of a chair and, using the strongest knee, push themselves up into the chair.

Teach home safety. Provide the patient or resident with information about how to prevent falls in the home (see Section Three, Part C for "Discharge Teaching Sheets"). In addition, patients or residents with mobility impairment should receive a home safety evaluation from physical or occupational therapists and instruction on home medical equipment required (e.g., walkers, wheelchairs, toilet and bathtub devices). Remember that equipment used in the hospital or nursing facility may not be adequate to support safe mobility in the home.

ENDNOTES

1. Lauritzen, J.B., Peterson, M.M., & Lund, B. (1993). Effect of external hip protectors on hip fractures. *Lancet, 341*(8836), 11–13.
2. Ekman, A., Mallmin, H., Michaelsson, K., & Ljunghall, S. (1997). External hip protectors to prevent osteoporotic hip fractures. *Lancet, 350*(9077), 563–564.
3. Hubacher, M., & Wettstein, A. (2001). Acceptance of hip protectors for hip fracture prevention in nursing homes. *Osteoporosis International, 12*(9), 794–799.
4. Cryer, C., Knox, A., & Stevenson, E. (2008). Factors associated with hip protector adherence among older people in residential care. *Injury Prevention, 14*(1), 24–29.

5. Coussement, J., De Paepe, L., Schwendimann, R., Denhaerynck, D., Dejaeger, E., & Milisen, K. (2008). Interventions for preventing falls in acute- and chronic-care hospitals: A systematic review and meta-analysis. *Journal of the American Geriatrics Society, 56*(1), 29–36.
6. Becker, C., Kron, M., Lindemann, U., Sturm, E., Eichner, B., Walter-Jung, B., & Nikolaus, T. (2003). Effectiveness of a multifaceted intervention on falls in nursing home residents. *Journal of the American Geriatrics Society, 51*(3), 306–313.
7. Schwendimann, R., Buhler, H., De Geest, S., & Milisen, K. (2006). Fall prevention in an acute care setting reducing multiple falls. *Journal of Gerontological Nursing, 32*(3), 13–22.
8. Barrett, J.A., Bradshaw, M., Hutchinson, K., Akpan, A., Reese, A., Metcalfe, L., Wong, H., & Maxwell, M.J. (2004). Reduction of falls-related injuries using a hospital inpatient falls prevention program. *Journal of the American Geriatrics Society, 52*(11), 1969–1970.
9. Krauss, M.J., Tutlam, N., Constantinou, E., Johnson, S., Jackson, D., & Fraser, V.J. (2008). Intervention to prevent falls on the medical service in a teaching hospital. *Infection Control and Hospital Epidemiology, 29*(6), 539–545.
10. von Renteln-Kruse, W., & Krause, T. (2007). Incidence of in-hospital falls in geriatric patients before and after the introduction of an interdisciplinary team-based fall-prevention intervention. *Journal of the American Geriatrics Society, 55*(12), 2068–2074.

Chapter Five

Environmental Modifications

Older adults residing in hospitals and nursing facilities differ in their functional capacity: Some have no limitations, whereas others experience partial to severe loss of function. For people with diminished physical capacity, the physical environment takes on greater significance. It can either contribute to hazardous mobility and increase the risk of falls or it can be used as a resource to compensate for individual mobility problems and reduce the risk of falls. For example, poor lighting increases the degree of functional visual loss and adversely affects ambulation, but it can be improved to provide a level of illumination that facilitates safe walking. Low-seated chairs without armrests can cause unsafe transfers in people with diminished muscular strength. Furniture can be made more supportive with the addition of seat cushions and armrests.

For patients and residents with decreased mobility, environmental modification can be a powerful adaptive strategy to promote mobility and reduce the likelihood of falling. Thus, the design of institutional environments and any subsequent adjustments must transcend appearances and be based on activity-based standards: Function must take precedence over aesthetics. Put plainly, in structure and design, floor surfaces and coverings, lighting, and furnishings should maximize or support ambulation and transferring function and be aesthetically pleasing. This chapter focuses on aspects of the hospital and nursing facility environment that are most likely to contribute to unsafe mobility and that suggest corrective modification.

LIGHTING

Lighting can be described in terms of numerous factors, including illumination, location, quality, changes in intensity, access, and glare reduction.

Illumination

The proper amount of illumination in the environment depends on the visual needs of patients and residents. As a rule, older people need two to three times more light than do younger people because of the aging-related decline in visual functioning. However, this is a generalization. In some cases, lower levels of lighting may be more appropriate than higher levels. For instance,

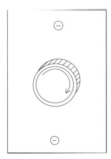

Figure 5-1. Rheo-static light switch.

people with cataracts or glaucoma tend to be sensitive to bright light. For these people, any increase in lighting may impair their vision and increase their fall risk.

Under ideal circumstances, the control of lighting levels should rest with the individual so that he or she is able to regulate and maintain a level of illumination that is both visually comfortable and safe for mobility. Rheostatic light switches allow a person to increase or decrease light levels as desired (Figure 5-1). However, patient or resident control of lighting may not always be possible, especially for those who have cognitive impairments or who are in wheelchairs. The best way to help determine the lighting needs of an individual is to observe the person in his or her environment and note any difficulties encountered. Correction may call for increasing, decreasing, or redistributing lighting levels.

Strategic Lighting

Extra lighting may be needed in certain locations, such as the bedroom, that represent high fall risk. The path from the bedside to the bathroom may be difficult to visualize, especially at night, when patients and residents may get up to go to the bathroom. In an attempt to provide adequate illumination and safe passage, staff members sometimes leave the bathroom light on throughout the night. However, the bright bathroom light may interfere with sleep or may temporarily blind the person with a sudden flooding of bright light when he or she enters the bathroom. Conversely, leaving a bright bathroom and walking into a dark bedroom can cause similar problems because older eyes readjust to lighting levels more slowly than do younger eyes.

A bedside lamp with a secure base that will not tip over, a light attached to the headboard within easy reach, or a night-light can be used to provide adequate illumination and facilitate safe ambulation (Figure 5-2). A light can be installed under the apron of a bedside table or nightstand to provide night

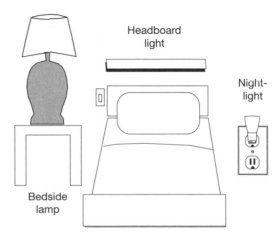

Figure 5-2. Lighting sources that increase illumination.

lighting, or night-lights can be positioned close to the floor along the path leading from the bedroom to the bathroom. Motion-sensor lighting located in the bathroom is also a good solution.

Effective Lighting Sources

In addition to an adequate quantity of illumination, the quality of available lighting is important for safe ambulation. Full-spectrum fluorescent lighting is much more effective than incandescent lighting for overall illumination in the environment. Blue fluorescent light simulates natural sunlight, providing light that is spread evenly and is continuous and free of shadows. However, the best effects are produced by a bulb emitting light that is in the yellow spectrum. Halogen lamps produce light that is more like natural sunlight and freer from glare than either fluorescent or incandescent fixtures. Halogen lamps are particularly effective for task lighting, illuminating specific areas in the bedroom and bathroom. Because these lamps get quite hot, however, safety precautions should be observed.

Lighting Changes

The ability of the eye to adapt to changes in illumination decreases with age. Any sudden change in light intensity, as occurs when a person moves from a dark to a bright area and vice versa, should be avoided because it can lead to momentary visual loss and increase the risk of falls. Perhaps the most common example involves traveling at night from a darkened bedroom into the bathroom and turning on the light. Rheostatic light switches that vary the amount of available light can ensure an even distribution of light and prevent the sudden and pronounced shifts in illumination that may occur with toggle light switches. Another alternative is to use compact fluorescent bulbs in transition areas or in rooms and areas where older people encounter dramatic changes in light levels. These bulbs take approximately 1 minute to heat to full brightness, minimizing the adjustment from darkness to light. Night-lights can be used in the bedroom and bathroom as well but are not as effective. Also, night-lights can produce frightening shadows or create an illusion of steps or edges where light and shadows meet.

Lighting Access

All environmental lighting should be physically accessible to patients and residents. Light switches should be positioned approximately 32 inches off the floor and located directly on the outside or inside of doorways to help people avoid walking across a darkened room to turn on a light (Figure 5-3). The color of the switch plates should contrast that of the wall to improve visibility. If the wall and switch plate colors are identical, the switch plate should be painted in a contrasting color, or adhesive tape in a contrasting color should be placed around the borders of the switch plate to

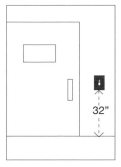

Figure 5-3. For ease in reaching, the light switch should be located 32 inches above the floor.

enhance its visibility. A small light located within the switch or an illuminated switch plate will improve visibility and access at night. Pressure-plate controls are easier to use than standard toggle switches. The pull cord that controls bedside lighting should be long enough for users to avoid excessive reaching and risk loss of balance. In addition, the pull cord should be in a contrasting color so that it can be seen easily by the older user.

Glare Reduction

Glare from sunlight shining through windows, skylights, or other light sources such as fluorescent lights reflecting directly on polished waxed floors, on furnishings such as laminated tabletops, and on plastic chair seats produces discomfort and can impair a person's vision. Draperies or adjustable Venetian blinds can be used to block sunlight from windows. Unfortunately, they reduce the amount of available light and may not present the best solution to glare. Furthermore, horizontal and vertical blinds, with their tilting capability, cause sunlight to be deflected, creating light patterns on the floor that can be visually confusing. Polarized window glass or tinted Mylar shades can eliminate glare without loss of ambient light. Another solution is translucent light-filtering pleated shades or sheer draperies, which diffuse light and offer some degree of light and glare regulation.

Floor glare can be controlled by using carpeting or nongloss floor waxes and finishes that diffuse rather than reflect light and eliminate glare. Also, wall-mounted valances or covered lighting fixtures that conceal the source of light and spread it indirectly on the ceiling and floor serve the same purpose. Matte or dull finishes on tabletops and nonreflective material on chair seats can help prevent surface glare.

FLOOR SURFACES

Floor surfaces can be dangerous for people with gait and balance impairments. By identifying dangerous flooring conditions and applying some simple modifications to make floor surfaces safer, staff can reduce the risk of falls and injury greatly.

Ceramic and Linoleum Surfaces

Highly polished or wet flooring can contribute to slip-related falls. In addition, highly buffed and polished flooring can cause reflected glare, the result of lighting sources shining directly on it. Glare can give floors the appearance of being wet or slick, creating a fear of falling or injury in some older people and leading to uncertainty or a reluctance on the part of the patient or resident to walk on the floor surface. Floor surfaces that inhibit ambulation can be viewed as a form of passive restraint, a condition resulting in restricted mobility.

Two modifications are helpful in eliminating these hazards by making bathroom and other floors skid-resistant: unglazed tile or adhesive strips and antiskid acrylic coating or no-wax vinyl flooring. First, ceramic tiles and linoleum floors must be slip-resistant, particularly when wet. Unglazed tiles,

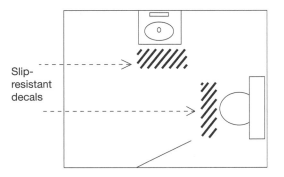

Figure 5-4. Slip-resistant adhesive strips are applied to the floor by the sink and toilet.

which are nonslip by design, can be used in the bathroom, or slip-resistant adhesive strips can be applied to the floor next to the sink and toilet, locations that are prone to water and urine spillage (Figure 5-4). Because the purpose of adhesive strips is to help render the floor slip-resistant, it is not necessary for them to be visible. The color of the adhesive strips should match that of the floor surface to prevent easy visualization. Older people, especially those with altered depth perception or dementia, may misinterpret color-contrasted floor strips, perceiving them as ground elevations or depressions that they may attempt to avoid. They may try to step over the strips, thereby increasing their risk of falls because of alterations in gait and balance. Sheet rubber flooring in the bathroom can be used as an alternate method of slip resistance.

The second modification is to make linoleum floors slip-resistant by applying antiskid acrylic coating or by using no-wax sheet vinyl flooring. If tile and vinyl flooring are waxed, minimal buffing after waxing helps to reduce slipping and eliminates glare. Using nongloss wax as opposed to high-gloss finishes on flooring also corrects glare.

All flooring should be flush and even to prevent patients and residents from tripping on it. Doorway thresholds, such as those on the floor between the bedroom and bathroom, should be avoided or eliminated. Thresholds create a problem for older people who have poor eyesight or difficulty lifting their feet to clear obstacles.

Carpeting

Carpeting offers several advantages in hospital and nursing facility settings: It provides a slip-resistant surface and cushion that helps to reduce the risk of injury in a fall. In particular, indoor–outdoor carpeting in the bathroom is beneficial in that it traps water or other liquids, such as urine, and dries quickly, thereby reducing the likelihood of slipping. As compared with vinyl flooring, a carpeted bedroom floor greatly reduces the risk of injury from a fall by providing a much softer surface on which to land.[1] Carpeting also has acoustic value in that it reduces echo resulting from shoes striking tile and linoleum flooring.

Carpeting has disadvantages as well. Older adults who use wheeled walkers and wheelchairs may experience difficulty rolling these assistive devices over carpeted surfaces, especially those that are thick. People who push along pick-up walkers rather than lift up and put down the walker with each step also may experience problems with carpeting. The legs of the walker can catch on the carpet, causing an older person to lose his or her balance and fall. In addition, those who walk with a shuffling gait may find that thick carpeting impedes safe mobility and increases the risk of tripping.

Despite concerns about carpeting, institutions should not be discouraged from using it; when it is properly chosen, its advantages far outweigh any disadvantages. Uncut, low-pile carpeting is the best choice for institutional settings because this surface is least likely to interfere with walking and using walkers and wheelchairs. Deep-pile carpeting should be avoided. Aside from interfering with safe ambulation, dense carpets can cause a loss of proprioceptive feedback and balance, which are gained from the feet striking the ground. Carpet tiles are usually not recommended in institutional settings because the number of seams between the tiles creates an opportunity for liquids to seep into the underlayer. The greatest concern is that of urine seepage, the odor of which can become offensive to patients or residents, staff, and visitors alike.

Carpets made of nylon fibers provide a smooth walking surface and possess excellent strength and durability, beneficial features in areas subject to heavy traffic and soiling. The color of the carpeting should contrast with that of the walls to help older people, especially those with impaired depth perception, to define the boundary between the floor and wall. A person's balance may be affected adversely when this distinction is not made clear. Patterns such as floral or checkered configurations, although pleasing to look at, should be avoided because they can lead to misjudgment of spatial distances. Misperception is heightened in people with a visual dysfunction, such as cataracts and poor depth perception, and dementia (i.e., patterns seem to move, leading a person to feel increasingly confused and unbalanced). Plain, unpatterned carpeting is less confusing, both visually and intellectually. All carpeting should be checked periodically for curled edges and excessive wear in order to guard against tripping.

Transitions from one type of floor surface to another must be as smooth and level as possible (i.e., no more than ¼ inch) to accommodate wheelchairs, shuffling feet, and ambulation assistive devices. Changes in floor surfaces should be avoided in areas prone to shifts in lighting because older adults' eyes need time to adjust to changing light levels, and these people may not recognize changes in surfaces in time to adjust their gait. Transitions in floor surfaces should occur only in locations where lighting is sufficient and constant.

HALLWAYS

Hallways can present an obstacle for patients and residents. Long hallways are a particular problem because they require older people with mobility problems to travel a long distance to reach the nurses' station, dining rooms, and so forth. As a result, patients and residents may be reluctant to walk distances, especially if they become fatigued easily, experience balance problems, or fear falling. One solution to this problem is to move the patient or resident to a bedroom that is located closer to the nurses' station and other commonly used areas. However, relocation may not be safe or easy to achieve; for example, new environments may be disorienting for people with dementia. A more realistic and perhaps better solution is to provide "rest stops," or chairs strategically placed every 20–30 feet along long hallways. These rest stops allow older adults to rest whenever they become tired or unsteady and to continue their journey when they feel better.

Hallways and traffic lanes can become cluttered with medicine, laundry, and food carts, cleaning equipment, wheelchairs, unused walkers, and poorly placed furniture, which present obstacles and interfere with safe ambulation. Clutter should be avoided as much as possible. Because many older people lose peripheral vision, they can easily bump into objects located in their path and may trip or lose balance as a result. Moreover, cluttered hallways can obstruct a person's view of handrails or access to them.

Handrail Support

In all areas used by ambulating patients and residents, handrails should be installed to provide support (e.g., enhance balance, encourage movement, allay fear of falling). Handrails are especially helpful in areas with poor footing (e.g., polished or slick flooring) or if abrasive wall finishes or coverings are present that can cut into fragile aging skin easily if walls are relied on for mobility support (i.e., hand or shoulder support) and brushed up against. Handrails are most effective for gripping if they are round rather than flat. Round handrails allow a person's thumb and forefingers to meet; flat handrails are difficult to grasp, particularly for people with arthritic hands, and are less effective than round handrails for maintaining support. In addition, the color of the handrails should contrast with that of the walls to promote easy visibility; they should be nonslip (e.g., with a wraparound cover of textured vinyl) when

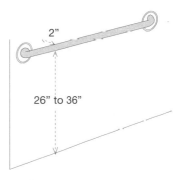

Figure 5-5. Handrail support should be located 2 inches from the wall and 26–36 inches in height from the floor.

grasped and should be located approximately 2 inches from the wall and 26–36 inches above the floor for easy access (Figure 5-5). Handrails that are well designed and well placed allow older people to grasp the rails and glide along them. They also allow people to lean on their forearms for added support.

BEDS

For patients and residents with diminished mobility, modification of the bed and its surrounding area can support safe mobility.

Bed Height

Bed height is defined as the distance from the floor to the tip of the mattress. Bed height is appropriate when a person is able to sit on the edge of the mattress with the knees flexed at 90° and plant both feet firmly on the floor (Figure 5-6). A bed height that is safe enough to support transfer activity can be obtained with the use of height-adjustable "hi–low" beds. Because the "hi–low" bed can be lowered to any level desired, it can provide a greater sense of security and confidence to patients and residents, which promotes independence and ease of transfers. If the bed is still too high despite the use of this mechanism, a thinner mattress may be used to achieve the desired height. Because bed height may be altered routinely in order to change linens or perform routine nursing care, staff should check the height periodically to ensure that it is maintained at a level that is appropriate for the patient or resident. Also,

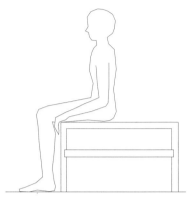

Figure 5-6. Bed height is appropriate when the person is able to sit with the knees flexed at 90° and both feet planted firmly on the floor.

if the beds are controlled manually with crank handles, staff should check that the handles are recessed underneath the bed at all times so that they do not constitute a tripping hazard.

Institutional bed design has changed dramatically over the past several years. This change probably occurred in response to the persistent problem that falls from bed represent for hospitals and nursing facilities and to a general dissatisfaction with the type of beds available. As a result, the types of beds on the market fit various needs. Apart from a new generation of "hi–low" beds, which can be positioned at varying heights ranging from near-floor level to elevations higher than standard beds, several models of fixed low-deck beds are available. These beds have a mattress deck height of 5½–7 inches above the level of the floor and are designed to eliminate the use of mechanical restraints for patients and residents at risk of falling from bed. The use of a low-deck bed can replace the common practice of placing the older person's mattress or double mattress directly on the floor to eliminate falls from bed. Although placing the mattress on the floor is effective, family members can become upset about seeing their loved one lying on the mattress, especially if the floor or carpet is not clean. In this case, families may find fixed low-height beds a better alternative. In addition, these beds are equipped with casters, which permit the bed to be moved when the floor is cleaned.

Bed Supports

Sometimes patients and residents with poor bed or walking mobility may use the footboard as an aid in transferring in and out of bed or in ambulating about the bedroom. To provide adequate support, the footboard should be easy to grasp and slip-resistant. Nonslip adhesive strips placed along the top of the

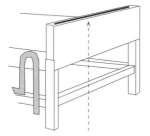

Figure 5-7. Nonslip adhesive strip is placed along the footboard to support mobility.

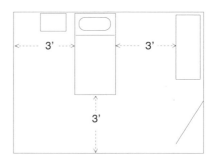

Figure 5-8. Bedroom circulation space.

footboard prevent hands from slipping (Figure 5-7). A color-contrasted strip on the footboard can help a person to recognize it more easily, calls attention to the board itself, and helps prevent the person from bumping into the bed.

In addition, an adequate amount of space between the bed and other furnishings should be created to allow safe ambulation and transferring, particularly if walkers are used. A circulation space of at least 3 feet provides enough room for patient or resident movement with or without ambulation devices (Figure 5-8).

Mattresses

Patients and residents with poor sitting balance may be at risk for falling from bed if mattress edges sag or slouch. An overly soft mattress does not provide the support necessary for safe bed transfers, particularly if one relies on hand support to accomplish them. All mattresses should be firm enough to support older adults securely when they are seated in an upright position. Mattress edges that are rolled offer older adults a good grasping surface when transferring (Figure 5-9).

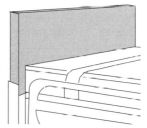

Figure 5-9. Rolled mattress edge.

Bedside Rails

Bedside rails have both disadvantages and advantages. As mentioned previously, bedside rails in the raised position can contribute to falls and physical injury. For example, patients and residents who are agile may climb over the top of the rail and become entangled in it. However, if they are used properly, bedside rails offer real benefits, providing safety and assistance in bed transfers. When positioned at least 14 inches above the top of the mattress, full-length bedside rails can help prevent people under sedation from rolling and falling out of bed unexpectedly. With one full-length bedside rail up on the opposite side of the bed, patients and residents are reminded of the side of the bed from which they should exit. However, full-length rails should not be used for people who are able to get out of bed. A better choice is to use half-bedside rails, which do not interfere with exiting but help prevent older adults from rolling out of bed inadvertently.

Many patients and residents are accustomed to sleeping on a wider bed surface at home, and in the hospital or nursing facility they must adjust to sleeping in a smaller bed. The standard hospital bed has several inches or, sometimes, several feet less space than what older adults are used to, increasing their risk for rolling out of bed. People with dementia or confusion may not be able to make the adjustment to a smaller bed surface, so they are at particular risk. Also, nurse call bell cords that are out of reach can cause rolling or falling out of bed because people may lose their balance while attempting to reach the call bell.

Placing a pillow or rolled blanket under the mattress edge to create a lip or "bumper" guard can be used to prevent people from rolling out of bed, but this intervention may lead to transfer problems. Some staff have adopted the practice of placing a mattress on the floor alongside the bed to prevent injuries if a fall from bed occurs. However, this strategy may cause additional problems; for example, older people and even staff members may trip over the mattress if it is left in place when the bed is not occupied. In addition, staff may need to place and remove the mattress several times a day, which can lead to noncompliance with this strategy. A specially designed soft vinyl and foam floor mat (approximately 35 inches wide, 70 inches long, and 2 inches thick) has been used in some settings as an alternative to accommodate the sudden impact of a fall from bed. The mat can be walked on and left in place while direct care is provided. However, a certain amount of caution must be taken when floor mats are used. Patients and residents with loss of proprioception can encounter balance problems and fall risk when walking on the mat.

Appropriately placed half-bedside rails can function as assistive or enabling devices, supporting people who have poor sitting and transfer balance, such as those with Parkinson's disease or those who have had a stroke (Figure 5-10). Also, the rails can help older adults build confidence in their ability to

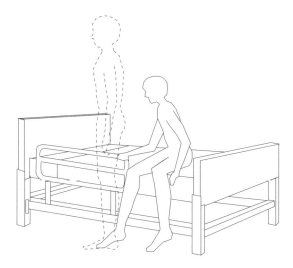

Figure 5-10.   Half-bedside rail is used as an assistive device.

safely transfer from bed, thus reducing their fear of falling. When used as enabling devices, conventional bedside rails have some design problems. Some bedside rails are hard to grasp securely, especially for people with upper extremity dysfunction; also, bedside rails may not be secure enough to support bed transfers. As an alternative, transfer handles are available: They mount to metal bed frames, providing good stability, which allows older adults to pull themselves up and out of bed. If bedside rails or transfer handles are used in transfers as safety devices rather than as restraints, it is a good idea to document this use in the chart. When bedside rails are not in use and are in the down position, they should recess completely underneath the bed to prevent people from climbing on the rails to enter or leave the bed.

Routine bedside rail use has long been considered standard practice in hospitals and nursing facilities. However, even half-rail use should not be ordered routinely without asking staff a few questions: "What do you hope to achieve with the use of bedside rails (e.g., will they prevent or facilitate the patient's or resident's physical and cognitive function)?" "Does the older person want you to use bedside rails?" (Patients and residents have the right to refuse bedside rails. If patients and residents cannot make their preferences known, family members should be consulted.) (See Section Three.)

Bed Wheels

Bed wheels constitute a special hazard because they may roll or slide away during patient and resident transfers. Although all beds, including those with adequate wheel-locking systems, are unsteady to some degree, a combination swivel-and-wheel brake provides the most stability. Even when bed wheels lock properly, the bed may slide, especially if the wheels are resting on a slippery linoleum floor. To prevent sliding, the flooring can be rendered slip-resistant by placing nonslip adhesive strips or decals on the floor directly underneath the wheels (Figure 5-11). Beds that are equipped with immobilizer legs—the wheels recess when the legs are down on the floor—are an acceptable alternative to sliding bed wheels or malfunctioning locking systems (Figure 5-12).

A slippery floor surface surrounding the bed area can cause the feet of older adults to slide during bed transfers. Slippage can be prevented: Placing nonslip adhesive strips on the floor along the length of the bed provides the

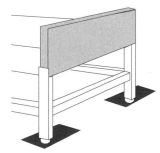

Figure 5-11. Nonslip adhesive strips placed underneath the bed wheels prevent slippage.

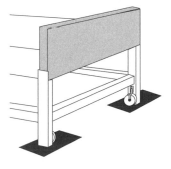

Figure 5-12. Bed with immobilizer legs.

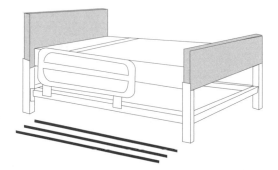

Figure 5-13. Nonslip adhesive strips are placed on the floor to prevent falls.

feet with a slip-resistant surface (Figure 5-13). The color of the nonslip strips should blend with the color of the floor so that people with altered depth perception do not misinterpret the strips as hazards. In addition, patients and residents should wear slip-resistant footwear when transferring in and out of bed. Some older people may not take the time to put on slippers when exiting bed. For these people, socks with nonslip or traction soles are a good choice.

Fall Alarm Systems

Even after comprehensive bed modifications are implemented, a certain number of patients and residents remain at risk for falls. People with cognitive dysfunction (e.g., dementia, depression, delirium) are at particular risk. Cognitive losses can cause errors in judgment, such as an inability to recognize a difference between safe and hazardous bed transfers. People with neuromuscular disorders (e.g., Parkinson's disease, stroke) and poor bed mobility who do not ask for staff assistance are also at risk. In an effort to avoid the use of mechanical or chemical restraints, some institutions use nursing assistants or family members as in-room sitters for patients and residents at risk for bed falls. In other institutions, nurses conduct hourly "bed rounds," usually at night, checking on the safety of patients and residents while in bed. Both interventions are costly because they require extra nursing staff. Fall alarm systems can be used as alternatives to in-room sitters and bed rounds and help staff avoid the use of mechanical restraints to prevent bed falls. Fall alarms are designed to warn nursing staff that patients or residents who should not attempt to leave their bed unassisted are doing so.

A variety of fall alarm systems are available, some of which attach to both the bed and the patient or resident, some to the person alone, and others to the bed alone (Table 5-1). All systems function similarly and allow people to maintain a free-movement zone or an area adequate for normal bed activity. If the patient or resident leaves the bed and exceeds the free-movement zone, an alarm sounds in the bedroom, the nurses' station, or both, indicating that the person is about to transfer from the bed. According to reports, all systems are user-friendly, safe for patients and residents in that they cause no adverse effects, and easy to install, operate, and maintain. Some institutions use

Table 5-1. Types of Fall Alarms

Pressure Pad Alarm

Consists of a thin pad (placed on top of or underneath a bed mattress; on a chair or wheelchair seat) and a control unit (typically mounted on the bed or chair). The pad senses changes in weight and pressure; if the person gets up from a bed or chair, the alarm sounds. Pad alarms are also available for use on toilet seats to detect unsafe egress.

Pull-String Alarm

Consists of an adjustable-length cord and garment clip that is attached to the person's clothing. The end of the cord is attached to the control unit by a small magnetic disc or ball. The alarm is activated when the person exits the bed, chair, wheelchair, or toilet and the cord detaches from the control unit. Pull-string alarms equipped with a prerecorded voice message (i.e., instructing the person to not get up until help arrives) are available. (Some alarm companies have also incorporated prerecorded voice messages into pressure pad alarms.) These alarms activate automatically when the cord detaches from the control unit.

Leg Band Alarm

Alarm consists of a small, lightweight control unit that attaches to the person's thigh by means of a washable fabric band. When the person changes position (i.e., getting up from bed, chair, wheelchair, or toilet) the alarm is activated.

Postural Change Alarm

Alarm is attached directly to the person (by means of an adhesive sensor patch to the thigh) and is activated by changes in position. When the person attempts to stand from bed, chair, wheelchair, or toilet (i.e., the person's leg becomes weight-bearing) the adhesive patch sends a signal to a receiver unit, which activates an alarm.

Floor Mat Alarms

Alarm consists of a pressure pad mat placed on the floor alongside the bed, chair, wheelchair, or toilet. The alarm unit is activated when foot pressure is applied to the mat.

Infrared Alarm

Alarm consists of directional infrared sensors that send a beam over the top or alongside the bed. The alarm is activated when the beam is broken (i.e., person sits up in bed and puts a leg over the side of the bed).

Built-In Alarm

Some bed manufacturers have equipped their beds with fall alarms. These alarms function very similarly to pressure pad alarms.

---

homemade fall alarm devices such as baby monitors or motion detectors, which alert staff to the person stirring from sleep or leaving the bed; and nurse call light cords or personal security alarms with pull cords fastened to bed clothing, which sounds an alarm when the person exits the bed. Although these devices are less costly than commercially available systems, they may not be as effective: They sometimes fail to work by not sounding an alarm or detecting bed movement, and they break down easily.

Nurses in hospitals and nursing facilities perceive fall alarms as capable of reducing the risk of falling and the need for mechanical restraints. Fall alarms, which do not require active participation by patients or residents to trigger, are preferable to nurse call systems, which demand active participation to activate. Institutions that use fall alarm systems as part of an overall fall prevention program have reduced bed falls by up to 85%.[2, 3] Without exception, concerned family members of patients and residents prefer alarm systems to the use of restraints, citing the preservation of dignity and autonomy that they offer.

The use of fall alarms should be based on a set of criteria that indicate that the patient or resident is at risk for bed falls:

- Patient or resident experiences fall(s) from bed.

- Patient or resident experiences fall(s) while ambulating in bedroom or bathroom shortly after leaving bed or is found on floor after an unwitnessed fall.

- Patient or resident demonstrates unsafe bed transfers.

- Patient or resident has a history of cognitive or communicative problems (e.g., forgets to use call bell or ask for assistance with bed transfers).

- Patient or resident has a history of nocturia (i.e., excessive urination at night).

Once a decision has been made to use an alarm system, individual patient and resident characteristics should determine which type is the most appropriate. A number of factors may determine choice; for example, people with dementia may become confused and agitated by the use of systems that attach to their bodies. It may be better to use pressure-sensitive systems that rest on or lie underneath the mattress and out of view. Pressure-sensitive systems that have a built-in alarm time delay are useful for people who shift positions frequently during sleep. This system prevents the false alarms that can occur when people simply move on or off the pressure sensor pads repeatedly. Some alarm systems are equipped with a prerecorded voice message (i.e., instructing the person to remain in bed until help arrives), which activates automatically when the person leaves his or her bed. One potential problem with this type of system is that patients or residents with dementia might become increasingly confused because they don't understand the concept of hearing a voice without seeing a face.

An alarm system that attaches to the bed or to the person is also useful under certain circumstances. For example, the weight of the person can be a factor. People who weigh less than 100 pounds may not be able to apply sufficient weight to activate certain pressure-sensitive systems. In addition, antidecubitus pads added to the mattress may prevent activation with some alarm systems.

All fall alarm systems, even when appropriately selected, raise some common concerns that need to be addressed. The efficacy of any alarm system depends on the response time of the nursing staff. One of the leading concerns is that by the time the alarm sounds, staff may not be able to respond quickly enough to prevent a fall, particularly if the person's bedroom is distant from the nurses' station. Other than attempting to relocate this person to a bed closer to the nurses' station, a solution to this problem is to make it difficult for the patient or resident to get out of bed. A decubitus preventive water mattress filled to one half capacity, placed on the bed in combination with full-length bedside rails, is effective in limiting quick bed exits even in the most agile person and thus can give nurses adequate response time (Figure 5-14).

Skeptics contend that fall alarm systems are expensive in terms of initial cost and labor because additional nurses are needed to assist patients and residents. However, they are cost-effective in that they prevent falls, and they allow staff to avoid using restraints. When measured against the cost of

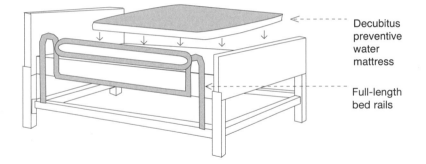

Figure 5-14. A bed with water mattress prevents decubiti, and full-length bedside rails prevent falls.

injuries sustained in bed falls and nursing time spent in caring for people recovering from the complications of falls and restraints, the cost of fall alarms is worthwhile. Most devices can be billed to diagnosis-related groups and to other third-party payers by charging a daily monitoring fee or budgeting the expense under the category "capital equipment." In addition, questions may be posed about legal liability and fall alarm use. Despite the use of these systems, the risk of bed falls and injuries continues. Although not challenged by the courts, hospitals and nursing facilities would do well to assume a defensive position in order to protect themselves. Assuming such a position would entail documenting the use of fall alarm devices in patients' or residents' charts and recording the rationale. Also, the risks and benefits of alarm systems should be explained to patients and residents, if competent, and family members; written consent should be obtained as well.

Legislation eliminating the use of mechanical restraints has contributed to a proliferation of fall alarm device manufacturers. The result is positive but confusing: Although improved devices are introduced routinely, the variety of choices makes it difficult to know which product to select. Bed alarm systems should meet a basic set of criteria:

- The system emits a distinctive alarm that is loud enough to be heard at the nurses' station and other locations.

- The system is silent in the patient's or resident's bedroom and emits a loud alarm at the nurses' station so that sleeping patients or residents are not aroused by the alarm.

- The system does not interfere with patient or resident care.

- The system is easy to use and maintain.

- The system is durable; warranty and service contracts are included.

- The system has performed reliably, and users, both nursing staff and patients or residents, are satisfied with the product. The customer should request a list of clients.

When purchasing the system, staff should ask the manufacturer whether its devices meet these standards.

SEATING

Modification of chairs can support independent and safe transfers in older adults with diminished transfer skill. Before seating can be modified, however, knowledge of seating standards is essential.

Seating Criteria

The criteria for proper seating in hospitals and nursing facilities are governed by one simple rule: Proper seating should meet the seating needs of patients and residents. To this end, chairs should assist in and not impede self-initiated transfers and provide comfort. Several methods are available to assess proper seating. Perhaps the most common is to select chairs that match the anthropometric, or body, measurements of older adults. For example,

- Seat height (Figure 5-15) is obtained by measuring a person's lower leg length, the distance from the foot on the floor to the knee or popliteal area behind the knee, generally 15–17 inches.

- Seat depth (Figure 5-16) is obtained by measuring upper leg length, the distance from the plane of the back to the popliteal area, generally 16–20 inches.

- Seat width (Figure 5-17) is obtained by measuring the distance across the widest point of the person's hips or thighs—generally 14–16 inches—and adding another 2 inches (i.e., 1 inch on each side of the hip) to prevent the body from rubbing or resting against the side of the chair.

- The height of the armrest from the seat is generally 7–7½ inches.

- The length of the armrest is generally 18–20 inches.

- The seat slope, or angle of the backrest, is generally 10–20 degrees.

- The height of the backrest from the seat is generally 17 inches or higher.

Anthropometric seating criteria are useful for purchasing chairs in quantity, which is a common practice for most institutions because of the economic

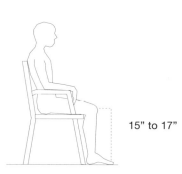

Figure 5-15. Seat height is appropriate when it is 15–17 inches from the floor.

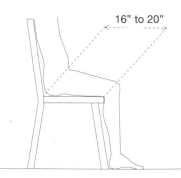

Figure 5-16. Seat depth is appropriate when it is 16–20 inches from the popliteal area to the buttocks.

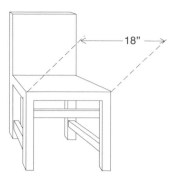

Figure 5-17. Seat width is appropriate when it is at least 18 inches.

advantages offered. Appropriate seating requires more than simply selecting a chair or sofa that is anthropometrically correct, however. Even if these criteria are met, a person may experience problems with seating mobility. Therefore, the best method of assessing optimal seating is to observe the person actually using chairs in the environment to determine whether any difficulty is experienced. The person performing the assessment must take into account the variability of individual anthropometric indices and the effects of different disease conditions as they affect chair mobility. The assessor must watch the person sit down and rise from the chair and check that the task is performed safely and independently, and ask whether the seat is comfortable when the person is seated.

Seating Height

Seat height, or the distance between the floor and the front edge of the chair, is critical to mobility. If the seat height is too low or too high, it can interfere with safe transfers. Seats that are too low require the body to move a great distance between sitting and standing positions: Greater knee flexion and leg muscle strength are necessary to initiate the upward thrust needed to rise and to support the downward motion needed to sit. This extra effort is especially hard on people whose range of motion in the knees and hips is limited and whose muscle strength is reduced. Conversely, it is much easier to transfer on and off higher seats. High-level seating requires the body to exert less joint flexion and muscle strength for both transfer functions.

In an effort to compensate for low seating, people usually add cushions or a pillow to the seat or select a higher chair on which to sit. However, compensation can be problematic. If the feet do not rest flat on the floor, the person is forced to slide from the seat to reach the floor when attempting to stand and to climb onto the seat when attempting to sit. Both movements can compromise safety. If loss of balance occurs, the person risks a fall. Seat height is appropriate when it allows the patient or resident to sit with both feet planted firmly on the floor and the knees flexed at 90° (Figure 5-18). The front of the seat should be low enough to allow a small space between the thighs and seat (Figure 5-19). The ability to pass the flat of the hand freely between the seated person's thigh and edge of the seat is a good indication of the space that is needed between the seat and the body. Patients and residents should be provided with chair seat heights that are functionally suited to the individual. If these heights are not available, a seating

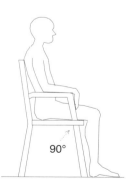

Figure 5-18. Seat height is appropriate when the person is able to sit with the knees flexed at 90° and both feet are planted firmly on the floor.

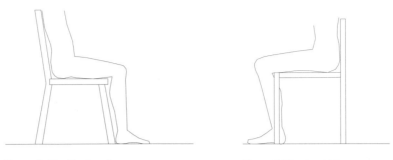

Figure 5-19. Front seat space.   **Figure 5-20.** Leg kick space.

cushion can be added to an existing chair. Its thickness should be determined by how much height is needed to achieve independent mobility.

Leg Space

To facilitate rising from a chair, the provision of a kick space below a seat is essential (Figure 5-20). Proper kick space allows the person to slide one foot underneath the chair and one foot forward to obtain the leverage necessary for the lower extremities to exert maximum thrust upward. Cross-bars or cross-rails on chair legs, used to provide structural support, may interfere with rising if they are positioned too low or too far forward on the chair (Figure 5-21). Cross-bars or cross-rails should be positioned high enough or set back far enough to ensure that they do not interfere with the biomechanics of rising (Figure 5-22). The presence of armrests or seats that are somewhat higher may compensate for poorly positioned cross-rails.

Armrests

All chairs used by older people should be equipped with armrests. Older people, much more than younger people, depend on armrests for assistance in propelling the body weight forward and maintaining balance when standing. The support offered by armrests is also advantageous because it helps reduce

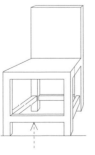

Figure 5-21. Cross-bars positioned too far forward or too low can interfere with safe rising from a seated position.

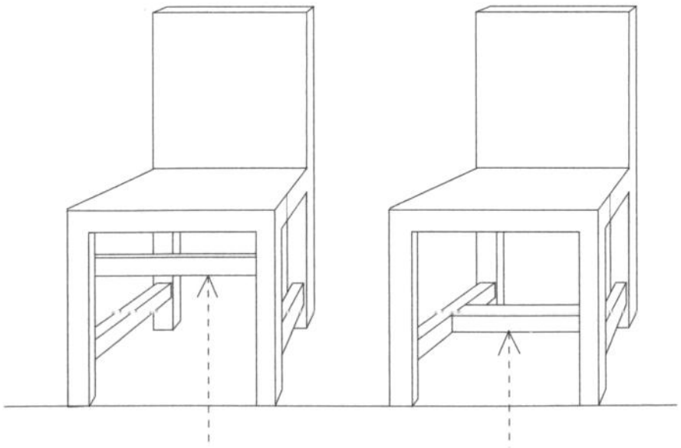

Figure 5-22. Appropriately positioned cross-bars.

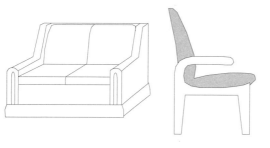

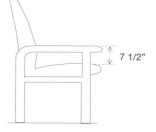

Figure 5-23. Nonsupportive armrest positions. (Left) Too low; (right) set back too far.

Figure 5-24. Appropriate armrest height.

pressure on the knee joints. Armrests also play a supportive role in helping a person to sit. A point is reached, particularly for people with decreased strength in the lower extremities or limited range of motion in the knee, when older adults' leg muscles and knee flexion no longer function effectively to help them sit down easily. As a result, they drop their body weight onto a seat. Armrests help arrest this quick downward thrust of the body by assisting in its gradual descent.

Armrests that are too low, too high, or set too far back may inhibit both rising from the chair and sitting in it. Low-level armrests force a person to lean forward when rising and thus threaten balance. Armrests that are too high or set too far back cannot provide a sufficient angle of leverage for the upper extremities when rising from a seat (Figure 5-23). To achieve optimal function in providing assistance, armrests should be of the correct height, positioned horizontally 7–7½ inches above the seat (Figure 5-24). They should extend at least to the seat's edge or, ideally, 1–2 inches beyond the front edge (Figure 5-25). This position allows for maximum leverage when rising because it enables people to engage their stronger lower body muscles in the task of rising to a standing position and continues to provide support until stability in standing is achieved (Figure 5-26). In addition, armrests should be nonslip, easy to grasp, and sloped slightly, more to the back than to the front, for maximum comfort.

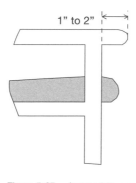

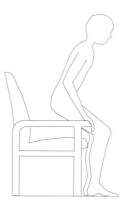

Figure 5-25. Appropriate armrest length.

Figure 5-26. Armrest support during transfer activities.

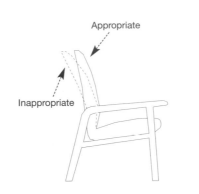

Figure 5-27. Chair seat or back rest angles.

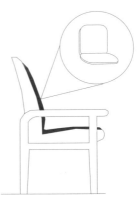

Figure 5-28. Appropriate seating cushion.

Seat Depth and Backrest Angle

In general, the deeper the seat (i.e., the distance measured from the popliteal area to the buttocks), the greater the effort needed for the person to move the body forward to the edge of the seat to rise. In addition to length, seat depth is affected by the angle of the backrest. The greater the angle or slant, the deeper the seat depth and the greater the distance a person must negotiate to pull himself or herself up (Figure 5-27).

The seat depth or backrest slope should always be considered in relation to the ability of the person to rise independently and should support the lower back. If the seat is too deep or the angle of the backrest is too great, a seating cushion placed along the length of the backrest usually can correct the deficiency (Figure 5-28).

To facilitate rising from a chair, the seat should slope gently backward no more than 1 inch from the front edge of the seat to its back edge (Figure 5-29). Seating that angles too far backward may present problems with rising because the person's knees will be positioned at a higher level than the buttocks (Figure 5-30). A seating angle that is tilted too far forward places the person's knees at a level that is lower than that of the buttocks and contributes to a slouched sitting position, which encourages sliding out of the chair (Figure 5-31). A wedge cushion can correct both problems (Figure 5-32). The

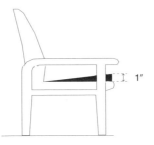

Figure 5-29. Appropriate angle for a seat slope.

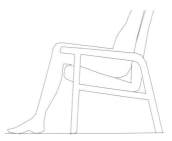

Figure 5-30. Inappropriate backward seating angle.

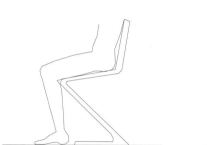

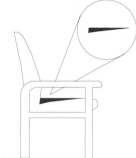

Figure 5-31. Inappropriate forward seating angle.

Figure 5-32. Appropriate wedged cushion.

wider part of the cushion should be positioned either in front of the seat to prevent sliding or at the back to assist people who experience difficulty in rising from their seat. In addition, the front edge of the seat should curve gently to avoid placing pressure on the back of the person's knees (Figure 5-33), which restricts blood flow and causes the development of leg swelling or phlebitis.

Seating Cushions

Cushions on chairs should provide comfort and absorb the impact caused by a person sitting in a seat, but they should not be too soft. People tend to sink into overly soft cushions, making it difficult to get out of them (Figure 5-34). Moreover, overly soft cushions reduce effective seat height because they are compressed by the seated person, thus lowering the seat. Therefore, it is difficult to rise in one fluid motion. Also, overly soft cushions prevent people from shifting their buttocks, a natural protective motion that helps them avoid developing decubiti.

The best type of seating cushion for chairs is the one that is flat and firm, has some resilience, and does not bottom out when a person sits on it. A suitable cushion should give way when a fist is pressed firmly into it yet resist if

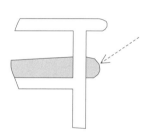

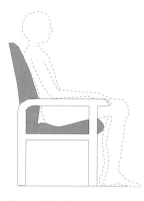

Figure 5-33. Appropriate curved seat edge.

Figure 5-34. Inappropriate seat cushion (too soft).

further pressure is applied. A cushion consisting of latex provides pliancy sufficient for comfort and firmness, without excessive compression. Foam cushions should be avoided because they lose resilience over time and tend to bottom out. The color of the seat cushion should contrast that of the chair so that it can be seen during seating. To prevent sliding, the seat covering should be manufactured of a slip-resistant material.

Seating Stability

The stability of a chair is crucial to a person's safety. If the chair tips forward, sideways, or backward during the act of transferring, the risk of loss of balance and falling increases greatly. Chairs with a seat edge that overhangs the position of the legs should be avoided. The design can cause the chair to tip forward when a person moves to its front edge or sits on the edge rather than in the middle of the seat (Figure 5-35). Casters or metal tips attached to the ends of the chair legs can be dangerous, especially on slick linoleum flooring. The weight of the body can cause chairs that are equipped with these devices to slide when the person sits, rises, or leans on the chair for balance support. Dining room chairs, in particular, can be precarious. Although dining room chairs must pull away easily from the table, casters are too unstable for most frail

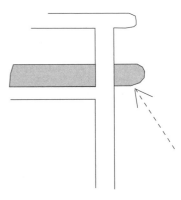

Figure 5-35. Inappropriate elongated seat cushion.

older people to use safely. In general, casters and metal tips should be removed. As an alternative, chairs can be placed against the wall, which prevents them from sliding away during transfers.

Chairs are most stable when the chair legs are straight and positioned well forward of the seat's leading edge but not so splayed as to invite tripping, and the edge of the seat does not extend too far forward beyond the chair legs. In addition, some people with balance problems use chair backrests for mobility support. Therefore, backrests should be placed high enough on the chair to provide adequate support. In general, a height of approximately 32 inches, the distance from the floor to the top of the backrest, is sufficient for this purpose (Figure 5-36). The backrest must be nonslip for safe grasping: A nonslip adhesive strip placed along the backrest prevents slipping. A good test of a chair's stability is for a staff member to grasp and lean into the chair and slide and tilt it forward, backward, and sideways.

Seating Alternatives to Restraints

Patients and residents who experience poor mobility and remain at fall risk, despite adaptation of existing chairs, may benefit from one of several different types of seats. A deep-seated, soft-cushioned lounge chair or recliner with a seat that slants downward toward the back; a wedge cushion, the

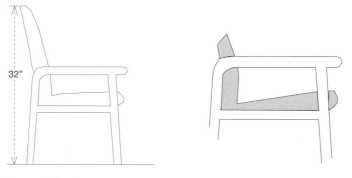

Figure 5-36. Appropriate back-rest height.

Figure 5-37. A wedge cushion that slants backward prevents independent rising.

widest part of which is placed toward the front of the seat (Figure 5-37); or a beanbag chair filled with Styrofoam pellets may be alternatives to mechanical restraints. These furnishings work by keeping a person's buttocks at a level that is lower than that of the knees, making it exceedingly difficult for the person to rise. Their purpose is to prevent the person who cannot ambulate safely from getting up independently or from sliding off a seat. Caution is advised because this seating position places increased pressure on the buttocks, particularly on the buttocks of thin people, placing them at risk for developing decubiti. Although these seats are considered by some critics to be restraints because they prevent independent movement, they can help people avoid many of the harmful effects of mechanical restraints (see Chapter Six).

If these seating choices are unsuitable, a chair alarm system may be an option. A fall alarm system is a battery-powered, portable device that consists of either a cord that attaches to the person's gown or a pressure-sensitive pad that rests on the seat or against the backrest. When a patient or resident slides to the edge of the chair or attempts to stand, the device sounds an alarm that alerts the nursing staff. The indications for a fall alarm are as follows:

• Patient or resident experiences fall(s) from a chair or wheelchair.

• Patient or resident experiences fall(s) while ambulating (shortly after rising from the chair) or is found on the floor next to the chair or wheelchair (unwitnessed fall).

• Patient or resident demonstrates unsafe chair or wheelchair transfers.

Fall alarms are effective, but only to a point. By the time a nurse comes to assist a patient or resident, the person already may be standing, or he or she may be lying on the floor. Placing pressure-sensitive pads against the chair backrest and keeping the length of clothing-attached cords short helps staff detect early departure from chairs.

In order to be heard by staff, fall alarms are generally loud, which can have a negative impact on patients and residents (e.g., the loud sounds may frighten them) and lead to a fear of leaving the chair.

BATHROOM

For older adults with poor walking and transferring balance, bathrooms can be especially hazardous places. Modifications of the existing bathroom can support safe mobility and reduce the risk of falls and injury.

Fixture Support

Patients and residents with balance dysfunction and people who are unable to use their walkers in the bathroom because of space limitations often resort to the use of sink tops, towel bars, and wall surfaces for support. These structures are poor alternatives and may contribute to falls, particularly if the person's hand slips. Moreover, towel bars are often located too high on the wall to provide adequate support. Several modifications to eliminate this hazard are available: A grab bar placed horizontally in place of the towel bar or a grab rail that runs around the perimeter of the bathroom wall can be used to provide balance support (Figure 5-38).

The color of the grab bars should contrast that of the wall for visibility; they should be slip-resistant (vinyl coating offers a better gripping surface than do standard metal bars) and should be positioned no more than 1½ inches from the wall to keep a person's arm from slipping between the bar and the wall. It is important that grab bars be attached securely to wall studs so that they do not give way easily. A wide variety of grab bar lengths and angles are available, which allows health care providers to tailor grab bars to specific patient and resident needs.

Nonslip adhesive strips placed along sink tops prevent hands from sliding (Figure 5-39). The color of strips should be similar to that of the sink top to eliminate visual confusion. In addition, grab bars can be mounted on the face of vanity tops to provide an additional support surface.

Toilets

Toilets that are low in height often cause problems in transferring. To circumvent such problems, corrective modifications should be made, which can include raised toilet seats and grab bars. Raised toilet seats are available in two

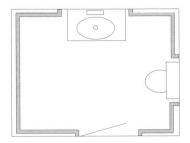

Figure 5-38. Bathroom grab rails.

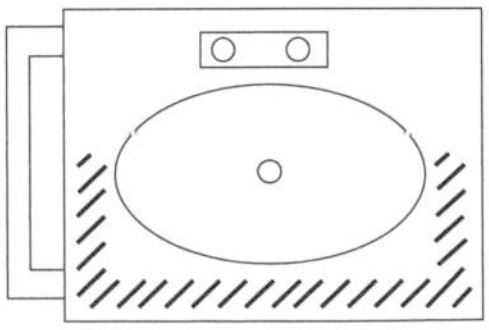

Figure 5-39. Nonslip adhesive strips placed on a sink.

types: fixed and adjustable height. Several sizes of fixed-height toilet seats should be available to accommodate individual needs. Raised toilet seats should be constructed of materials that are sturdy enough to provide support. The seats themselves should be made of soft vinyl or plastic to provide patients or residents with an absorptive cushion. An absorptive cushion reduces the risk of pelvic or hip fracture in people who tend to drop onto the toilet seat. The color of the toilet seat should contrast that of the toilet tank and bowl and the surrounding area to facilitate proper seating placement, particularly in people who depend on visual cueing. Contrasting the color of bathroom walls with that of the toilet can help people visualize the toilet as well.

The installation of grab bars on the wall next to and behind the toilet or a double armrest grab bar system, commonly called a toilet safety frame, that attaches to the toilet can be used by patients and residents to maintain their balance during toileting transfers. The type and height placement of grab bars mounted to the wall depend on the individual, his or her disability, and the surrounding environment. For example, people with hemiplegia find it difficult to use grab bars placed on their dysfunctional side, people of short stature or limited reach find grab bars placed at heights that are convenient for the average person unsatisfactory because they are beyond their reach, and people in wheelchairs experience transfer problems with conventional grab bars and find wall-mounted "swing-up" or "hinged-arm" grab bars easier to use. (This type of grab bar folds flat against the wall directly behind the toilet when not in use and can be moved to the horizontal position when in use.)

An alternative to wall-mounted grab bars is the toilet safety frame, or double armrest system (Figure 5-40). Many older people find this grab bar easier to use because the maximum amount of force exerted during transfers is completed in a straight downward movement of the arms, which provides optimum transferring support. Conversely, wall-mounted grab bars provide less support because, when transferring, the person must reach to the side and bend forward in order to grab the bar. As a result, the direct benefit of a downward thrust offered by the double armrest system is lost. The double armrest system is convenient for staff because it is easy to attach and can be readily adjusted for an individual patient or resident. As a cautionary measure, nonslip adhesive strips in a noncontrasting color should be placed on the floor in front of the toilet to prevent the person's feet from slipping during transfers. Nurse call alarms located in the bathroom and toilet paper holders must be accessible to guard against falls from the toilet.

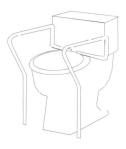

Figure 5-40. Armrest toilet riser.

Patients and residents who are unable to toilet autonomously may be able to maintain independence by using a bedside commode. Bedside commodes that are height adjustable for individual variation and fitted with armrest support to aid safe transfers should be chosen. Commodes that are equipped with wheels should be avoided because they can roll away easily during transfers.

TABLES AND NIGHTSTANDS

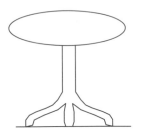

Figure 5-41. Pedestal table.

Many patients and residents with balance disorders use the edge of tabletops and nightstands for transferring and walking support. If these furnishings are unstable or the tops are slippery when grasped, they may fail to provide balance support. Furnishings that are not supportive can cause people to develop a fear of falling as well. It is best to avoid pedestal-style tables, which tend to tip over easily when a person's weight is applied to the edge (Figure 5-41). Nightstands that are used to assist with bed transfers may slide away, particularly if they are equipped with wheels or metal casters. Over-the-bed tables are similarly dangerous.

All tables and nightstands in the institutional environment should be stable when leaned on or grasped. They should have nonslip surfaces. Stability can be achieved by selecting tables with four legs that are free of wheels or casters and have a slip-resistant matte surface that promotes grasping. Tabletops with a contrasting border help patients and residents identify the edges of the table, thus promoting proper hand placement and support and averting "bumping into" accidents. Table edges that are rounded or bull nosed prevent bumping injuries that result from contact with sharp edges. Dining tables with spill-free edges, which restrain spilled liquids, are useful because they guard against wet floors and slippage. Dining room tables and chairs should work together: The arms of the chairs and wheelchairs should fit under the table to allow older people to move in as close as possible for dining and to avoid fluid spillage. To accommodate wheelchairs, tables must be approximately 34 inches high. Because the height may be exclusively for people dining in regular chairs, tables with adjustable height bases to accommodate both populations should be purchased. In addition, the position of tables and nightstands in the institutional environment should not obstruct ambulation.

STORAGE AREAS

All closets and dressers used by patients and residents must be accessible without the need for excessive reaching and bending. Frequently used items such as day and night wear and footwear should be placed on shelves or in drawers that lie between the person's eye and waist levels. This height accommodates the functional reach of most older people, thus minimizing the risk of balance loss.

ENDNOTES

1. Drahota, A., Gal, D., & Windsor, J. (2007). Flooring as an intervention to reduce injuries from falls in healthcare settings: An overview. *Quality in Ageing Policy, 8*(1), 3–9.
2. Kelly, K.E., Phillips, C.L., Cain, K.C., Polissar, N.L., & Kelly, P.B. (2002). Evaluation of a nonintrusive monitor to reduce falls in nursing home patients. *Journal of the American Medical Directors Association, 3*(6), 377–382.
3. Widder, B. (1985). A new device to decrease falls. *Geriatric Nursing, 6*(5), 287–288.

Chapter Six

Reducing Mechanical and Chemical Restraints

Until the 1990s, the sight of an old, frail person being restrained in a bed or chair was a familiar scene in hospitals and nursing facilities throughout the United States. Anywhere from 25% to 85% of older adults—more than half a million people—in these institutions were placed in mechanical restraints each day.[1] Concerns about their lack of effectiveness, safety, and serious consequences have been expressed in the U.S. health care community and among sensitive laypeople. As a result, a nationwide effort has been under way for a number of years to reduce and eventually eliminate the use of restraints as a fall prevention measure. The impetus stems from consumer advocates, health professionals, and government regulators who are concerned about the negative effects of restraints and lack of effectiveness of restraints in preventing falls. As a result, policies aimed at eliminating mechanical restraints have been developed. The most prominent policy is the Omnibus Budget Reconciliation Act (OBRA) of 1989 (PL 101-239).[2] OBRA represents a legislative concern about the quality of care in nursing facilities in general and the widespread use of restraints in particular. One of OBRA's strongest mandates was that nursing facilities examine their use of mechanical restraints and begin to find alternatives. As a consequence of OBRA regulations, the use of restraints in nursing facilities has declined dramatically, from a prevalence rate of 41% in 1988 to a level at the beginning of the 21st century of just under 20%. The movement to reduce restraints has affected acute care hospitals as well. The Joint Commission on Accreditation of Healthcare Organizations (JCAHO) has put into place restraint reduction initiatives for hospitals modeled after OBRA.

RATIONALE

The reasons for the use of mechanical restraints in hospitals and nursing facilities are often multifactorial, encompassing both patient and resident (host-related) and institutional factors:[3]

Patient- or resident-related factors

- Restraints prevent falls and related injury.

- Restraints decrease fall risk resulting from mobility problems, unsafe wandering, confusion, or agitated behaviors.

- Restraints correct seating alignment.

- Restraints prevent unsafe wandering.

- Restraints prevent interference with medical treatment.

Institutional factors

- Frail patients and residents are at risk for falls, injury, or both if not restrained.

- Inadequate staffing necessitates the use of restraints.

- Institutions have a moral duty to protect patients and residents.

- Failure to restrain places employees and the facility at legal risk.

- Restraints allow nurses to provide efficient and timely care.

- Families request and demand "risk-free" care, which includes restraint use.

- Few alternatives to restraints exist.

Although restraints are designed to protect patients and residents from falls and harm, they are not the best choice, nor do they represent the best solution, except possibly under extreme circumstances. All the firmly entrenched beliefs mentioned in the list that support their continued use are based on myth because no documented evidence exists that restraints are effective in accomplishing the purposes for which they are used. Many studies conclude that restraints seldom eliminate the risk of injury from falls and that, conversely, they can precipitate or exacerbate the problem. Most researchers concur that people in restraints are subject to the same or even greater fall risk as are people without restraints. Among facilities that do or do not use restraints, little difference exists in the extent of fall occurrences.[4] Moreover, facilities that do restrain experience a higher incidence of serious injury after falls.[5] When restraints are removed, there may be an increase in the number of falls but not in the number that result in significant injury.

Some nurses continue to believe that rendering care to patients and residents is easier and more efficient when restraints are used. Although it may appear that providing daily care to people with mobility problems is achieved more quickly when they are restrained, this strategy is ineffective. People in restraints rapidly develop immobility and associated morbidity, which creates greater dependency and need for custodial care from the staff and heightens the risk of falls. Aside from concerns about effectiveness, the use of restraints to "protect and safeguard" patients and residents is suspect. Although restraints have been applied in some instances for protective reasons (e.g., to prevent falls in people who are confused and wander when an immediate and clear threat of injury exists), the risks associated with restraints outweigh the benefits. The arguments supporting restraint use in protecting patients and residents at risk for immediate harm are questionable because alternatives have been used successfully to serve the same purpose and do not subject patients and residents to harm.

Rather than protecting older adults, restraints place them at risk for numerous detrimental physical and psychological consequences. Restraints that are too restrictive or applied too tightly can cause circulatory obstruction of the lower extremities, edema, skin abrasions, respiratory difficulties, and unintentional death by strangulation. Hospital patients who are restrained have twice the length of institutional stay of those who are free from restraints; they are also more likely to be transferred to nursing facilities for care and are at higher risk for early death. Much of the resulting mortality is the consequence of restraint use and its concomitant immobility.

The psychological consequences of restraints are many and help refute the belief that older people are not bothered by their use. Often, application triggers one of several emotional reactions: People feel either fear and a sense of panic, which can result in belligerent behavior, or a sense of humiliation and abandonment, which can result in aggressive behavior, a loss of self-image, depression, withdrawal, or low social functioning. In addition, self-esteem decreases because, typically, others view people who are in restraints as disturbed, dangerous, or mentally incompetent, which can be demoralizing. Moreover, when older adults are not informed about the decision to apply restraints or are not allowed to refuse their use, they are denied their right of self-determination. This violation of personal rights constitutes a restriction of a person's autonomy, including the freedom to make choices about engaging in activities. When a person is restrained and denied the ability to get up, sit down, or walk about with undue interference, his or her quality of life and psychological well-being are impaired.

Health care professionals are not immune to the effects of restraints. Nurses, who are often responsible for initiating restraint orders in hospitals and nursing facilities, struggle with the burden brought on by this decision. On one hand, they feel a professional duty to safeguard people who are at risk for falls. This obligation is often heightened when nursing allocations are scarce and monitoring of problematic patients and residents is difficult. To avoid the risk of legal sanctions, some nurses believe that they have no alternative but to apply restraints. On the other hand, nurses find the act of restraining older people stressful and emotionally taxing, often provoking in themselves anxiety, dissatisfaction, and guilt. They recognize that restraints deprive people of their autonomy and dignity, and they sympathize with them, conceding that they themselves would not want to be placed in a similar position.

Although nurses perceive themselves as less vulnerable to legal sanctions if restraints are used, particularly in the event of injury, the fear of legal liability is ill founded. Despite the fact that lawsuits for damages resulting from falls are common, few have been successful against facilities and their employees based solely on the failure to restrain. In cases involving injury to people without restraints, a preponderance of other factors usually constitutes negligence, including improper assessment and documentation of the patient's or resident's condition, failure to assess and monitor the person at risk for falls, and failure to respond to falls and injury in a timely manner. Rather, the use of restraints may increase the risk of litigation. Lawsuits involving the improper application of restraints that results in patient and resident injury (e.g., falling out of a bed or chair with restraints either intact or removed by the person) have been successful. In addition, facilities and staff may be held liable when restraints are used for convenience, for example, during staffing shortages.

Family members are also affected by restraint decisions and react in various ways to finding their relatives restrained. Some express dismay at the sight of a relative in restraints and demand their removal, even if the action places the person at fall risk. Others, although not accepting of the practice, come to accept restraints as a necessary evil, believing that they will keep their relative from being injured in a fall. This notion is reinforced when family members are not informed by staff of the harmful effects of restraints and of the available alternatives for safeguarding their relative.

Much of the justification for using mechanical and chemical restraints is based on the misapprehension that no alternatives are available. Many hospitals and nursing facilities in the United States have deliberately reduced restraint use without experiencing a concomitant rise in serious injury. Such facilities have adopted a policy of non-restraint use that is common in several European countries. These countries place greater emphasis on structuring the physical environment and the activities of patients and residents in such a way that restraints are rarely, if ever, needed or used.

MANAGEMENT

The challenge for health care professionals in hospitals and nursing facilities is reducing the use of mechanical and chemical restraints while decreasing the risk of falls. To achieve this objective, hospital and nursing facility staff can take a number of steps in their facilities:

Step 1

Examine current restraint practices, the attitudes of employees toward their use, and institutional policies that govern the use of mechanical and chemical restraints. The intent of this exercise is to determine the prevalence of restraint use; the availability, use, and effectiveness of restraint alternatives; and whether policies are viable and provide staff with appropriate direction in the use of restraints. Inquire about the following:

- To what extent are restraints used?

- Under what circumstances or conditions are restraints ordered and why?

- Are restraints the first or last choice in treatment?

- Are restraints effective in controlling the risk of falls?

- Are restraints used continuously, intermittently, or on a short-term basis? Under what conditions?

- Are patients and residents (if able) and family members consulted on the need for restraints and given the right of refusal?

- If either party refuses the use of restraints, what procedures are in place to ensure the patient's or resident's safety?

- Are people who are restrained observed or monitored for nutritional or toileting needs and adverse effects? How often? By whom?

- If people experience adverse effects, are restraints discontinued? If not, why? If so, what forms of management are used to replace restraints?

- Are restraint alternatives ever considered as an initial choice of treatment? Under what circumstances?

- What types of alternative treatments are available? Are they effective in controlling the problem indicated? If not, why?

- Are institutional policies clear as to the types of conditions or situations in which restraints can and cannot be used, the types of restraint alternatives available, the assessment procedure for restraint use and discontinuation, and who has the responsibility of ordering, monitoring, and documenting restraint and non-restraint use?

- Are institutional policies updated periodically? Are staff members aware of the content of policy statements?

Step 2

Establish an ongoing program of in-service education aimed at assessing restraints (Table 6-1) and assessing and managing the problems (e.g., dysmobility, falls, confusion, wandering, poor sitting posture) that are commonly cited as indications for restraints. These problems should not be viewed as end-stage processes but as signs of an underlying medical or environmental condition. Ordering a restraint as initial treatment is inappropriate; rather, these problems should trigger further investigation and treatment aimed at eliminating the underlying conditions responsible. If the problem persists, alternatives to the use of restraints should be explored (Table 6-2). Restraints, if necessary, should be considered only as a temporary measure to be used under extreme emergency conditions or as a last resort when the advantages to the patient or resident clearly outweigh the disadvantages. To this end, attention to staff education regarding selection of appropriate restraints and their proper application is warranted. In general, the restraint chosen should be the one that is the least restrictive and safest. Both the patient or resident and the restraint should be checked frequently.

Step 3

Hospitals and nursing facilities should develop and implement restraint reduction policies. The purpose of these policies is to provide staff with step-by-step guidelines related to mechanical restraint decisions and care for patients and residents. These documents also can serve as defense against potential legal liability because they illustrate an attempt by the institution and staff to practice reasonable standards of restraint practice. The policy statement should be clear and simple to follow and should address the following points specifically:

- Define what a mechanical restraint is and describe the types of restraining devices available.

- Define and categorize the types of situations in which restraints may or may not be used.

- Define the assessment procedure for the application and discontinuation of restraints.

- Define who has the responsibility for ordering and discontinuing restraints.

- Define the procedure and staff responsibilities for documenting restraint use.

- Define the procedure for monitoring restraint use.

Table 6-1.   Content for educational in-service training on restraints

I. Overview of restraints
- A. Prevalence
- B. Reasons for restraints
  - 1. Avoidance of falls
  - 2. Control of wandering behavior
  - 3. Control of agitation/behavioral problems
  - 4. Correction of seating/positioning problems
- C. Ineffectiveness of restraints in managing patient or resident safety

II. Adverse effects of restraints
- A. Physiological consequences
- B. Loss of autonomy
- C. Loss of dignity
- D. Agitation/depression
- E. Family and staff discomfort

III. Legal
- A. Current OBRA and JCAHO regulations concerning restraint use
- B. Institutional policies regarding restraints
- C. Staff liability issues

IV. Restraint alternatives
- A. Assessment
  - 1. Identify causes of fall risk
  - 2. Identify causes of wandering
  - 3. Identify causes of agitation/behavioral problems
  - 4. Identify causes of seating problems
- B. Non-restraint management
  - 1. Modify underlying problems discovered
    - a. Fall risk
    - b. Wandering
    - c. Agitation/behavioral manifestations
    - d. Poor seating
  - 2. Review available restraint alternatives
    - a. Approaches/methods to support seating
    - b. Approaches/methods to guard against falls
    - c. Approaches/methods to permit safe wandering
    - d. Approaches/methods to manage behavioral manifestations
    - e. Approaches/methods to support mobility

- Define the types of circumstances under which restraint alternatives should be considered.

- Define the types of restraint alternatives available.

- Define the procedure to follow when patients and residents or family members refuse restraints.

- Define a procedure for ensuring that all staff are aware of the institution's policy and that the contents of the policy are updated periodically.

Table 6-2. Alternatives to restraints

Caregiving

Additional nursing supervision/observation of activities

Assistance of family members/volunteers
(companionship, supervision of activities)

Daily ambulation, structured activities

Exercise; gait/balance training

Instruction on safe chair/wheelchair transfers

Maintain regular toileting schedule

Evaluate adverse medication affects

Correct sensory deficits
(e.g., eyeglasses, hearing aids)

Provide safety when patient or resident judgment is impaired

Environmental

Orient patient/resident to environment

Arrange for patient/resident to be near nursing station

Provide adequate lighting, night-lights

Maintain obstacle-free environment

Provide ambulation devices

Employ strategic seating

Make available a variety of seating options
(different heights, seat angles)

Provide alternative seating
(wedge cushions, seating props, slanting chairs, beanbag chairs)

Provide nonslip floor surfaces

Supply/encourage appropriate footwear

Provide bed and chair alarms, accessible call buttons

Lower bed height, mattress on floor

Remove bed wheels

Provide accessible call light

Avoid full-length bedside rails

Use half-bedside rails to support transfers ("enablers")

Provide commode at bedside

Provide perimeter alarms, safe wandering areas

Provide Merry Walker
(designed walker that permits independent ambulation for individuals
with dementia or confusion)

Reducing mechanical restraints may be difficult to achieve in all instances, perhaps more so in the acute care hospital than in the nursing facility. It is important to recognize that, with respect to fall prevention efforts, good care consists of helping patients and residents achieve maximum independence while attempting to reduce the likelihood of falls. It is clear that there are few justifications for the use of mechanical restraints and that restraints are more likely to cause falls than prevent them.

Health care providers also must be cognizant of the misuse of psychoactive medications as chemical restraints and eliminate this practice. The most common categories of psychoactive medications include antipsychotics (i.e., neuroleptics or major tranquilizers), anxiolytics (i.e., antianxiety or minor tranquilizers), sedatives and hypnotics (i.e., sleep inducers), and antidepressants. Often, these drugs are prescribed to control mood, mental status, or behaviors—acute confusional states, agitated or violent behaviors, anxiety, depressive states, or wandering—that place patients and residents at risk for falls or other harmful consequences. Drugs are considered inappropriate chemical restraints when they are

- Given without specific indications

- Prescribed in excessive dosages, which affect an older adult's ability to function properly

- Used as sole treatment without investigating nonpharmacological or behavioral interventions

- Administered for purposes of discipline or convenience of the staff.

Many cases of inappropriate psychoactive drug use result either from the mistaken belief that these medications are the only way to manage behaviors or from the fact that they are used as a substitute for adequate treatment.

Whether psychoactive medications are used as therapeutic agents or as restraints may be difficult to determine. For example, a psychoactive drug may be prescribed to treat agitated behavior, and its use results in an increased fall risk. The psychoactive drug is considered a therapeutic agent if it controls the person's behavior and eliminates the risk of falls without restricting his or her ability to function; it is deemed a restraint if the person's activities (e.g., getting out of bed, going to the bathroom, engaging in social activities) are inhibited. Other medications used by older adults may be considered chemical restraints. For instance, some medications such as nonsteroidal anti-inflammatory drugs (analgesics), antihypertensives, and cardiotonics (cardiac drugs) prescribed for physical ailments can produce side effects such as disorientation, confusion, dizziness, and orthostatic hypotension, or low blood pressure. In addition, polypharmacy (i.e., taking four or more medications) is common among older people. Any adverse interactions between drugs, such as increased sedation or loss of coordination, can result in cognitive and mobility impairments.

The side effects of psychoactive drugs are particularly taxing on the physiological systems of older people. These side effects may include increased drowsiness, delirium or disordered thinking, low blood pressure, and Parkinsonian symptoms such as muscle rigidity in the limbs and gait disturbances. Such conditions may not only lead to further disruptive behavior but also increase the risk of falls and hip fractures. Also, psychoactive drugs may produce paradoxical agitation (i.e., rather than calming down a person, the drugs can sometimes increase agitation) in some older adults, which clouds the issue of whether to increase or decrease drug dosages. Any increase of medication is likely to result in a vicious circle of higher dosages and decreased functional ability.

Health care providers must take several steps before using psychoactive medications in patients and residents who present with cognitive or behavioral disturbances; they must identify the disturbance or specific symptom, and, if possible, discover the cause of the disturbance. Assessment of the underlying conditions responsible may eliminate the need for psychoactive medications. For example, confusion leading to disoriented behavior, agitation, or falling episodes may result from an underlying infection or pharmacotoxicity. Therefore, giving an antibiotic to clear the infection or stopping the medication is more appropriate than giving a psychoactive. Other common causes of disturbed behavior and changes in cognitive function in older people are the presence of pain, fecal impaction, metabolic abnormalities, and acute exacerbation of chronic diseases. Also, simple events such as a wet bed, a room that is too hot or too cold, and hunger or thirst should not be overlooked as causes of behavior disturbances. Attempts should be made to reverse or eliminate the underlying cause through nonpharmacological approaches. In many instances, intervention with corrective behavioral or environmental strategies eliminates the need for psychoactive drugs. For instance, a succession of stressful events such as declining health, episodes of falling, admission to a hospital or a nursing facility, and the possibility of long-term institutional placement can bring about a complete breakdown of coping mechanisms, causing confusion. In such a situation, the provision of proper psychosocial counseling to deal with the underlying stress may be beneficial in reversing the confusion. Likewise, allowing patients and residents to wander and providing a safe walking area may be all that is needed to alleviate agitated behaviors.

During the period in which the underlying cause is being investigated, the patient or resident may continue to exhibit disturbed behaviors. To protect the person from injuring himself or herself or others, it may be necessary to use a psychoactive drug in order to gain control over anxiety or aggression. In addition, if alternative approaches to eliminating the disturbed behavior are unsuccessful, psychoactive drugs may be needed to improve the older person's quality of life. Under such circumstances, obtaining a comprehensive drug history to guard against additive adverse effects and conducting laboratory studies to detect any hepatic or renal abnormalities that may influence the metabolism and excretion or elimination of drugs must precede the use of psychoactive drugs. When a psychoactive is initiated, the prescriber should start with a low dosage to test the person's responsiveness. Then the dosage should be increased slowly until the desired level of control is achieved without unwanted side effects. To ensure that psychoactive medications are used properly, staff should monitor patients and residents frequently for drug effectiveness and evidence of side effects. If drug therapy is unsuccessful or if the person experiences adverse effects from the therapy, the medication should be discontinued and the plan of care revised. Also, staff must evaluate continually whether the person's disturbed behaviors have ceased or decreased in severity. In such an instance, staff should consider stopping the medication or reducing the dosage of the drug in order to avoid the risk of chemical restraint.

In summary, institutionally based health care providers play a major role in keeping patients and residents free of mechanical and chemical restraints. To meet this objective, providers should avoid the use of mechanical restraints to control falls and, instead, attempt restraint alternatives. Staff should not expose older adults who have never used psychoactive medications to these drugs unless they have a specific condition that calls for the medication. In addition, staff should reduce the dosage for people already using psychoactive drugs with the intent of stopping the drug, unless such a course is contraindicated clinically.

ENDNOTES

1. A mechanical restraint is defined as any mechanical device, material, or equipment attached or adjacent to the person's body that the person cannot remove easily and is used to inhibit free, independent movement. These devices include vest and chest jackets or harnesses, waist belts and sheets, leg ties, full-length bedside rails, wheelchair safety bars, and geri-chairs with fixed tray tables.
2. Omnibus Budget Reconciliation Act (OBRA) of 1989, PL 101-239, 42 U.S.C. §§ 1396 et seq.
3. All such rationales supporting the use of mechanical restraints are based on myth, not reality.
4. Mohr, W.K., Petti, R.A., & Mohr, B.D. (2003). Adverse effects associated with physical restraint. *Canadian Journal of Psychiatry, 48*(5), 330–337.
5. Tinetti, M.E., Liu, W.L., & Ginter, S.F. (1992). Mechanical restraint use and fall-related injury among residents of skilled nursing facilities. *Annals of Internal Medicine, 116,* 369–374.

Fall Prevention Practice

Chapter Seven

Key Process Steps and Interventions

PROCESS + STRUCTURE = OUTCOME

The goal of any fall prevention program is to achieve a reduction in falls and injury. The success of a fall prevention program depends on process and structure. The process is what caregivers do every day while providing care. It includes the multidisciplinary professionals' activities in assessing the risk of falls, implementing multidisciplinary interventions designed to reduce risk, monitoring patients or residents at risk, and evaluating falling episodes. In other words, the process is the clinical framework of fall prevention. However, an effective fall prevention program depends on a greater commitment. The structure consists of the organizational or administrative components needed to help staff achieve effective process. The outcome represents the effects of the process and structure. In the end, a good structure increases the likelihood of a good process, and a good process increases the likelihood of a good outcome.

Chapters 7, 8, and 9 cover a wide range of topics, including:

- Key process steps and interventions

- Key organizational factors and strategies influencing fall prevention

- Staff education (e.g., in-service training, newsletters, e-mail blasts)

- Fall prevention guidelines and protocols.

This chapter covers the following process topics:

Process Topics

Risk Assessment

—Implementing an Institution-Based Fall Risk Assessment Program

—Fall Risk Assessments and Targeted Care Plans

—Fall Risk Assessment: Help, My Tool Doesn't Work!

—Fall Risk Assessment Tools: How to Validate Low and High Fall Risk Scores

—Admission Fall Risk Assessment

RISK ASSESSMENT

Implementing an Institution-Based Fall Risk Assessment Program

Falls are complex events caused by multiple intrinsic factors related to mobility, sensory perception, cognitive function, medications, and comorbidities and extrinsic or hazardous environmental conditions. In order to reduce falls, institutions need to take a number of steps. First, the staff must understand the conditions under which falls occur and the most common factors associated with fall risk. This information will enable the staff to identify patients or residents at risk and explore appropriate solutions aimed at reducing fall risk. Second, the staff must have in place a formal fall risk assessment program, which consists of assessing risk, communicating risk, and reducing risk.

Where, When, and Why Falls Occur

Falls that occur from or near the bed account for up to half of all falls. Another common fall location is the bathroom, especially near the toilet. Most falls occur during the first 72 hours after admission, at night, and just after meals. Bed and chair transfers are the most frequently cited activity at the time of falling. Other activities commonly associated with falls include toileting and getting up from bedside commodes and wheelchairs.

Common Fall Risk Factors

The most common fall risk factors include past history of falls, cognitive impairment, elimination or special toileting needs, impaired mobility, and medications.

These risk factors form the basis of risk assessment tools. An assessment program must be acceptable and user-friendly to both staff and patients or residents, and, most importantly, the program must result in reduced falls.

Fall Risk Assessment Program

Assessing Risk   Because most institutional falls are caused by preventable factors, the use of fall risk assessments and tools to identify patients or residents at risk of falling plays a crucial role in minimizing the number of falls. The rationale for this assessment is that if patients or residents at fall risk can be identified, then appropriate interventions can be instituted to minimize this risk. Assessment tools may also assist in stratifying or targeting the urgency and types of interventions needed and play a role in raising staff awareness of the risk of falls.

To be effective, assessment tools must be sensitive (correctly identify those at high risk) and specific (correctly identify those not at risk) and, perhaps most importantly, be easy for staff to use; embedding a fall risk assessment tool into existing nursing assessments promotes acceptance of the tool or process (Table 7-1) (Oliver et al., 2004; Vassallo et al., 2005).

Baseline fall risk assessments should be completed within 2 hours of admission. Because older adults are subject to changes in acuity of illness, medications, mobility, and cognition, fall risk factors are subject to change as well. As a result, fall risk assessment is an ongoing process, repeated whenever patients experience a change of condition or medication, daily or with every shift change in certain high-risk patients or residents, and immediately after a fall. The purpose of the postfall assessment is to identify the circumstances or causes of the fall, identify the presence of new risk factors, and plan appropriate interventions to prevent further falls. Postfall assessments are beneficial in detecting and eliminating precipitating factors for falls.

Table 7-1.   Fall risk assessment tools

Several assessment tools meet the aforementioned criteria:
- The Morse Fall Scale
- The STRATIFY tool
- The Hendrich II Fall Risk Model
- The Schmid Fall Risk Assessment Tool

See page 125 for resources validating the outcomes of each assessment tool. (Coker & Oliver, 2003; Hendrich, Bender & Nyhuis, 2003; O'Connell & Myers, 2002; Perell et al., 2001)

Communicating Risk   Once a person's risk of falling has been assessed, his or her risk status must be communicated to everyone involved (e.g., therapists, nurses, nursing assistants, other staff members, and even family members). Remember that fall prevention is everyone's responsibility. Fall risk can be communicated by means of colored decals (placed on the patient's or resident's chart or in his or her bedroom), colored wristbands, and daily shift reports. Formalizing and incorporating the process of risk communication into risk assessment protocols or guidelines can be very helpful. In this way, everyone in the facility knows that anyone wearing a colored wristband has a higher risk of falling or potential for injury.

Reducing Risk   An assessment program is useful only if an effective treatment or intervention is available for patients or residents identified as being at risk. Thus, once assessments are complete and risk factors identified, preventive strategies must be implemented. To be effective, interventions must include a number of different strategies. Interventions are most effective when they are designed to reach those with the greatest risk of falling and combine personalized attention, environmental changes, and medication review.

For those at low fall risk, universal fall precautions should still be used. This measure acknowledges that all older adults, even low-risk ones, are potentially at risk of falling (e.g., in new environments, with new routines and new people). Universal precautions include such strategies as setting the bed at low level, ensuring that patients or residents have necessary items such as call bells within easy reach, and assessing and eliminating potential environmental hazards.

For patients or residents at risk, interventions must be more specific and based on identified risk factors (e.g., maintaining regular toileting, reorienting confused people, and assessing the need for side rails, ambulatory aids, fall alarms, hip protectors, hourly rounds or one-to-one nursing, or room relocation close to a nursing station). It is important to remember that as risk factors change, interventions may have to change as well.

In summary, preventing falls is really about carefully identifying and assessing the needs of each patient or resident. A fall risk assessment program that assesses, communicates, and attempts to reduce risk on a regular basis can be very effective in preventing falls.

Fall Risk Assessments and Targeted Care Plans

It is becoming clear that falls in older adults result from a small number of risk factors. Previous falls, cognitive impairment, elimination problems or frequent toileting, use of sedative–hypnotic drugs, and mobility impairment are consistently cited as significant fall risk factors. When several of these risk factors occur together, risk can be significant. Consequently, fall risk assessment tools, particularly those based on significant risk factors, can predict the risk of falling with reasonable accuracy. However, risk assessments are useful only if an effective targeted intervention or strategy is available for those identified as being at risk. Once fall risk factors have been identified, the implementation of preventive strategies is imperative. Unfortunately, this does not always occur. According to root cause analysis of falling episodes in the institutional setting, the failure to initiate interventions aimed at reducing fall risk in a timely manner is one of the most common reasons for falling.

Combining the fall risk assessment and initial care plan into one tool can be an effective way of implementing preventive strategies, especially for interventions that may have an immediate impact on reducing falls (Table 7-2).

There are several potential benefits of combining the fall risk assessment and initial care plan:

- Providing a list of specific immediate interventions, which are targeted to specific risk factors, reminds nursing staff what interventions are available and what can be done right away to reduce the person's risk of falling or injury.

- Incorporating the assessment and care plan into existing forms, such as the nursing admission assessment and postfall protocol, reminds nursing

Table 7-2. Fall risk assessment and care plan

Risk Factors	Care Plan Interventions
Cognition	Consider:
Delirium	Physician referral (evaluate mental status)
Dementia	Fall alarm
Depression	Nursing observation rounds
Uncooperativeness	Anticipatory care (one-to-one nursing)
Inability to follow directions	Sitter program
	Relocating close to nursing station
Medications	Consider:
Sedative–hypnotic	Physician or pharmacist review (evaluate drugs)
Psychotropic	Care plan for anticipated medication side effects, such as
Diuretics	monitoring for low blood pressure (a risk factor for several of the drugs listed)
Elimination	Consider:
Incontinence	Physician referral (evaluate bladder status)
Frequency	Bedside commode
Nocturia	Toileting schedule
	Fall alarm
Mobility	Consider:
Impaired ambulation	Physician referral (evaluate mobility status)
Impaired transfers	Side rail or transfer bar (enabler)
Balance impairment	Physical therapy referral (safety of walker or cane)
Assistive aid (walker, cane)	Assisted transfers and ambulation
	Low bed
	Floor mat
	Fall alarm
	Hip protector

staff to assess for fall risk and about the need for preventive strategies, especially during times when falls are most likely to occur.

- Having a menu of specific risk reduction strategies available at the time of risk assessment makes nursing staff aware of basic preventive precautions and increases the likelihood that interventions will be applied and documented.

Fall Risk Assessment: Help, My Tool Doesn't Work!

Every week, I receive several e-mails from nurses around the country with the following complaint: "I work at a hospital and see a lot of older adults. I was wondering whether you have a fall risk tool that you would suggest. The fall risk tool we are currently using does not work; our patients keep falling."

Fall risk assessment is an important component of fall prevention; its purpose is to

- Identify people at increased risk of falling before they fall
- Identify intrinsic and extrinsic risk factors
- Design targeted risk reduction strategies.

The most important fall risk factors include the following:

- History of falls
- Dementia or depression
- Dizziness
- Bladder dysfunction
- Gait or balance impairment
- Altered mobility
- Psychotropic medications.

The purpose of using a fall risk assessment tool is to

- Identify patient or resident problems (rational basis for deciding whether risk exists)
- Trigger further fall-related assessments (multidisciplinary)
- Guide patient or resident care (care planning)
- Evaluate treatments and interventions.

Fall risk assessment tools exist that show good validity and reliability. However, few tools are tested more than once or in more than one setting. No single tool can be recommended for use in all settings or for all subpopulations in each setting (Scott et al., 2007).

In the event of a fall, a host of other reasons must be explored other than possible shortcomings of the risk assessment tool used; these include the following:

Care Plan Development

Using information from the assessment and evaluation process, the care plan summarizes the results and lists all multidisciplinary interventions for the best strategy and course of action. After identifying a patient or resident at fall risk, a multidisciplinary team should be involved in conceiving the care plan, engaging medical, nursing, pharmacy, and physical or occupational therapy staff to develop interventions aimed at fall reduction. A proper care plan includes the following:

1. A list of the patient's or resident's risk factors.

2. Short-term goals focusing on immediate safety needs.

3. Long-term goals focusing on what you hope the interventions will accomplish. All short- and long-term goals should be SMART: specific, measurable, achievable, realistic, and timely.

4. Interventions addressing the causes and consequences of the patient's or resident's current status, problems, and risks. Departments and individual staff members responsible for implementing interventions should be named.

Monitoring and Follow-Up

Ongoing monitoring and follow-up of goals and interventions listed in the care plan are critical (Table 7-5). Did the patient or resident respond as expected?

Table 7-5. Example of care planning process for a person at fall risk

Assessment results	Increased fall risk due to • Urinary frequency • Degenerative joint disease • Mobility impairment
Evaluation	• Increased fall risk during toileting as a result of urinary frequency (hurries to toilet) and mobility impairment • Mobility impairment caused by degenerative joint disease • Urinary frequency caused by urinary tract infection
Care plan	Short-term goals: • Provide bedside commode and mobility support with toileting activities Long-term goals: • Reduced falls during toileting activities • Improved mobility • Optimal medical management of degenerative joint disease • Reduced urinary frequency Interventions: • Anticipate toileting needs (nursing) • Assist with toileting and mobility needs (nursing) • Medical evaluation and management of degenerative joint disease and urinary frequency (physician) • Management of mobility impairment (physical therapy)
Monitoring (follow-up)	• All goals and interventions have been achieved

Were goals achieved? Did new problems arise? Review progress toward defined goals and adjust interventions as needed. A lack of success with interventions or a significant change in condition (e.g., acute illness, functional impairment) must be addressed by revisiting the care planning process from the beginning.

CAREGIVER COMMUNICATION

Using the SBAR Tool to Communicate Fall Risk

A hospital patient is sent to the radiology department for an x-ray, but the nurse forgets to tell the radiology technician about the patient's confusion and fall risk. During a change of shift, a nursing home caregiver does not mention that the resident is at high risk for a fall injury. In both instances, the lack of communication resulted in a fall. Whenever patients or residents are handed off from one health care provider to another, it is a dangerous time. In fact, the failure to communicate fall risk is one of the major root causes of falls. Consequently, to ensure that a patient's or resident's risk status is transferred from one staff member or caregiver to the next, hospitals and nursing homes should have an approach to handing off or communicating fall risk.

An effective handoff of fall risk provides a snapshot of pertinent information that enables immediate provision of seamless care (i.e., written information from one caregiver or health care provider to another so that important care or service needs and the person's current condition and any recent or anticipated changes are communicated accurately). SBAR is an easy-to-use tool that allows communication between members of the health care team about a patient's or resident's fall risk status and plan of care (Table 7-6). SBAR stands for

- *Situation:* What is going on with the patient or resident (i.e., current risk status)?

- *Background:* What is the patient's or resident's clinical background (i.e., identified fall risk factors)?

- *Assessment:* What is the patient's or resident's current situation (i.e., current risk conditions and fall precautions)?

- *Recommendation:* What is being done to reduce risk (i.e., current care plan)?

POSTFALL ASSESSMENT

What Is a Fall?

Although falls occur frequently in acute hospitals and nursing homes, staff may not always report them. One of the main reasons for underreporting falls is that staff may not always know what to report. Unfortunately, because no universally accepted definition exists, falls are defined and reported in different ways. Having a clear fall definition allows organizations to accurately

Table 7-6. SBAR tool: Fall risk*

S	Situation
	• Jane Doe
	• High fall risk (provide current fall risk assessment score or risk level)
B	Background
	• Cognitive impairment
	• Mobility impairment (impaired transfers)
	• Bladder impairment (incontinence or nocturia)
	• Insomnia
	• Sleep medications
A	Assessment
	• Incontinence and nocturia; patient does not use call bell or ask for toileting assistance and attempts unsafe bed and chair transfers
	• Increased fall risk at night secondary to sleep medication
R	Recommendations
	• Scheduled toileting every 2 hours while awake
	• Bedside commode to assist with toileting
	• Fall alarm on 24 hours to detect unsafe bed and chair exits

*The handoff should ideally occur during shift change, temporary transfer of care during staff absence (e.g., lunch and other breaks, when the patient's or resident's caregiver leaves the unit), transfer of patient or resident between departments and floors or units, and so on.

count falls and consistently trend fall data and fall rates. Moreover, accurate fall reporting and postfall assessments, to discover why the fall occurred, are the best way to prevent future falls. As a result, it is important for each organization to establish a fall definition. Although many organizations have their own definitions of a fall, there are many definitions of falling to consider:

• *Observed falls.* These occur when a patient or resident experiences a loss of balance during walking or transferring and lands on the floor or another object such as a bed, chair, or wheelchair; or when a patient or resident comes to rest on the ground without intending to so.

• *Assisted falls.* These occur when a staff member lowers the patient or resident to the floor or when a patient lowers himself or herself to the floor because he or she feels dizzy or weak.

• *Unobserved falls.* These occur when a patient or resident is found on the floor and neither the patient or resident nor anyone else knows how he or she got there. Until proven otherwise, assume that this is due to a fall. This type of fall is often referred to as being "found down" or "found on the floor." Most falls occurring in the institutional setting are not observed. When a patient or resident is found on the floor, the facility is obligated to investigate, try to determine how he or she got there, and intervene to prevent this from happening again.

• *Near falls.* These occur when a patient or resident experiences a sudden loss of balance that does not result in a fall or other injury. For instance, a person may slip, stumble, or trip but is able to regain balance control, thereby avoiding a fall to the ground. Sometimes patients or residents experience a loss of balance but prevent a fall by grabbing hold of furnishings or walls for balance support. An episode in which a patient or resident lost his or her balance and would have fallen, were it not for staff intervention, is a fall. In other words, an intercepted fall is still a fall.

The presence or absence of a resultant injury is not a factor in the definition of a fall. Also, the distance to the next lower surface (i.e., the floor) is not a factor in determining whether a fall occurred. If a patient or resident rolls off a bed or mattress that is close to the floor, this is a fall.

Definitions of Injurious Falls

- *None* indicates that the patient or resident did not sustain an injury secondary to the fall.

- *Minor* indicates injuries necessitating a simple intervention.

- *Moderate* indicates injuries necessitating sutures or splints.

- *Major* injuries are those that necessitate surgery, casting, or further examination (e.g., for a neurological injury).

- Deaths may result from injuries sustained in a fall.

Classification or Types of Falls

According to Morse (2002), falls can be classified into three categories:

- *Accidental falls* (derived from extrinsic factors, such as environmental considerations). These occur when a person trips or slips (e.g., over a low-lying object or furnishing, on a wet floor).

- *Anticipated physiologic falls* (derived from intrinsic physiologic factors, such as confusion). These occur in patients or residents who have already been flagged as being at risk of falling. They are expected to fall again because the fall risk assessment has identified their high risk (e.g., caused by impaired gait or balance).

- *Unanticipated physiologic falls* (derived from unexpected intrinsic events, such as a new-onset syncopal event or a major intrinsic event such as stroke). These occur when a patient or resident falls for a physiological reason that has not been identified by the fall risk assessment. Examples of causes of these falls are fainting, seizures, or a pathological hip fracture.

Morse claims that by using this classification, approximately 78% of the falls related to anticipated physiologic events can be identified early, and therefore safety measures can be applied to prevent the fall.

Guide to Postfall Assessment

When a fall occurs, often the only immediate response is to rule out any injury or life-threatening conditions that might have resulted from the fall.

However, many people with falls have multiple underlying risk factors (e.g., postural hypotension, drug side effects, dehydration, cardiac problems). If the staff concentrates only on the consequences of falling, the causative factors responsible for falling or risk factors for further falls will go undetected. In order to reduce the risk of future falls, a proactive postfall assessment that investigates not only the possibility of injury but also the cause of the fall must be completed. The purpose of a postfall assessment is to prevent subsequent falls and to discover what caused the last fall (Tideiksaar, 2006). Effective postfall assessments consist of the following components:

- Rule out injury and life-threatening medical problems.

- Determine the circumstances of the fall (symptoms, location, and activity) to detect important clues and possible patterns of falling. Inquire about the following: Does the person know what caused the fall? Was the person feeling dizzy or weak? Did the person trip or slip? Did his or her legs give out, or did the person feel dizzy? Did the fall occur in bedroom or bathroom? What was the person doing at the time: Getting out of bed? Going to the bathroom? Ask about fear of falling. Fear of falling again is common and can lead to reduced mobility, loss of muscle strength or balance, and increased risk of subsequent falls. Interview staff and family members who may have witnessed the event; people around a fall can usually see a fall just before it happens and provide valuable details.

- Assess for and modify any environmental factors or hazards that may have contributed to the fall (e.g., slippery or wet floors, unstable furnishings, room clutter).

- Reassess fall risk, including a review of the person's medications, functional status, ambulation device use, and cognitive status.

- Implement immediate interventions to prevent further falls (e.g., if the person fell out of bed, a fall alarm might be appropriate for the short term).

- Analyze the fall, including root cause analysis to discover why the fall occurred. It is important to review the status of any medical conditions and medications that predispose to falls and any process issues that may have contributed to fall. In those with recurrent falls (two or more falls in a 30-day period), the use of a multidisciplinary fall evaluation team can be beneficial, providing more eyes and minds to look at possible causes and to think of possible solutions.

- Revisit the plan of care, based on items identified after the fall, implementing needed changes in the care plan, including communicating the patient's or resident's risk status to other staff members and other shifts.

Remember that falls are often the first sign of underlying acute and chronic medical problems that warrant attention. A comprehensive postfall assessment can be extremely helpful in identifying treatable causes of falls and reducing the risk of subsequent falls. A 10-step approach or guide to postfall assessment is shown in Table 7-7.

Table 7-7. Postfall assessment

Steps	Process
1. Rule out injury.	Evaluate person immediately to assess for injuries and provide treatment as appropriate. Perform neuro checks (if head trauma, reduced consciousness, or unwitnessed fall occurred).
2. Determine the causes and circumstances of the fall.	Obtain a fall history: • Symptoms before and at time of fall. • Previous falls. • Location at the time of fall. • Activity at the time of fall. • Time of fall. At the time of fall, was the person alone or being assisted? At the time of fall, was the person on fall precautions?
3. Determine fall risk factors.	Conduct a fall risk factor assessment and compare with most recent assessment (i.e., determine presence of new risk factors).
4. Determine presence of any environmental hazards.	Conduct a quick environmental assessment (e.g., flooring, lighting, equipment, call bells, ambulation aids, bed, chair, footwear) to discover any environmental conditions that may have contributed to the fall.
5. Determine causes of the fall.	Based on the information gathered in steps 1–4, conduct a quick root cause analysis (i.e., determine reasons for the fall). (See Guide to Root Cause Analysis on page 119.) Consider all intrinsic and extrinsic factors identified. If the patient or resident was previously at-risk, determine whether fall prevention strategies were appropriate and implemented.
6. Refer patient or resident for further evaluations.	Refer to interdisciplinary team members (e.g., medical staff, physical or occupational therapists) for further assessments and interventions.
7. Initiate short-term interventions, as appropriate.	While waiting for feedback from interdisciplinary referrals, consider possible nursing strategies that can be implemented to address the extrinsic and intrinsic factors that contributed to the fall (e.g., providing anticipatory care, increased observation or use of a sitter, safety equipment, such as a fall alarm, low bed, hip protector, or bedside commode).
8. Communicate risk status.	It is crucial that all staff involved in care (e.g., nurses, nursing assistants, occupational and physical therapists, physicians, other relevant staff members and family members, as appropriate) are aware that the person has fallen and is at risk of falling again. Communication of risk can be achieved by means of • Visible identification of at-risk people (e.g., colorful identification wristband or sticker affixed by the patient's or resident's room, above the bed, and to his or her ambulation device). • Use of daily shift reports that indicate the person's risk factors, ambulatory status, and care plans.
9. Determine and implement a new or revised fall prevention plan.	Soon after the fall, the interdisciplinary team should meet and review the care plan, and implement appropriate fall and injury prevention strategies as needed. Because falls often have multiple causes, the entire interdisciplinary team (e.g., physicians, nurses, therapists) must be involved in the process.
10. Initiate observations and monitoring.	Observing the patient or resident for several days after a fall is helpful in detecting • Any change in the person's condition that might precipitate another fall. • Any change in the person's gait and balance or transfer abilities that may indicate a new health problem or a potential problem with the environment.

Guide to Root Cause Analysis

Despite the best efforts by acute hospitals and nursing homes to prevent falls, many facilities continue to experience high fall rates. Root cause analysis (RCA) is a method that can be used to help identify the cause of falls. By evaluating a particular person's fall risk factors and circumstances surrounding their falls (e.g., symptoms, location, activity, environmental hazards), staff can identify the most likely causes of the falls. Simply put, RCA repeatedly digs deeper by asking, "Why did this person fall?" until no additional logical answers can be identified.

Once causes are identified, interventions to prevent future falls can be designed. Usually, a lack of success in reducing falls is blamed on intervention failures (i.e., either the intervention is not appropriate for a particular person or the intervention is of insufficient intensity or duration). However, in addition to well-designed interventions, fall risk reduction also depends on an organized system and process of care. System components include staff, equipment, and environmental factors, and process components include risk assessments, evaluations, care planning, and follow-up.

Similar to investigating the cause of individual falls, RCA can also be used to help identify system or process failures that may be the cause of falls and point out targets for change. In this instance RCA asks, "Did steps in the process—e.g., assessment and problem identification; evaluation, diagnosis, and cause identification; care planning; interventions and risk management; and monitoring and follow-up—occur, and did the steps occur in a timely and multidisciplinary fashion?" In essence, RCA tries to establish why falls happen by identifying failures occurring before, during, and after the fall; staff involvement (including actions taken); environmental factors; and other relevant information. Some of the most common root causes of falls related to system and process are shown in Table 7-8.

Typically, finding a root cause related to the system or process—resulting in a discontinuity of risk management care—should lead to corrective actions of the system or process failures identified. Any change contemplated should be generalizable to the entire facility. Furthermore, all facility staff members need to be informed about any change or changes in policy or procedure. Finally, follow-up is essential to ensure that corrective actions have been implemented and are preventing recurrence. Table 7-9 presents a step-by-step approach to conducting RCA.

Table 7-8.   Root causes of falls related to system and process

System	Process
Incomplete orientation and training of staff with respect to fall risk reduction policies and procedures	Inadequate assessment or reassessment of patients or residents
Inadequate staffing levels to care for and supervise high-risk patients or residents	Failure to document risk or changes in the patient's or resident's condition
Unavailability or delayed multidisciplinary referrals or care for at-risk patients or residents	Failure to communicate risk status across settings or between shifts
Malfunction or misuse of safety equipment (e.g., bed exit monitors, side rails, wheelchairs)	Inadequate attention to multidisciplinary evaluations and care plannings

Table 7-9. Conducting root cause analysis

Step 1: Fall assessment	Collect details of the fall, including the following: • Circumstances of the fall (SPLATT): **S**ymptoms before and after fall. **P**revious falls (patterns). **L**ocation of fall. **A**ctivity at time of fall. **T**ime of fall. **T**rauma associated with fall. • Fall risk factors (new or additional). • Presence of environmental hazards.
Step 2: Root cause analysis (patient or resident)	Based on assessment information, determine the following: • What happened? • Why did it happen? Ask "why?" questions until all logical causes can be identified. Possible contributing causes of falls include the following: • Patient-related or internal factors. • Patient-related mobility or activity being undertaken at time of fall. • Environmental factors or equipment.
Step 3: Root cause analysis (staff and organization)	Corresponding processes and systems or organizational factors are identified that can be related to falling. In this step, the focus is on the clinical process and organization, not the patient or resident. Ask "why?" questions until all logical causes can be identified. **Clinical Process Factors** • Risk assessments are incomplete or inaccurate. • Risk is not communicated. • Falls are underreported. • There is no care plan or follow-up. **Organizational Factors** • Lack of policies and procedures. • Communication problems. • Staff related (lack of education or lack of staff). • Lack of resources (equipment or restraint alternatives).
Step 4: Chart audits	To determine clinical process factors, conducting chart audits can be helpful. **Purpose** • Helps to separate what you think is happening from what is really happening. **Objectives** • Evaluate staff compliance with fall prevention program. • Recommend further actions for improvement.
Step 4: Organizing and planning	• Once all possible "why" questions are answered, then the possible root causes, processes, and systems are evaluated to determine whether they contributed to the fall. • Factors that contributed to the falls are analyzed to determine how they can be improved. After this is complete, a plan for improvement is implemented and evaluated to verify that any changes put in place have produced the desired outcomes.
Step 5: Achieving success	• Involve all stakeholders (e.g., staff nurses, management staff, pharmacists, physicians, and other people directly related to the occurrence). • Create a blame-free culture in which staff are not afraid to discuss safety issues and leaders will support and implement any necessary changes. • Devote adequate time to conduct a root cause analysis.

Incident Reports

Incident reporting, a process intended to document falls, is an important component of any risk management program aimed at fall reduction. Added benefits of incident reporting include an awareness of falls and a learning culture among nursing staff that ensure that action is taken to minimize future falls. Incident reporting also documents departures from normal or usual care that might result in an injurious fall for which the facility and staff might be liable.

Unfortunately, many falls occurring in hospitals and nursing homes go unreported. A number of factors influence whether falls or incidents are reported. Nurses are more inclined to report incidents that will almost certainly be detected, such as injurious falls, rather than get caught not reporting the incident. Underreporting of falls can be attributed to confusion about which falls to report (e.g., a noninjurious fall may not be reported because it is believed that the incident is insignificant). Another factor preventing staff from reporting fall incidents is the belief that managers and other administrative staff do not act on incident reports, and the report is only an exercise in additional paperwork. Finally, staff may be hesitant to report a fall because they fear disciplinary action from supervisors (e.g., finger-pointing, blaming individual nurses for falls).

Because falls are an early warning sign for future events that could result in more serious injuries, the failure to report all falls is dangerous. The actual needs and fall risk factors of the patient or resident are masked, and the interventions necessary to reduce fall risk are not developed or implemented. Therefore, nurses and other health care providers should be encouraged to report all fall incidents. The best way to ensure that falls are reported is to have a written policy for incident reporting. A policy for incident reporting should clearly describe the following:

- What events constitute a reportable fall (e.g., an unanticipated event, usually of sudden onset, in which the patient or resident engages in an activity that results in balance loss and a subsequent fall, with or without injury).

- What actions to take in the event of injury or acute illness.

- Fall precaution measures to follow in order to prevent immediate recurrence (e.g., fall alarms, sitters, frequent nursing rounds and observation).

- A step-by-step procedure to follow for completing the incident report.

- A step-by-step process to follow after the incident report is completed (e.g., documenting the incident in the patient's chart, forwarding a copy of the incident report for administrative review to the medical and nursing director, quality assurance staff, or safety committee).

- A process to inform all staff involved in the patient's or resident's care that a fall has occurred, necessitating a review of the care plan.

- A process to inform all staff involved in patient or resident care of the current policy (e.g., during orientation, during in-service educational activities).

- A time period in which policy statements are updated to reflect institutional attempts to practice reasonable standards of care related to fall prevention.

Postfall Management

Compared with people who fall without injury, people who have cognitive impairment, those who have mobility impairment necessitating staff assistance, and those who use psychotropic medications are more likely to suffer recurrent falls and injury after a fall. These risk factors or predictors of injurious falls may be amenable to prevention and should be considered in the development of postfall care plans.

Targeted interventions that may reduce the risk of injurious falls include the following:

• RCA of the fall, evaluating both patient or resident and system issues. RCA provides a greater understanding of fall causation and helps in identifying specific interventions aimed at preventing falls and injury.

• Medication review and modification, as appropriate.

• Staff assistance with transfers and ambulation.

• Supervised or assisted toileting schedules (i.e., many falls occur when patients or residents ambulate unassisted during elimination-related activities).

• Keep ambulation devices (e.g., canes, walkers) to support mobility at the bedside, as appropriate.

• Physical therapy sessions to teach transfer and ambulation skills and modify the patient's or resident's environment to support safe mobility.

• Hip protector, low bed, or floor mat aimed at preventing hip fractures and other injuries.

• Fall alarms to help staff detect unsafe bed and chair egress. Also, alarms can be used to monitor activity (i.e., identify times when patients or residents are attempting to leave the bed or chair), which can help identify needs and interventions.

• Communication of the patient's or resident's injurious fall risk status and postfall interventions to all relevant caregivers.

Preventing Injurious Falls

Although the majority of older adults who fall suffer no physical injury, about 10%–15% experience injurious falls. Bone fractures make up the largest group of injuries, with bruises and contusions second, and head and spinal cord injuries third. Injurious falls can lead to permanent impairment in functioning, resulting in loss of independence, and can also precipitate a cascade of events leading to death. Understanding the factors that contribute to injurious falls is essential to designing effective intervention strategies. The risk factors for injurious falls are similar to those of noninjurious falls (e.g., one or more prior falls, cognitive deficits, polypharmacy, mobility impairment); however, a number of factors place people at greater risk for injurious falls:

- The greater the number of falls or injurious falls experienced, the greater the risk of injury. A history of fall injury is a powerful risk factor for serious fall injury.

- Osteoporosis or decreased bone mineral density, especially among people who also have the ability to move about independently (i.e., mobility and osteoporosis work together to dramatically increase risk of injury), doubles the risk of an injurious fall.

- Neuromuscular disorders (e.g., Parkinson's disease, stroke, arthritis, diabetic peripheral neuropathy) are associated with decreased proprioception and quadriceps strength, which can result in gait, balance, and functional impairment.

- Dementia includes a loss of protective reflexes and an inability to stop a fall in progress, or loss of the "catching yourself" capacity. It also impairs decision-making processes for distinguishing hazardous from safe actions.

- Visual impairment is associated with increased risk of slips, trips, and injury. Low contrast acuity and contrast sensitivity, narrower visual fields, greater need for light, and difficulty adjusting between light and darkened environments lead older adults to miss visual cues for floor level changes and other environmental hazards.

- Psychotropic medications (e.g., sedatives, anxiolytics, antipsychotics, and antidepressants) are associated with cognitive and balance impairments.

- Slippery footwear (e.g., socks, slippers with vinyl soles) and linoleum or tile floors create the potential for slips.

- Use of physical restraints and full-length bedside rails increases the risk of injurious falls.

- Assisted ambulation, with an ambulation device or with caregiver assistance, increases the risk of injurious falls.

- Immobility directly contributes to falls and injuries by reducing muscle mass, strength, joint flexibility and vasomotor stability.

Interventions

The risk of injurious falls can be decreased by tailoring treatment to individual risk factors. In general, multifaceted and overlapping strategies that target both intrinsic and extrinsic risk factors are the most effective (Table 7-10). These include the following:

- Manage neuromuscular and other conditions associated with injurious falls.

- Treat osteoporosis with medications to increase bone mineral density.

- Reduce medications whenever possible. Overmedication, especially with psychoactive medications, should be avoided.

- Implement exercise programs, particularly those with a balance and strength training component.

- Provide safe footwear. Footwear should have nonskid, thin soles (which allow the wearer to detect shifts in balance) and have no more than a 1-inch heel. Nonskid socks provide good traction on slick linoleum and tile floors.

- Use hip protectors, which absorb the impact of falls against hard floor surfaces, protecting the hip and decreasing the risk of hip fractures.

- Maintain a low bed height or place a mat on the floor alongside the bed to reduce the risk of an injurious fall. Physical restraints and side rails do not reduce the risk of injurious falls and should be avoided whenever possible.

- Teach safe bed transfers.

- Reduce environmental hazards, such as slippery floors, and pay attention to lighting, especially nighttime lighting.

- Equip bathrooms and toilets with grab bars. Teach patients or residents safe toilet transfers.

It is unreasonable to think that all injurious falls can be avoided, but early risk assessment and targeted interventions can prevent many injurious falls.

Table 7-10.   10 strategies to improve the effectiveness of fall prevention practices

To improve staff compliance with fall prevention practices in your facility, consider the following strategies:

1. Keep fall prevention an active and visible topic; make fall prevention a routine part of care plan conferences and nurse or nurse assistant shift reports.
2. Use visual cues such as color-coded signs on bedroom doors and color-coded wrist bands to indicate which people are at risk.
3. Keep fall prevention supplies (e.g., hip protectors, fall alarms, gait belts, floor mats) in an area that is easily accessible to staff; make sure that fall prevention supplies are adequate.
4. Conduct admission staff huddles* to discuss a patient's or resident's fall risk and targeted interventions.
5. Conduct blame-free postfall huddles* to discuss the root cause analysis of the fall and interventions to guard against future falls.
6. Be proactive with rounds. Make routine toileting rounds, and return randomly for those who decline assistance.
7. Assess environment for broken equipment and furnishings (e.g., toilets, grab bars, showers, stretchers, beds, chairs) and other hazards; develop plans for modifying hazardous conditions and replacing broken equipment and furnishings.
8. Ensure that multidisciplinary team members receive updates on fall risk status and interventions.
9. Incorporate ancillary services, such as housekeeping and maintenance, in fall prevention discussions.
10. Involve the patient's or resident's family; educate visiting family members about specific risk factors and what they can do to assist staff with fall prevention efforts.

*The term *huddles* refers to an interdisciplinary approach in which various members of the care team discuss identified fall risk factors, causes, or precipitating factors and potential interventions.

REFERENCES

Coker, E., & Oliver, D. (2003, January–March). Evaluation of the STRATIFY falls prediction tool on a geriatric unit. *Outcomes Management, 7*(1), 8–14; quiz, 15–16.

Hendrich, A.L., Bender, P.S., & Nyhuis, A. (2003, February) Validation of the Hendrich II fall risk model: A large concurrent case/control study of hospitalized patients. *Applied Nursing Research, 16*(1), 9–21.

Morse, J. (2002). Enhancing the safety of hospitalization by reducing patient falls. *American Journal of Infection Control, 30*(6), 376–380.

Morse, J.M., & Morse, R.M. (1988, December). Calculating fall rates: Methodological concerns. *QRB Quality Review Bulletin, 14*(12), 369–371.

O'Connell, B., & Myers, H. (2002, January). The sensitivity and specificity of the Morse Fall Scale in an acute care setting. *Journal of Clinical Nursing, 11*(1), 134–136.

Oliver, D., Daly, F., Martin, F.C., & McMurdo, M.E. (2004, March). Risk factors and risk assessment tools for falls in hospital in-patients: A systematic review. *Age and Ageing, 33*(2), 122–130.

Perell, K.L., Nelson, A., Goldman, R.L., Luther, S.L., Prieto-Lewis N., & Rubenstein, L.Z. (2001, December). Fall risk assessment measures: An analytic review. *Journal of Gerontology, 56*(12), M761–M766.

Scott, V., Votova, K., Scanlan, A., & Close, J. (2007). Multifactorial and functional mobility assessment tools for fall risk among older adults in community, home-support, long-term and acute care settings. *Age and Ageing, 36*(2), 130–139.

Tideiksaar, R. (2006). *After the fall* [CD-ROM]. Baltimore: Health Professions Press.

Vassallo, M., Stockdale, R., Sharma, J.C., Briggs, R., & Allen, S. (2005, June). A comparative study of the use of four fall risk assessment tools on acute medical wards. *Journal of the American Geriatrics Society, 53*(6), 1034–1038.

Chapter Eight

Organizational Requirements

Chapter 7 covered the *process* component of fall prevention in the "process + structure = outcome" pathway. This chapter discusses the *structure* component through the following wide range of organizational and administrative topics:

Structure Topics

Organizational Fall Risk Factors

Fall Prevention Guidelines

Achieving a Culture of Safety

 —Leadership and Commitment

 —No Blame, No Shame

 —Effective Communication

 —Staff Empowerment

 —Fall Data and Trends

Unit-Based Fall Champions

Unit-Based Fall Prevention

Fall Rates and Clinical Benchmarking

Quality Indicators for Fall Prevention

Interdisciplinary Fall Team

Reducing Post-Hospital Falls

Nursing Factors Affecting Fall Prevention Programs

 —Educational Strategies

 —Targeting Strategies

 —Environmental Strategies

 —Support Strategies

Patient and Resident Education: Educational and Behavioral Approaches

 —Education During the Stay

 —Discharge Teaching

Family Role in Safety

What Is Restraint?

ORGANIZATIONAL FALL RISK FACTORS

A root cause analysis of falls is used to determine the most fundamental reason a fall occurred. The organizational factors included in such an analysis for hospitals and nursing homes are as follows.

Clinical Process Deficits

- Risk assessments and reassessments are incomplete or inaccurate

- Risk status is not communicated between staff, patients or residents, and family members

- Falls are underreported by staff

- Staff do not document changes in conditions

- Plans of care or follow-up are incomplete

- Staff underestimate or overestimate fall risk.

Administrative Deficits

- Lack of fall preventive policies, procedures, and guidelines

- Lack of staff education

- Incomplete orientation of new staff

- Inadequate staffing

- Lack of resources (safety equipment and restraint alternatives).

In order to implement an effective fall prevention program, hospitals and nursing homes need to assess organizational factors contributing to falls.

Guide to Assessing Organizational Risk Factors

1. Gather data and review potential areas of risk.

   - Previous institutional survey reports

   - Quality assurance or quality indicator reports

   - Occurrence and incident reports

   - Staff feedback

   - Patient or resident and family feedback

   - Litigation claims.

2. Review facility practices.

   - Review the charts of patients or residents at fall risk or with falls (e.g., for complete assessments, adequate care plans, and targeted and updated interventions).

- Review facility procedures, protocols, and guidelines related to fall prevention and restraint reduction activities; determine whether they are up to date and reflect everyday practice.

- Review staff education and orientation training activities related to fall prevention; determine whether they are consistent with procedures, protocols, and guidelines.

3. Identify risk exposure (root cause analysis).

- Based on Steps 1 and 2, determine presence of clinical and administrative deficits or shortcomings.

4. Assign a level of risk exposure and prioritize all problems identified that require corrective action.

Regardless of how a hospital or nursing home ultimately chooses to approach the creation of a risk reduction program, the time and effort invested to assess risk exposure and develop a facility action plan are beneficial in reducing falls. Once organizational factors or deficits have been identified, the following key ingredients can reduce risk exposure:

A Safety Culture

- A culture of safety permits staff to acknowledge the occurrence of error and encourages open and complete reporting of falls.

- The emphasis is on prevention, not punishment.

Operational Approaches

- Fall-related protocols, procedures, and guidelines must be current and include a step-by-step approach to help staff with fall prevention activities.

Education

- Educate all staff members about reasons for falls and interventions available to prevent falls. Follow-up education on specific problems identified from root cause analysis (both individual and aggregate falls) is also important.

- Educate all staff members on protocols, procedures, and guidelines related to fall prevention activities; ensure that staff are familiar with them. Protocols, procedures, and guidelines help reinforce what should be done and when it should be done.

- Educate patients or residents and family members on fall risk and what steps the facility is taking to prevent falls.

Audits

- Conduct regular audits or checks to monitor and discover clinical process and administrative deficits.

- Any deficiencies observed can help to identify emerging trends and patterns that may contribute to falls.

FALL PREVENTION GUIDELINES

As a rule, hospitals and nursing homes must demonstrate that falls did not occur because of staff error or that a fall occurred because of some unavoidable or unpredictable problem. In other words, despite reasonable attempts to anticipate or prevent falls, the fall occurred anyway. The best way to avoid staff error is to have guidelines for preventing falls. Guidelines are a simple tool that identifies the strategies and practices that produce the best outcomes for a particular patient or resident population and facility. Simply put, guidelines describe what works. Guidelines help to reduce system variables and variability that affect outcomes by systemic cueing and monitoring of the process. In essence, guidelines include whatever steps are necessary to maximize the chance that the right thing is done at the right time. Although guidelines may be similar from one facility to another, what works for one hospital or nursing home will not necessarily work for another. To be successful, the development and implementation of a guideline must involve the clinicians and others who will be carrying it out.

Guidelines should include the following:

- Purpose of guideline

- Procedure or steps for staff to follow in implementing guideline.

The following outlines the essential components of a fall risk guideline.

Purpose

- To identify people at fall risk

- To prevent or reduce falls or injurious falls.

Procedure

1. Obtain a fall risk assessment for all patients or residents (Table 8-1).

    - Assess patients or residents at admission, with a change in condition, when a new medication is started, and after a fall. Reassess fall risk during each shift and as needed.

    - The presence of one or more risk factors places the patient or resident at fall risk.

2. Document which patients or residents are at fall risk.

    - Place a yellow armband ID on the patient's or resident's wrist.

    - Place a fall precaution decal on the bedroom door frame.

    - Chart the patient's or resident's risk status in medical and nursing records.

3. Implement an individualized plan of care to reduce risk factors (Table 8-2).

4. Document the plan of care in medical and nursing records.

Table 8-1. Fall risk assessment

Components	Fall Risk Factors
Diseases and conditions	☐ History of falls (past 30 days)
	☐ Sensory impairment (vision or hearing)
	☐ Urinary problems (special toileting needs)
	☐ Muscle weakness
	☐ Gait or balance impairment
	☐ Dizziness
	☐ Mobility impairment (e.g., poor bed, chair, and toilet transfers)
	☐ Orthostatic hypotension
Medications	☐ Polypharmacy (more than 5 medications)
	☐ Psychotropic medications
	☐ Medication side effects
Mental status	☐ Dementia
	☐ Depression
	☐ Delirium
	☐ Impaired safety judgment
	☐ Disruptive behaviors
	☐ Non-English speaking
Situational conditions	☐ New admission
	☐ Floor-to-floor (or unit-to-unit) transfer
	☐ Postfall
	☐ Change of condition or new medication

Table 8-2. Interventions to reduce fall risk

Fall Risk Factors	Available Interventions
New admission or relocation	• Orientation to unit and staff • Safety education
History of falls	• Obtain circumstances surrounding falls • Refer to physician for evaluation
Visual impairment	• Adequate lighting, night-lights • Avoid clutter; remove low-lying furniture
Lower extremity dysfunction/ Mobility impairment (bed, toilet, and chair transfers)	• Teach safe bed and chair transfers • Keep bed in low position • Toilet durable medical equipment • Staff supervision • Fall alarm
Gait or balance disorder/ Uses cane or walker	• Strength and flexibility exercises • Ambulation device evaluation • Nonslip footwear • Monitor environment for safety (floors dry and free of clutter and obstacles; assistive devices accessible) • Staff supervision
Elimination disorder	• Regular voiding schedule • Consider bedside commode • Toilet durable medical equipment
Polypharmacy (5 drugs or more)/ Psychotropics	• Eliminate or reduce dosages (if feasible) • Monitor for drug side effects

5. Educate the patient or resident and family members about fall risk and fall preventive measures.

6. Develop a follow-up care plan to ensure that all fall precautions and interventions are in place.

Finally, make sure that guidelines are complete (i.e., that they contain all information needed by staff to reduce falls) and that everyday staff practices match your guidelines. Staff who understand and follow guidelines are likely to be successful in preventing falls. Adherence to effective guidelines prevents many falls; on the other hand, failure to follow existing guidelines is a major cause of falls. Consequently, it is important to maintain updated guidelines and to make sure that all staff are familiar with them.

ACHIEVING A CULTURE OF SAFETY

Developing a culture of safety is one of the most important steps that acute hospitals and nursing homes can take to ensure that their fall prevention efforts are effective. Adopting such a culture shapes the way staff members think, behave, and approach fall prevention. The following outlines the crucial components needed to achieve a culture of safety.

Leadership and Commitment

Strong leadership and organizational commitment from top management (e.g., administrators, department directors) are essential in establishing a culture of safety. The primary role of leaders is to make fall safety a top priority. This includes setting goals for the facility, allocating resources, and having clearly defined policies to support fall prevention activities.

No Blame, No Shame

Staff should not be blamed or shamed when a patient or resident falls. Rather, having a no blame, no shame environment provides an open atmosphere in which staff members can report falls, errors, and safety concerns without fear of punishment. An important element of a blame-free environment is to reward rather than discourage reporting of falls and errors and to create a system in which nurses and other staff members do not fear retribution for raising concerns or reporting errors.

Punishing staff for making mistakes stems from the misconception that people are entirely to blame for mistakes, without looking beyond the problem to underlying process malfunctions. Facility managers and staff need to understand that most errors occur as result of ineffective, flawed systems. Few errors are due to carelessness or misconduct of a single person.

Effective Communication

Effective, open communication is crucial to achieving a culture of safety. An open style of communication means that facilities support discussion about patient or resident safety, and direct care staff are encouraged to report full details of unsafe conditions without fear of punishment. Errors are recognized and valued as opportunities for improvement.

Staff Empowerment

Engage front line staff. No one knows the pitfalls better than they do. Make staff feel that they own the program and that their input will drive changes to correct safety problems. Emphasize that safety initiatives will focus on fixing systems, not people.

Fall Data and Trends

Provide all staff with fall data and trends. Monthly reports of falls should be openly shared by the administration, and staff feedback should be used to make program improvements.

UNIT-BASED FALL CHAMPIONS

The need for an ongoing education and training program in support of fall prevention programs is clear. Despite training, many hospitals and nursing homes still struggle with high fall rates. One of the major barriers to achieving a successful fall prevention program is staff noncompliance with fall risk and postfall assessments and interventions aimed at reducing falls. The identification of a unit-based fall champion or coordinator (i.e., a staff nurse who receives additional education and mentoring on fall prevention strategies) who can support and follow through with fall prevention initiatives can help ensure success of fall prevention programs. In essence, the fall champion pulls together a unit's fall prevention program, takes responsibility for making things happen, and sees what needs to be changed and improved. A fall champion's tasks may include the following:

- Raise awareness about the importance of preventing falls.

- Provide ongoing education of staff and training of new staff.

- Oversee staff compliance with fall prevention procedures.

- Ensure that communication of fall risk occurs between staff and between shifts.

- Provide guidance in individualizing and targeting care plans.

- Collect unit-based fall data and evaluate outcomes.

- Review fall cases and postfall outcomes.

- Provide supportive feedback to staff regarding falls and prevention activities.

- Maintain equipment (e.g., fall alarms, hip protectors, ambulation aids, fall mats) and serve as the main connection with equipment vendors.

- Maintain and update fall prevention guidelines, policies, and protocols.

- Eliminate roadblocks and communication problems between staff members.

- Notify administration of resource needs (e.g., staff, equipment).

Appointing a fall champion to provide constant oversight is often an important component of an effective fall prevention program.

UNIT-BASED FALL PREVENTION

Although many institutions have facility-wide fall prevention programs, unit-based programs that are targeted to specific populations are the most effective. Successful unit-based fall prevention programs are developed as follows:

1. Determine your unit's fall incidence or baseline fall rate.

   - Fall rate is the most reliable and best measure of fall incidence and is a good indicator or internal benchmark as to whether your fall prevention program is achieving success.

   - Fall rate is calculated by the following formula: Number of falls × 1,000/Total number of patient or resident days.

2. Decide what risk assessment, postfall tools, and other tools and interdisciplinary interventions you will use.

   - No matter what risk assessment and other tools are selected, they should be specific and sensitive to the population being assessed. For instance, cognitive impairment, altered elimination, loss of balance, decreased mobility (transfers), and psychotropic medications are the major fall risk factors; however, some units may have unique risk factors that must be included.

   - Interventions must be targeted and specific for the population cared for (e.g., interventions appropriate on an orthopedic floor may not work on a cardiac unit).

   - Staff members should participate in planning the unit-wide interventions and implementing their use.

3. Educate staff members. The purpose of education is to increase fall risk awareness across all disciplines. It is important that staff members know what tools are involved in the unit's fall prevention program and where they are kept. Most importantly, make sure that staff understand how to use the tools. Guidelines that address how to use tools can be very helpful.

4. Involve staff members of each unit. It's important to involve staff members early in planning. Listen carefully to their ideas and suggestions and incorporate as many as possible into the fall prevention program.

5. Pay consistent attention to environmental hazards.

- Conduct a walk-through of your particular unit, including each room, targeting environmental factors that must be changed to make it a safer place. Do hallways need rails on the walls to help the unsteady patient or resident walk? Are the paths from beds to bathrooms obstructed? Should some of the furniture be removed? Is the lighting adequate?

- Efforts to reduce environmental hazards are most helpful in patients or residents with altered mobility (e.g., gait, balance, and transfer impairment).

6. Evaluate outcomes.

- Evaluate your program after the first month and every quarter thereafter. Compare fall and injury rates with your baseline data. If they have not decreased, find out why. Reexamine the tools you are using. Do they require modification to your unit? Are there unique characteristics to the falls documented on your unit? Staff consultation and documentation are extremely important at this stage.

- If your fall rate has increased, do not panic. Often, the rate of falls will increase because staff grow more aware of falls and therefore tend to document them better.

- Reevaluate your intervention strategies. Are there additional modifications that would improve safety? Do not be afraid to make ongoing changes.

- Ongoing evaluation should also include accuracy of assessments, initiation of interventions, and care guidelines.

FALL RATES AND CLINICAL BENCHMARKING

Many organizations rely on clinical benchmarks to monitor the process and outcomes of care. With respect to fall prevention, comparing fall rates (the rate at which patients or residents fall during their stay), by means of external (with different facilities) or internal (within a facility) benchmarking, allows an organization to evaluate the effectiveness of its fall prevention program.

Although comparing fall rates between various organizations, facilities, or institutions may be helpful, it also raises some important concerns. Certain methodological problems make external benchmarking or comparison of fall rates difficult:

- Definitions of what constitutes a fall differ. Organizations use different definitions; some include near falls and "found down" in their definition, whereas others do not.

- Staff may not report or document all falls that occur, so calculated fall rates may not be accurate.

- Some organizations collect only data on first falls, not subsequent falls. This can result in inappropriately low fall rates.

- Methods for calculating fall rates differ. Fall rate can be measured in different ways (falls per bed, per patient or resident, per patient or resident day, per patient or resident year), and these methods are not equivalent. Organizations also express fall rates in numerous ways, which leads to confusion. The recommended method for calculating fall rate is the rate per 1,000 patient or resident days (Total number of falls × 1,000/Total number of patient or resident days). This measure is best for computing rates in facilities with varying case mix, lengths of stay, and occupancy. Consistent application of the numerator (total falls are included, not just all patients or residents who have fallen) is important as well.

- Differences in populations. Some organizations include all inpatient units, whereas others confine their data collection to specific services, such as units where patients or residents are considered at higher risk of falling than the total hospital population (e.g., geriatrics, psychiatry, rehabilitation). This can lead to inappropriately high fall rates.

- Resistance to reporting. Not all organizations like to report their fall rates, often to hide problems; organizations do not like to report errors any more than individuals do.

The main reason for benchmarking is to gain a better understanding of processes (to identify what works and what does not). Benchmarking should provide a systematic way of evaluating services and practices between organizations and learning from each other's organizations (where everyone is encouraged to improve the way things are done). Given some of the methodological problems described, comparing fall rates externally is difficult.

The difficulties of external benchmarking are demonstrated by the wide range of fall rates reported in the literature. In acute hospitals, fall rates of 0.6 to 2.9 falls annually per bed, 0.3 to 19 falls per 1,000 bed days, and 3.1 falls per 1,000 patient or resident days are commonly cited. Data from the California Nursing Outcomes Coalition, a large ongoing nursing quality measurement research project that gathers data on patient falls from California's acute hospitals and develops benchmarks, shows a wide variation in fall rates (ranging from less than 1.0 to more than 13 per 1,000 patient days). The Maryland Hospital Association Quality Indicator Project, another large data-gathering project, reports rates of 3.8 falls per 1,000 patient days. Moreover, fall rates for certain hospital units are higher than in the general acute care population (e.g., neurology, 5.2 per 1,000 patient days; psychiatry, 4.1; rehabilitation, 7.6–12.6; geriatrics, 7.8). Likewise, in nursing homes, up to 75% of residents fall each year (the average fall incidence is 1.5 falls per bed per year), and more than 40% experience recurrent episodes. Reported fall rates in nursing homes range from an annual incidence of 650 to 1,200 falls per 1,000 beds and 1,650 to 3,000 falls per 1,000 residents per year.

These wide-ranging fall rates make it difficult to compare falls rates between hospitals and nursing homes and to establish meaningful national benchmarks. The most reliable and useful approach for an organization or facility to take is to examine its own data over time (internal benchmarking). Comparisons with external organizations may help institutions set target goals (i.e., clinical indicators and expectations) (Table 8-3).

Table 8-3. Organizations providing information on fall rates

- Maryland Hospital Association Quality Indicator Project: http://www.qiproject.org
- California Nursing Outcome Coalition: http://www.CalNoc.org
- American Society for Healthcare Risk Management: http://www.ashrm.org
- National Database of Nursing Quality Indicators: http://www.nursingquality.org/
- Long-Term Care Minimum Data Set: http://www.cms.hhs.gov

QUALITY INDICATORS FOR FALL PREVENTION

Routinely counting falls each month and measuring fall rates can be very helpful in assessing the overall care delivered to vulnerable patients or residents with respect to preventing falls, thus allowing staff to measure the extent to which they have met or failed to meet their objectives. But at the patient or resident level, relying on fall rates to pinpoint or identify clinical areas in need of improvement is insufficient because fall rates reveal no details about why falls are occurring.

In order to understand why fall rates are high, why programs have failed, or why changes have to be made, it is necessary to evaluate the day-to-day process of how fall prevention measures are implemented. There are a number of specific steps or quality indicators in the process or chain of care that can help to determine how well various services and components are provided and coordinated and whether fall prevention practices are effective. These include the following:

1. *A history of falls.* Documenting falls is a strong indicator of underlying, treatable risk factors.

2. *Assessment of fall risk.* Risk assessment should be completed at the time of admission for all patients or residents. At a minimum, risk assessments should include an inquiry about previous falls, cognitive status, and urinary function; an observation of mobility (e.g., gait, balance, and transfers); and an evaluation of assistive device use, if any. These factors are consistently associated with a high probability of falls.

3. *Reassessment of fall risk.* Risk assessment should be completed whenever patients or residents experience a change of condition, a change in medications, or a fall.

4. *Addressing risk factors.* All fall risk factors identified from the assessment should be included in the care plan with targeted multifactorial intervention strategies. In addition, evidence that the strategies listed in the care plan have been implemented should be recorded.

5. *Monitoring risk reduction strategies.* Follow-up of all risk reduction interventions listed in the care plan should be performed to determine their effectiveness. In addition, there should be evidence of redesigning any intervention found to be ineffective or an explanation as to why doing so is not indicated.

6. *Postfall assessment.* An assessment of all falls should be implemented. At a minimum, assessment should include an analysis of fall circumstances (i.e., why the fall occurred), a reassessment of fall risk factors, immediate strategies to avoid further falls, and a reevaluation of the care plan.

Process quality indicators set minimum standards for care that, if not met, almost ensure that the care related to preventing falls is inadequate. Continuous evaluation of the care process is beneficial in helping to determine whether staff are delivering appropriate and effective fall preventive care.

INTERDISCIPLINARY FALL TEAM

In many high–fall risk patients or residents, especially those with multiple falling episodes, an interdisciplinary or integrated team approach is often beneficial in achieving a comprehensive and effective fall prevention plan.

Aim of an Interdisciplinary Fall Team

- Develop a coordinated response to patients or residents with falls.

- Ensure that patients or residents with falls receive a comprehensive assessment and appropriate interventions to reduce risk of falls.

- Develop standards of fall prevention activities and practice within the facility.

Setting Up an Interdisciplinary Fall Team

- Because risk factors and causes of falling are often multifactorial, team members need to include representatives from administration, nursing, medicine, rehabilitation, pharmacy, activities, and social services. It is also important to include maintenance, custodial, or housekeeping personnel in the team process because a facility's layout and environmental factors such as lighting levels, floor conditions, and broken equipment (e.g., wheelchair brakes, bed wheel brakes) contribute to falls.

- Within the team, identify a fall coordinator and a team leader. The falls coordinator should be a person with knowledge and experience in falls, one who is able to provide the team with guidance and literature resources. The team leader should be a person who is well respected in the facility, such as the director of nursing or medical director, and one who can help move activities forward within the facility.

Interdisciplinary Fall Team Functions

- Review and analyze institutional falls (i.e., incidence of falls and injurious fall frequency, fall and injurious fall circumstances); this will help determine causes of falls and potential actions that can be taken to prevent falls.

- Review and revise (as needed) the current fall prevention or risk reduction process (i.e., identification of fall risk, available care plan interventions, evaluation of outcomes, and fall reporting mechanism or incident reports).

- Identify patients or residents who will be evaluated by the team (i.e., all newly admitted patients or residents and those experiencing one or more falls within a 30-day period). Patients or residents most likely to benefit from an interdisciplinary team approach are those with multiple falls and disabilities in two or more assessment domains (e.g., physical health, mental status, functional status, and environmental safety). Because implementation of an interdisciplinary team entails a large time commitment by the team members, sometimes away from other daily clinical and administrative responsibilities, the financial cost of having a fall team must be considered.

- Conduct interdisciplinary assessments of patients or residents, including a review of common causes of falls and risk factors leading to falls (e.g., diseases, medications, environment, mobility, assistive devices, and safety activities). After completing interdisciplinary team assessments, the team develops recommendations to reduce fall risk (i.e., a plan of care with specific, individualized interventions with the goal of preventing falls and injury) and communicates the care plan to the primary care team to implement. The team should involve floor nurses, physicians, and other professionals who have day-to-day care responsibilities whenever patients or residents on their unit or floor are discussed. Finally, the team should evaluate the effectiveness or outcome of their recommendations.

- Educate staff about falls. Organize a staff orientation program on fall prevention, to include precautions to take and methods for preventing falls, and review potential fall hazards in the facility. Educate staff on fall-related policy, procedures, and protocols. Also, the team should arrange in-service training on new safety technologies (e.g., low beds, fall alarms, hip protectors) and recognition and elimination of environmental hazards.

- Collect data on falls in the facility as part of a monitoring program. These data should be analyzed to look for patterns and trends. Also, monitoring falls will help determine the effectiveness of the interdisciplinary fall team (i.e., whether the rate of falls and injury in high-risk patients or residents has decreased since the implementation of the team).

REDUCING POST-HOSPITAL FALLS

Falls experienced shortly after discharge from hospitals is a major reason for unplanned rehospitalization. This is not so surprising. Acute hospitalization often leads to significant functional decline in older adults; up to 40% of people suffer a decline in function between admission and discharge. Almost half of hospitalized older adults need help with walking at discharge, compared with only one quarter of those needing assistance before hospitalization. Presumably, the effects of acute and chronic illness, treatments rendered, and activity (e.g., remaining in bed or at chair rest) contributes to the loss of function. As a consequence, the period immediately after hospitalization is associated with increased falls and rehospitalization. Major risk factors include declines in mobility, living alone or not having reliable caregiver support, use of assistive devices (i.e., canes and walkers are a marker of gait and balance impairment), and cognitive impairment. Other reasons for falls and risk of rehospitalization include the following:

- Short hospital stays, with acute disease process remaining active

- Recurrence of active or chronic illnesses

- Side effects from new medications or dosage increases of current medications

- Lack of durable medical equipment to support the patient's or resident's current functional needs (i.e., either the need for equipment was never recognized, or there is a time delay between discharge and arrival of the necessary equipment)

- Fear of falling or excessive confidence about one's mobility and capabilities

- Failure to order appropriate home care services

- Lack of recognition of fall risk by home care professionals.

Clearly, the transition between hospital discharge and the return home is an especially dangerous period for many frail older adults, one associated with an increased fall risk.

Both hospital and home care professionals can be instrumental in helping to reduce the frequency of post-hospital falls and risk of rehospitalization. Older adults at risk can be identified easily through a few simple screening questions and maneuvers incorporated into hospital discharge and home health admission care planning. Screening should elicit the following information:

- Recent falls, especially those associated with injury or significant downtime (i.e., inability to get up from the floor after a fall)

- Fear or concern about falling and any subsequent self-imposed mobility restrictions

- Current ambulation and transfer abilities and the use of assistive aids and durable medical equipment

- Current living situation (e.g., living alone or with a caregiver, such as a spouse, adult children, or formal care attendant)

- Caregiver status, as appropriate (i.e., are caregivers willing to provide care, available to provide care, and physically capable of providing care?)

- Polypharmacy, especially use of psychotropic medications

- Gait and balance, including all impairments.

Interventions aimed at reducing falls and risk of post-hospital readmission include the following:

- *Risk reduction.* Identify people at high risk of falling (e.g., impaired cognition, impaired gait and balance, diseases affecting mobility, medications affecting balance and orientation) and implement strategies aimed at reducing risk.

- *Caregiver education.* Educate caregivers about safety measures and fall prevention strategies; provide information on how to identify risk. Provide basic information on how to transfer older adults safely (use of gait or transfer belts as appropriate [see "Ambulation Device Utilization" in the Fall Prevention Guidelines section, page 207]) and on proper use of a cane or walker and durable medical equipment, as appropriate. If caregivers are unwilling or unable to provide care, consider the use of formal caregiver support.

- *Prevent downtime.* Provide older adults with a personal emergency response system (i.e., an electronic device designed to summon help in an emergency) or teach them how to get up from the floor by themselves after a fall (i.e., position themselves to a side-sitting position and then kneel with the support of a chair and push themselves up into the chair). Preventing downtime is especially important for older adults living alone without caregiver assistance.

- *Home safety.* Provide older adults and caregivers with information on how to identify and modify environmental hazards in the home.

NURSING FACTORS AFFECTING FALL PREVENTION PROGRAMS

Most fall prevention programs are based on identifying intrinsic and extrinsic risk factors and developing multidisciplinary risk reduction interventions. Despite the best efforts of hospitals and nursing homes, fall prevention remains a challenging issue. However, it is not helpful to approach fall prevention from a purely clinical perspective. Because nurses play a central role in managing fall prevention programs, the success of any program depends to a large degree on the effectiveness of the nursing staff. A number of nursing factors are associated with increased fall risk and falls:

- Chronic staff shortages
- Overload of nursing duties (attempting to do more with less staff)
- Constant changes in nursing staff
- Lack of time; staff spending more time on non-nursing activities (e.g., documentation and paperwork) and less time on care
- Poor performance or noncompliance with fall prevention activities because of low motivation or dissatisfaction with job
- Lack of awareness of fall prevention policy and procedures
- Long working hours (i.e., double shifts) or increased workloads, which can lead to fatigue and errors.

In contrast, organizations that support nursing staff are more likely to be successful with their fall prevention program. Important support activities include the following:

- *Resource support*, making sure that adequate numbers of nursing staff are available to care for patients or residents with complex needs.

Table 8-4. Consider method of delivery when developing training

An important aspect to consider when developing an education program is the delivery method (i.e., whether in person, by computer, or by some other means).

- In-person training allows staff to ask questions as the material is delivered, and a skillful trainer can identify confusion and explain or repeat information as needed. Ensure that the training is not delivered via a lecture format in which staff can easily tune out the trainer. A drawback is that the cost of in-person training is higher than other methods.

- Computer training can take many forms, from PowerPoint presentations to live sessions recorded for later replay. One of the big advantages to computer training is the consistency of its delivery, which ensures that the same message is given throughout the organization.

- *Culture of safety*, characterized by not blaming staff for falls but rather using falls as an opportunity to analyze possible staffing factors that may have contributed to falling and attempting to correct them.

- *Education*, including frequent in-service programs to increase staff awareness of the organization's fall prevention policies, procedures, and multidisciplinary interventions. Education is crucial for increasing compliance with fall prevention activities and improving the competence of staff (Table 8-4).

- *Guidelines*, including updated fall prevention policies and protocols that clearly state what is expected of staff (i.e., desired and undesired performance) to minimize the chances of staff errors.

- *Equipment*, including fall and injury prevention devices (e.g., fall alarms, low beds, floor mats, hip protectors). Using the right equipment can be extremely beneficial in the face of staff shortages.

Implementing a program of fall prevention means more than just knowing about falls and how to prevent them. It also includes focusing on nursing staff as a necessary and vital component of effective fall prevention. Toward this end, there are a number of key strategies to support nursing staff.

Educational Strategies

Success in reducing falls has a lot to do with nurses' attitudes and knowledge. The attitudes staff hold about patients or residents and whether they believe that fall prevention is even possible in frail older adults is an important factor in whether risk reduction strategies are implemented and completed in a timely manner. Also, nurses who care for vulnerable people must be knowledgeable about available strategies to prevent falls; interventions will not work if nurses do not know about them. As a result, it is important not only to educate nurses about falls and available interventions but also to promote positive attitudes toward patients or residents, especially those who are at risk.

Targeting Strategies

Several important patient factors contribute to falls: cognitive impairment, mobility impairment (especially recent changes), short-term memory changes, inability to use a nurse call bell, reluctance to ask staff for assistance, slow adaptation to environmental changes, complex medication regimens or polypharmacy, lack of awareness of elimination needs, and communication difficulties. In addition, most falls occur during the change of nursing shifts, within the first week after admission, and during the night. Major injuries are more likely to occur in the mornings, even when maximal staff are available (i.e., mornings are a time of high activity with toileting and treatment needs, and staff often take a morning break, which may make them less available and increase the risk of injury at that time). Finally, differences exist in fall demographics between units (i.e., who falls and when, where, and why falls occur). Therefore, it seems reasonable to assume that by knowing which patients or residents are at the highest risk and when most falls or injurious falls occur may help in determining appropriate staffing levels (i.e., targeting specific at-risk patients or residents who need close observation and considering different staffing levels at the times that may have a positive impact on fall rates).

Environmental Strategies

Important fall risk factors related to the physical environment are low visibility in the rooms of patients or residents, configurations that include private rooms rather than open units, and large units with long hallways. Locating nurses' stations near at-risk patient or resident rooms or relocating those prone to falls closer to nursing stations may help to reduce this risk.

Another fall risk factor relates to bed heights that do not meet the safe mobility needs of patients or residents (i.e., beds are too high, even in their lowest position). Height-adjustable low beds (approximately 8 inches above the floor in the low position and 34 inches above the floor in the high position) can be used to maintain a height suitable for safe egress. Also, the use of half side rails or bed transfer bars designed to support patient balance during transfers can be very helpful in preventing falls.

Because many falls in the hospital are unwitnessed and staffing levels do not allow constant patient surveillance, bed and chair alarms can be used to alert nurses when at-risk patients who should not get up on their own are doing so.

Support Strategies

Family members can help support busy staff. Many families are willing and able to report changes in their loved ones to the nursing staff. In order to use family members as a resource, it is important to let them know why the patient or resident is at risk, what they should look out for, and whom to communicate any changes or concerns to.

Likewise, nonclinical and administrative staff working in the hospital can let nurses know when at-risk patients do not look or act right. Identifying at-risk patients or residents with colored tags, bracelets, or nonskid socks is helpful in communicating to everyone which are at risk.

PATIENT AND RESIDENT EDUCATION: EDUCATIONAL AND BEHAVIORAL APPROACHES

Patient or resident education on fall prevention measures is an important component of a fall prevention program. The purpose of education is to change behavior, to help patients or residents adapt safe habits aimed at reducing falls while in the facility. Patients or residents who are aware of their risk of falling and take steps to avoid falls are less likely to fall.

Safety education begins at the time of admission, continues throughout the length of the hospital or nursing home stay, and includes discharge teaching as appropriate. Explaining to patients or residents and their families why falls are likely to occur and what they can do to reduce the likelihood of falls is important. Also, communicating this information helps patients or residents and their families appreciate that a number of factors (unrelated to staff negligence) can contribute to falls. Ordinarily, most facilities provide a safety tips sheet or brochure when a person is first admitted. The purpose of this material is to make patients or residents aware of some simple actions they can take to prevent falls. However, this is often a stressful time, and they may not be receptive to the material.

Patients or residents are more likely to pay attention to information when they need it. For example, after a fall risk assessment, several risk factors may be identified, such as impaired bed or toilet transfers or impaired gait or balance. Education under these circumstances would include teaching the patient or resident to call for assistance when getting out of bed or going to the bathroom, especially at night; to get out of bed and up from toilets slowly; to wear nonskid footwear; and to use canes or walkers. Patients or residents are more likely to exhibit a readiness to learn, follow directions, or engage in safe behaviors if they are aware of their risk factors. Those who receive planned or targeted education related specifically to their risk of falls tend to have better outcomes than those receiving routine or off-the-shelf education aimed at a wide variety of risk factors, which may or may not be relevant.

Education During the Stay

It is important to remember that fall risk is subject to change during the patient's or resident's stay. For instance, the onset of acute diseases or conditions and the addition of new medications or dosage changes may increase fall risk. Whenever patients or residents experience a change in their medical conditions or risk status, it is important to immediately educate them about their risk factors, such as asking them to call for assistance if they feel weak, dizzy, or lightheaded. Also, patients or residents should be advised to notify staff if their physical abilities deteriorate in any way.

Discharge Teaching

Discharge teaching is critical. Patients or residents and their families should be taught about self-management of diseases and medications and safe mobility in the home. Making patients or residents partners in managing their own health helps to avoid falls and institutional readmission.

Teaching must be adapted to the educational level of the patient or resident. Some patients or residents have limited formal schooling and are functionally illiterate (reading at a fourth-grade level or less). Therefore, staff must take special care in explaining health problems, risk factors, and safety instructions in very simple, direct language. For those who do not speak English or have a limited English vocabulary, the use of interpreters to communicate the information is vital. Poor compliance with education often results from an inability to understand instructions. In general, a combination of verbal instruction and demonstration is optimal. Education that focuses on what the patient or resident needs to learn, safety behaviors he or she needs to establish, and mastery of the information or behavior can be very effective in reducing the risk of falls.

FAMILY ROLE IN SAFETY

In hospitals and nursing homes, family members often become overly concerned and sometimes even angry about the safety of their loved ones when falls occur. As a result, families may ask staff to be much more attentive to the safety needs of their loved ones. For busy staff, however, spending the time needed to observe patients or residents at fall risk and making sure that their safety needs are met can be difficult. Involving family members in assisting with care can be tremendously helpful in monitoring fall risk and preventing falls. Also, getting family members involved may reduce some of their fear and anxiety.

One way of getting families involved is to provide them with educational leaflets about fall prevention. These materials are generally well received by family members and may influence patient or resident behavior, provided that the message is presented appropriately and that the patient or resident is able to understand and comply with the information. In many ways, a family's support, or lack of it, has a far greater impact on the degree to which patients or residents follow safety advice than information presented by health care professionals.

Yet general educational leaflets might not be sufficient to prevent falls from occurring because they often do not address the patient's or resident's specific risk factors and actions to manage risk. Another failure of educational materials is that they usually describe what patients or residents can do to prevent falls but not what family members can do to help. In order for educational interventions to be productive, families need to have specific information about their loved one's risk status and needs, including specific ways in which they can help prevent falls.

The best place to start in designing individualized family education is by identifying the patient's or resident's risk factors for falling. It is especially important to identify the person's mobility problems (i.e., inability to get up from a bed or chair without assistance, stand independently, walk without assistance, and recognize his or her limitations). It is easier for family members to understand these risk factors if they observe the assessment and the patient's or resident's ability or inability to perform mobility tasks. Once these risk factors have been identified, an individualized teaching plan can be developed. It is important for families to know

- That falling is not normal and that the risk of falling can be reduced

- That falls can be caused by certain medical problems, medications, and environmental hazards

- The importance of preserving mobility and not restricting mobility (including the adverse effects of restraints) in order to prevent falls

- General information about the patient's or resident's health problems and medications

- The patient's or resident's fall risk factors

- What interventions are in place to prevent falls

- The purpose and necessity of all interventions

- What family members can do to assist staff in preventing falls (e.g., observing safe cane or walker use, providing assistance with rising to prevent dizziness)

- How and when to communicate about their loved one with nursing staff (e.g., complaints of confusion, weakness, and balance instability should be reported immediately).

The use of case studies to illustrate what other families in similar circumstances have done to reduce fall risk is an excellent teaching strategy. Family caregivers are often very interested in how other caregivers have helped their loved ones and respond positively to learning through case examples. But most importantly, families need to have realistic expectations about preventing all falls in their loved ones. This point is critical. The problem is, nobody tells families what to expect. They want to believe that everything will go well and that nothing bad is going to happen. Some of the risks (e.g., falling or sustaining a fracture) are difficult or impossible to avoid because of the environment or the patient's or resident's condition. Families need to understand that falling and injury may be unavoidable. It is also important to remember that when family members assume the role of caregiver, they become part of the health care team. Therefore, health professionals need to legitimize the family's participation as team members. Health care professionals must learn to see family caregivers as true partners and to see themselves as health educators whose role it is to teach families how to help.

WHAT IS RESTRAINT?

No reliable research indicates that restraints keep patients or residents safe from falling. In fact, research shows quite the opposite. Restrained people are three times more likely to suffer injurious falls than those not restrained, and restraint reduction does not appear to increase the incidence of injurious falls. Although some patients will fall if they are not restrained, when they fall these people have less serious injury than those who are restrained. As a result, hospitals and nursing homes have successfully implemented programs of restraint avoidance. They have relied on regulatory definitions of restraint as any manual, or physical, or mechanical device, material, or equipment attached or adjacent to the body that the patient or resident cannot remove easily and that restricts freedom of movement or normal access to one's body, and they have acted accordingly to avoid their use. Common examples of restraints include vests that tie patients or residents to their chairs or beds and restrictive chairs, such as geri-chairs with lap trays or small wheels that limit mobility. Even bed rails, once considered a safety measure, are restraints when they are used to prevent patients or residents from getting out of bed. Without doubt, all these devices can put patients or residents in more danger than the actions they are designed to prevent, and their use should be contested. But what do we really mean by restraint? When we think about restraints, most of us automatically think about direct physical restraint (i.e., applying physical devices) and occasionally chemical restraints. But there are other ways we prevent patients or residents from doing what they want to do that might not be thought of as restraint. For example, does staff ever tell patients or residents to sit down, stay in bed, or stop what they are doing in order to prevent a fall? Are patients or residents ever told to wait if they ask to go to the bathroom or to their bedroom?

Sometimes, protecting patients or residents from harm may involve stopping them from doing something they appear to want to do. In some circumstances it is right to restrict their movement; it can keep them safe and may even improve their quality of life, despite some loss of independence. But stopping people from doing what they want to simply because we think they may fall is a form of restraint, no matter what the reasons are for doing so. Use of excessive verbal restraint, which restricts freedom of movement, may eventually harm them, reducing their confidence and making them fearful of attempting independent mobility. Some of these actions might have the same effect on other patients or residents, regardless of whether they are at risk. Moreover, persistent restraint may be an indication that risk of falling is not sufficiently controlled by existing interventions.

What should be considered when deciding how to protect patients or residents who are at risk without resorting to physical, chemical, or more subtle forms of restraint?

1. First, it is important to assess the behavior that is leading to restraint.

    *   What is the cause or meaning behind this behavior? Consider both patient or resident and caregiver factors.

    *   What actions precipitated the behavior?

    *   For whom is the behavior a problem: the patient or resident or the caregiver?

    *   What harm might there be for the patient or resident or the caregiver if the behavior persists?

    *   What risks might the behavior cause for other patients or residents and staff?

2. Second, once the causes or reasons behind the behavior are identified, consider solutions.

3. Third, put in place the appropriate interventions.

4. Finally, monitor the outcome.

   • Has the behavior been eliminated?

   • If not, what further actions are necessary to control the behavior? Weigh the pros and cons of each action or strategy.

Determining whether restraint is taking place is more than just assessing physical devices; it includes evaluating the actions we take on a daily basis to prevent falls and their effect on patients or residents. We should not settle for avoiding physical restraint only. We should avoid all forms of restraint that erode patients' or residents' independence.

REFERENCE

Mahoney, J.E., Palta, M., Johnson, J., Jalalluddin, M., Gray, S., Park, S., et al. (2000). Temporal association between hospitalization and rate of falls after discharge. *Archives of Internal Medicine, 160*(18), 2788–2795.

Chapter Nine

Evidence-Based Practice

One of the challenges in preventing falls and developing fall prevention pro-grams is taking data discovered in evidence-based research studies and apply-ing the information to everyday practice. The purpose of this chapter is to summarize the evidence for preventing falls in acute hospital and nursing home settings, summarize clinical practice recommendations for fall preven-tion based on the best evidence available, and summarize nursing best prac-tice guidelines for fall prevention.

Evidence-based fall prevention practice for hospitals and nursing homes generally focuses on four areas: assessment and evaluation, interventions, ed-ucation, and organizational components.

ASSESSMENT AND EVALUATION

Fall Risk Assessment

Fall risk assessment is an effective method for:

- Identifying fall-prone patients or residents

- Providing direction for fall prevention or reduction interventions.

Important components of risk assessment include the following (Table 9-1):

Review the Record for Evidence of Previous Falls

- Ask the patient or resident and caregiver or family whether the person has a history of falling.

- A history of one or more recent falls (within 90 days) should be listed as a problem in the patient's or resident's record.

- The potential for falling should be addressed in the care plan.

Document Risk Factors for Falling and Discuss the Patient's or Resident's Fall Risk in Care Conferences

- History of falls

- Fear of falling

Table 9-1. Assessment tools

Tools to assess fall risk include the following:
- Morse Fall Scale
- The STRATIFY risk assessment tool
- Hendrich II Fall Risk Model

To be useful, fall risk assessment tools must
- Be appropriate for the setting and for the specific population. Therefore, it is essential to assess the patient or resident population in order to select the tool most appropriate for the setting.
- Be both sensitive (low false negatives) and specific (low false positives).
- Be relevant to the population for which it is used.
- Be easily completed to facilitate staff adherence.
- Provide suggested care plan interventions for identified risk factors.

Tools to assess risk for falls may help increase staff attentiveness, but no single tool from the literature can be recommended for all practice settings.

- Bowel and bladder incontinence
- Cognitive impairment
- Mood
- Dizziness
- Functional impairment
- Medications
- Medical problems
- Environmental risks.

Each of these risk factors must be carefully considered and entered into a risk assessment tool to help determine the patient's or resident's degree of risk.

Time of Completion
- Admission fall risk assessment completed within 48 hours of admission
- If indicated, comprehensive fall risk assessment within 21 days after admission.

Frequency of Reassessment
- Upon a fall
- After a significant change of condition
- Quarterly for skilled nursing facilities and nursing facilities.

Injury Assessment

Risk factors for significant injury from falls should be considered during the risk assessment. Important risk factors include the following:

- Current use of anticoagulants such as warfarin; use of these agents increases the risk of bleeding after a fall.

- People who have a history of osteoporosis; they are at increased risk of fracture following a fall.

Medication Assessment

In consultation with the health care team, nurses should conduct periodic medication reviews to prevent falls. Patients or residents who are taking the following should be considered at high risk:

- Benzodiazepines

- Tricyclic antidepressants

- Selective serotonin reuptake inhibitors

- Trazodone

- More than five medications.

All medications should be reviewed for their potential to cause a fall. Medication review should be conducted periodically throughout the institutional stay.

Environmental Assessment

Important aspects of the environment to assess include the following:

- Physical room layout (see "High–Fall Risk Room Setup" in Section Three, Part C, Forms).

- Equipment and assistive devices are sturdy and in good repair.

- Room modifications (see "Strategies to Reduce Bedside Falls" and "Strategies to Ensure Bed Safety" in Section Three, Part C, Forms).

- Floor surfaces are free of spills, wet areas, and unevenness.

- Level of illumination is appropriate and lights (including night-lights) work correctly.

- Tabletops, furniture, and beds are sturdy and in good repair.

- Grab rails and grab bars are in place in the bathroom.

- Adaptive aids work properly and are in good repair.

- Bed rails do not collapse when used for transfers or support.

- Gowns and clothing do not cause tripping.

- Intravenous poles are sturdy if used during ambulation, and tubing does not cause tripping.

Environmental assessment is effective only in conjunction with follow-up and intervention, not in isolation.

Postfall Assessment

Important components of the fall assessment include the following:

- Define the nature, frequency, and causes of falls. Describe the situation accurately and in as much detail as possible, but distinguish facts from speculation. If the patient or resident was found on the floor without a witness to preceding events, describe the circumstances accordingly.

- When a patient or resident has just fallen or is found on the floor without a witness to the fall, a nurse should record vital signs and evaluate the person for possible injuries to the head, neck, spine, and extremities. If there is evidence of a significant injury such as a fracture or bleeding, provide appropriate first aid.

- If possible, begin to identify possible causes within 24 hours of a fall. Review the chain of events that preceded the fall and complete root cause analysis of each fall whenever possible.

- Notify the patient's or resident's attending physician and family promptly. For falls that do not result in significant injury or a condition change, the practitioner may be notified routinely (e.g., by fax or by phone the next office day) instead of immediately.

- Because of the known incidence of delayed complications, including fractures, observe all patients or residents for about 48 hours after an observed or suspected fall. Document relevant postfall clinical findings such as vital signs, pain, swelling, bruising, and decreased mobility in the record. It is also desirable to note the absence of such significant findings (i.e., pertinent negatives) to demonstrate that the patient or resident is being monitored appropriately.

Provide staff with a clear, written procedure that describes what to do when a patient or resident falls and observe patterns and trends in fall incidents in individuals and in those sharing common characteristics, diseases, or medications, which may assist in identifying patterns of falls.

INTERVENTIONS

Care Planning

Each person identified as being at risk for falls should have a care plan that is individualized to minimize his or her specific risk factors. Because most people's fall risks are multifactorial and the factors are intertwined, the most effective strategies are interdisciplinary. Important aspects of care planning include the following:

Develop a Plan for Managing Falls and Fall Risks

- Once fall risk factors are identified, targeted interventions aimed at reducing falls should be available (Table 9-2).

- Use a clear, consistent approach to select interventions to manage and prevent falling in individual patients or residents.

- It is appropriate to prioritize approaches to managing fall risk and falling. That is, if a systematic evaluation of a patient's or resident's fall risk identifies several possible interventions, it is reasonable to choose one of these interventions to try first.

- If falling recurs despite the initial intervention, additional or different interventions may be needed.

- Adjust the care plan as necessary to reflect the implementation of new or modified interventions to try to minimize the risk of falling and fall-related injuries.

- Briefly document the rationale for specific interventions to show that causes of the problem are being sought.

In summary, care plans should address the status of conditions that predispose the patient or resident to falling, specific fall prevention efforts, and the patient's or resident's response to each intervention.

Table 9-2. Interventions based on fall risk factors

Risk Factors	Risk Reduction Interventions
History of falls	• Identify the patient or resident as being at risk for falls; use sticker on chart or door to identify risk.
Fear of falling	• Strengthen self-efficacy related to transfers and ambulation by providing verbal encouragement about capabilities and demonstrating to patient or resident his or her ability to perform safely.
Bladder and bowel incontinence	• Determine type and severity of urinary or fecal incontinence and type-specific treatment. • Set up toileting program and regular voiding schedule (every 2 hours or as appropriate based on patient or resident need). • Monitor bowel function and encourage sufficient fluids and fiber (eight 8-ounce glasses daily and 24 grams of fiber).
Cognitive impairment	• Evaluate patient or resident for reversible causes of cognitive impairment or delirium and eliminate causes as appropriate. • Monitor patient or resident at least hourly; relocate so that staff can observe regularly. • Encourage family members to hire sitters. • Use monitoring devices such as bed and chair alarms.
Depression	• Encourage verbalization of feelings. • Encourage engagement in daily activities. • Refer to geriatric psychiatry as appropriate.
Dizziness	• Monitor lying, sitting, and standing blood pressure and evaluate for factors contributing to dizziness. • Encourage adequate fluid intake (eight 8-ounce glasses daily). • Set up environment to avoid movements that result in dizziness. • If diabetic, monitor and manage blood sugars.

(continued)

Table 9-2. *(continued)*

Risk Factors	Risk Reduction Interventions
Functional impairment	• Encourage participation in personal care activities at highest level (e.g., encourage walking to bathroom, if possible, rather than using bedpan). • Refer to physical therapist or occupational therapist as appropriate. • Facilitate exercise program and promote adherence to program when indicated. • Monitor appropriate use of assistive devices; refer to physical therapy for evaluation as appropriate.
Medications	• Review medications with primary care physician and determine need for each medication. • Ascertain that medications are being used at lowest possible dosages to obtain desired results. • Patients or residents who have fallen should have their medications reviewed and altered or stopped as appropriate. • Implement processes to effectively manage polypharmacy and psychotropic medications, including regular medication reviews; explore alternatives to psychotropic medication for sedation. • All attempts should be made to manage symptoms nonpharmacologically rather than initiating a new medication. • Monitor effects of medications that increase the risk of falling.
Medical problems	• Refer to primary care physician for evaluation and management.
Osteoporosis	• Refer to primary care physician for evaluation and management. However, medications used to treat osteoporosis do not reduce fall rates; therefore, consider other injury reduction strategies such as low bed, floor mats, and hip protectors.
Environmental risks	• Familiarize patient or resident with environment (e.g., identify call light, bathroom). • Maintain call bell in reach and have patient or resident demonstrate ability to call for the nurse. • Remove clutter and unused furnishings. • Make sure that furniture and assistive devices are in good condition. • Make sure that lighting is adequate for safe mobility. Use night-light. • Make sure that safety bars are available in bathroom. • Place bed in low position with brakes locked.

Manage Factors that May Cause Serious Consequences of Falling

• Some of the physical, functional, and environmental factors that predispose patients or residents to falling also increase the risk of serious consequences of these falls. Many members of the interdisciplinary care team, as well as staff in support services such as housekeeping and maintenance, can help to address these risk factors.

Monitor Falling in People with a Fall Risk or Fall History

• Monitor and document the patient's or resident's response to interventions intended to reduce falling or the risks of falling. If interventions have been successful in preventing falling, continue with current approaches or reconsider whether these measures are still needed if the problem that necessitated the intervention (e.g., dizziness, joint pain) has been resolved.

- If the patient or resident continues to fall, reevaluate the situation and reconsider current interventions. Amend the care plan as necessary to reflect the addition of new interventions and the need for continued monitoring.

- Document the presence of irreversible risk factors. Also, consider relevant interventions to try to minimize fall-related injuries (e.g., using hip protectors, treating osteoporosis).

- If falls continue despite initial interventions, the reason could be that different or additional causes exist, that the underlying causes are not readily correctable, that the cause cannot be identified, or that the interventions are insufficient. Consider other possible reasons for the falls besides those that have already been identified, or document why a further search for causes is unlikely to be helpful.

- Some consequences of falling, such as fractures and symptomatic intracranial bleeding, may become clinically apparent days or weeks after a fall. Be aware of, and ensure that staff respond to, delayed consequences of falling. Consider the possibility of late consequences if the patient or resident has a significant change in function, mental status, or level of consciousness within several weeks of a fall.

Universal Fall Precautions

Universal or standard fall precautions are recommended for all hospital patients and nursing home residents and include the following:

- Familiarize the patient or resident with the environment (e.g., identify the call light and bathroom; may need to label).

- Maintain a call bell in reach and have the patient or resident demonstrate ability to call for the nurse.

- Place the bed in low position with brakes locked.

- Ensure that footwear is fitted, nonslip, and used properly.

- Determine the appropriate use of side rails based on cognitive and functional status.

- Use night-lights.

- Keep floor surfaces clean and dry.

- Keep the room uncluttered and make sure that furniture is in optimal condition.

- Make sure that the patient or resident knows where personal possessions are and that he or she can access them safely.

- Provide adequate handrails in the bathroom, bedroom, and hallway.

- Establish a plan of care to maintain bowel and bladder function.

- Evaluate the effects of medications that increase the person's risk of falling.

- Encourage participation in functional activities and exercise at the patient's or resident's highest possible level and refer to physical therapy as appropriate.

- Monitor the patient or resident regularly.

- Educate the patient or resident and family about fall prevention strategies.

Postfall Medication Management

- Evaluate the patient's or resident's drug regimen carefully to identify medications that may precipitate falls. Falls that start after a change in medication regimen should trigger a review of the patient's entire medication regimen. Long-standing medications that may not have been problematic in the past should be reevaluated in conjunction with recent acute illnesses or general condition changes.

- If it is decided not to adjust medications that may be associated with falling, document how it was determined that the patient or resident did not have lethargy, dizziness, or postural blood pressure changes that might indicate that the medications had played a role in the falls.

Mobility Interventions

Exercise and Balance Training

- Patients or residents with recurrent falls may benefit from exercise programs and balance training. The optimal type, duration, and intensity of exercise remain unclear.

- Beneficial exercise programs include walking, balance training, resistance and strength training, aerobics, stationary cycling, and tai chi chuan. Those most likely to benefit are people with a history of recurrent falls or balance and gait deficit. Exercise programs should be individually prescribed and monitored by an appropriately trained professional.

- After a fall, address underlying causes and implement restorative or rehabilitative care to try to improve strength, balance, gait, and transferring ability.

The benefits of improving physical mobility and endurance through any of these interventions alone as a fall prevention intervention, without concurrent reduction of other fall risk factors, has not been documented.

Protective Devices and Other Interventions

Hip Protectors

- Nurses should consider the use of hip protectors to reduce hip fractures among patients or residents considered at high risk of fractures associated with falls; however, there is no evidence to support universal use of hip protectors. Use of hip protectors does not reduce the risk of falling.

Fall Alarms

- Bed and chair alarms may indicate a patient's or resident's efforts to arise from a bed or chair and may allow caregivers to reach the patient or resident before he or she falls.

- The use of fall alarm systems is indicated for people with a history of falls, unsafe bed mobility, cognitive deficits, or confusion; for those who are alone in the room; and for those who are unable to use the call bell.

- The efficacy of an alarm system depends on effective technology and the response time of nursing staff.

Low Beds

- Lowering a standard bed or using a low bed may help to reduce falls and may reduce the risk of serious injury when falls occur.

Sitters

- The use of sitters for confused patients or residents seems to be of benefit in reducing risk. Each institution must establish what the sitters may or may not do to keep patients or residents safe. Training and competency evaluation for these personnel must reflect the established expectations. It is also common for family members to stay with confused patients or residents in the hope that family will be able to provide a certain degree of safety. The ability of the volunteering family member to intervene must be determined, and at least some education should be provided and documented.

Restraints

- The indiscriminate use of physical restraints is no longer an accepted standard of care in hospitals or nursing homes. Federal regulations provide clear guidelines for the use of physical restraints, which stress the need to try less restrictive approaches first and to use restraints only to try to maintain or improve—not reduce—a patient's or resident's function.

- Restraint reduction programs do not seem to cause a significant increase in the total number of falls and may reduce the number or seriousness of injuries sustained during a fall.

- Nurses should not use side rails to prevent falls; side rails may cause serious entrapment injury or death. However, other client factors may influence decision making around the use of side rails.

- Organizations should establish a policy for least restraint that includes both physical and chemical restraints.

Home Hazard and Safety Intervention

- Patients discharged from the hospital should be offered a home hazard assessment and safety intervention and modifications by a suitably trained health care professional. This should be part of discharge planning and be carried out on a schedule arranged by the patient or caregiver and appropriate members of the health care team. Home hazard assessment is effective only in conjunction with follow-up and intervention, not in isolation.

EDUCATION

Nursing Education

Education on the prevention of falls and fall injuries should be included in nursing training and ongoing education, with specific attention to the following:

- Safe mobility

- Risk assessment

- Multidisciplinary strategies

- Risk management including postfall follow-up

- Alternatives to restraints and other restrictive devices

- Policies and procedures

- Documentation expectations.

Fall program in-service for nursing should occur:

- Upon orientation

- Semiannually

- After a fall.

Frequent and varied staff education and re-education are important to promote and sustain sensitivity to the risk for falls.

Multidisciplinary Education

Health care professionals involved in fall prevention should be educated about assessment of fall risks and potentially helpful interventions.

Patient or Resident and Family Education

All patients or residents who have been assessed as being at high risk for falling should receive education regarding their risk of falling. It is important to evaluate the patient's or resident's ability to concentrate and learn new information. Family members should receive information on specific risk factors and interventions.

Patients or residents at risk of falling and their family members should be offered information orally and in writing about the following:

- What they can do to prevent falls

- Where they can seek advice and assistance.

Education should occur:

- Upon admission

- After care plan meetings

- After a fall

- Quarterly in nursing home settings.

Patient education should include the following:

- Instructions and information about fall risks and safety awareness

- Proper use of call bells, walking devices, wheelchairs, and other assistive devices.

Family education should include the following:

- Reasonable expectations from the facility about falls

- How they can assist the patient or resident in reducing fall risk.

ORGANIZATIONAL SUPPORT

Important organizational or administrative actions to support fall prevention include the following.

Enhance Fall Prevention Activities

- Prioritize fall prevention within the facility.

- Ensure ongoing staff education and training.

- Ensure involvement of multidisciplinary teams; clearly define each team member's role in evaluating and preventing falls.

- Ensure sufficient staff and equipment, such as transfer devices, low beds, and alarms.

- Assign a designated fall coordinator from the staff and use ongoing consultation with a fall expert to support the fall prevention program.

Conduct Quality Improvement Activities

- Use quality improvement techniques to both monitor for and reduce falls that occur.

- Conduct aggregate review of falls throughout the facility; include analysis of falls in the facility's quality improvement studies.

- Develop reporting mechanism and track falls within the facility by time, location, and identified categories of causes.

  —Relate these data to care processes to ensure that everything reasonable is being done to identify risk factors for falling and take appropriate preventive measures.

—Use the information collected about falls to evaluate and adjust the fall prevention program.

—Identify recurring common characteristics of the falls (consider who, where, when, what diagnosis, and what equipment and medications were in use).

—Address common or recurring factors with changes in practice patterns, environmental changes, staff education, and introduction of new equipment.

SUMMARY

Whether in the nursing home or acute hospital setting, research shows that effective fall prevention programs depend on having in place a multipronged approach consisting of an organized clinical approach (i.e., risk assessment, care planning, monitoring, and postfall assessment), organizational support, a designated fall coordinator and interdisciplinary team, staff education and training, and ongoing consultation with a fall expert.

Acute Hospital Settings

The most beneficial evidence-based fall prevention practices in the hospital setting include the following:

- Provide educational activities for nurses and support staff.

- Include safety awareness of individualized risk factors in patient orientation.

- Identify a patient's fall history and fall risk with subsequent implementation of targeted modifiable risk factors.

- Implement postfall evaluation and review of prior falls (some patients fall repeatedly for the same reason).

- Improve environment by reducing physical obstacles in rooms, adding supplemental lighting and grab bars in bathrooms, and lowering bed rails and bed height.

- Improve transfer ability and mobility through physical therapy.

- Incorporate interventions for cognitively impaired patients by educating families, minimizing sedating medications, and locating confused patients close to nursing staff.

- Ensure that hospital units are staffed adequately so that nurses and assistive personnel are available to assist patients with transfers, toileting, and other basic physical needs.

Nursing Home Settings

The most beneficial evidence-based fall preventive practices in the nursing home setting include the following:

- Implement staff education programs.

- Identify fall risk factors through a comprehensive fall evaluation.

- Improve management of falls through staff education programs.

- Improve physical mobility through gait training and advice on the appropriate use of assistive devices and wheelchair use and maintenance by an occupational therapist.

- Review and adjust medications, including psychotropic medications.

- Modify the physical environment; improve room lighting, flooring, and footwear.

REFERENCES FOR EVIDENCE-BASED PRACTICE

American Geriatric Society, British Geriatrics Society, American Academy of Orthopaedic Surgeons. (2001, May). Guideline for the prevention of falls in older persons. *Journal of the American Geriatrics Society, 49*(5), 664–672.

American Medical Directors Association. (2003). *Falls and fall risk.* Columbia, MD: Author.

Gray-Micelli, D. (2008). Preventing falls in acute care. In E. Capezuti, D. Zwicker, M. Mezey, & T. Fulmer (Eds.), *Evidence-based geriatric nursing protocols for best practice* (3rd ed., pp. 161–198). New York: Springer.

Health Care Association of New Jersey. (2006). *Fall management guideline.* Hamilton, NJ: Author.

The John A. Hartford Foundation Institute for Geriatric Nursing. (2003). Preventing falls in acute care. In M. Mezey, T. Fulmer, I. Abraham, & D.A. Zwicker (Eds.), *Geriatric nursing protocols for best practice* (2nd ed., pp. 141–164). New York: Springer.

National Collaborating Centre for Nursing and Supportive Care, National Institute for Clinical Excellence. (2004, June). *Clinical practice guideline for the assessment and prevention of falls in older people.* London: National Institute for Clinical Excellence.

Registered Nurses Association of Ontario. (2005). *Prevention of falls and fall injuries in the older adult.* Toronto: Author.

University of Iowa Gerontological Nursing Interventions Research Center. (2004). *Fall prevention for older adults.* Iowa City: University of Iowa Gerontological Nursing Interventions Research Center, Research Dissemination Core.

REFERENCES SUPPORTING EVIDENCE-BASED PRACTICE

Agostini, J.V., Baker, D.I., & Bogardus, S.T., Jr. (2001). Prevention of falls in hospitalized and institutionalized older people. In A.J. Markowitz, K.G. Shojania, B.W. Duncan, K.M. McDonald, & R.M. Wachter (Eds.), *Making health care safer: A critical analysis of patient safety practices* (pp. 281–299). Rockville, MD: Agency for Healthcare Research and Quality, U.S. Department of Health and Human Services.

American Geriatrics Society, British Geriatrics Society, and American Academy of Orthopaedic Surgeons Panel on Falls Prevention. (2001, May). Guideline for the prevention of falls in older persons. *Journal of the American Geriatrics Society, 49*(5), 664–672.

Arbesman, M.C., & Wright, C. (1999). Mechanical restraints, rehabilitation therapies, and staffing adequacy as risk factors for falls in an elderly hospitalized population. *Rehabilitation Nursing, 24*, 122–128.

Blegen, M.A. (2006). Patient safety in hospital acute care units. *Annual Review of Nursing Research, 24*, 103–125.

Cameron, I.D., Murray, G.R., Gillespie, L.D., Robertson, M.C., Hill, K.D., Cumming, R.G., & Kerse, N. (2010). Interventions for preventing falls in older people in nursing care facilities and hospitals. *Cochrane Database of Systematic Reviews*, Issue 1.

Capezuti, E. (2004). Building the science of falls-prevention research. *Journal of the American Geriatrics Society, 52*, 461–462.

Capezuti, E., Evans, L., Strumpf, N., & Maislin, G. (1996, June). Physical restraint use and falls in nursing home residents. *Journal of the American Geriatrics Society, 44*(6), 627–633.

Capezuti, E., Maislin, G., Strumpf, N., & Evans, L. (2002). Side rail use and bed-related fall outcomes among nursing home residents. *Journal of the American Geriatrics Society, 50*, 90–96.

Capezuti, E., Wagner, L.M., Brush, B.L., Boltz, M., Renz, S., & Secic, M. (2008). Bed and toilet height as potential environmental risk factors. *Clinical Nursing Research, 17*, 50–66.

Coussement, J., De Paepe, L., Schwendimann, R., Denhaerynck, D., Dejaeger, E., & Milisen, K. (2008). Interventions for preventing falls in acute- and chronic-care hospitals: A systematic review and meta-analysis. *Journal of the American Geriatrics Society, 56*, 29–36.

Evans, D., Hodgkinson, B., Lambert, L., Wood, J., & Kowanko, I. (1998). *Falls in acute hospitals: A systematic review*. Adelaide: Joanna Briggs Institute for Evidence Based Nursing and Midwifery, National Library of Australia.

Evans, D., Wood, J., & Lambert, L. (2002). A review of physical restraint minimization in the acute and residential care settings. *Journal of Advanced Nursing, 40*, 616–625.

Gales, B.J., & Menard, S.M. (1995). Relationship between the administration of selected medications and falls in hospitalized elderly patients. *Annals of Pharmacotherapy, 29*, 354–358.

Gallinagh, R., Slevin, E., & McCormack, B. (2001). Side rails as physical restraints: The need for appropriate assessment. *Nursing Older People, 13*, 22–27.

Gallinagh, R., Slevin, E., & McCormack, B. (2002). Side rails as physical restraints in the care of older people: A management issue. *Journal of Nursing Management, 10*, 299–306.

Gluck, T., Wientjes, H.J., & Rai, G.S. (1996). An evaluation of risk factors for in-patient falls in acute and rehabilitation elderly care wards. *Gerontology, 42*, 104–107.

Gray-Miceli, D.L., Strumpf, N.E., Reinhard, S.C., Zanna, M.T., & Fritz, E. (2004). Current approaches to postfall assessment in nursing homes. *Journal of the American Medical Directors Association, 5*, 387–394.

Hanger, H.C., Ball, M.C., & Wood, L.A. (1999, May). An analysis of falls in the hospital: Can we do without bedrails? *Journal of the American Geriatrics Society, 47*(5), 529–531.

Haumschild, J., Karfonta, T.L., Haumschild, M.S., & Phillips, S.E. (2003). Clinical and economic outcomes of a fall-focused pharmaceutical intervention program. *American Journal of Health-System Pharmacy, 60*, 1029–1032.

Healey, F., Monro, A., Cockram, A., Adams, V., & Heseltine, D. (2004). Using targeted risk factor reduction to prevent falls in older in-patients: A randomized controlled trial. *Age and Ageing, 33*, 390–395.

Healey, F., Oliver, D., Milne, A., & Connelly, J.B. (2008). The effect of bedrails on falls and injury: A systematic review of clinical studies. *Age and Ageing, 37*, 368–378.

Hignett, S., & Masud, T. (2006). A review of environmental hazards associated with in-patient falls. *Ergonomics, 49*, 605–616.

Hill-Westmoreland, E.E., Soeken, K., & Spellbring, A.M. (2002, January–February). A meta-analysis of fall prevention programs for the elderly: How effective are they? *Nursing Research, 51*(1), 1–8.

Kim, E.A., Mordiffi, S.Z., Bee, W.H., Devi, K., & Evans, D. (2007). Evaluation of three fall-risk assessment tools in an acute care setting. *Journal of Advanced Nursing, 60*, 427–435.

Krauss, M.J., Evanoff, B., Hitcho, E., Ngugi, K.E., Dunagan, W.C., Fischer, I., et al. (2005). A case-control study of patient, medication, and care-related risk factors for inpatient falls. *Journal of General Internal Medicine, 20*, 116–122.

Krauss, M.J., Tutlam, N., Constantinou, E., Johnson, S., Jackson, D., & Fraser, V.J. (2008). Intervention to prevent falls on the medial service in a teaching hospital. *Infection Control and Hospital Epidemiology, 29*, 539–545.

Lake, E.T., & Cheung, R.B. (2006). Are patient falls and pressure ulcers sensitive to nurse staffing? *Western Journal of Nursing Research, 28*, 654–677.

Leipzig, R.M., Cumming, R.G., & Tinetti, M.E. (1999). Drugs and falls in older people: A systematic review and meta-analysis: I. Psychotropic drugs. *Journal of the American Geriatrics Society, 47*, 30–39.

Leipzig, R.M., Cumming, R.G., & Tinetti, M.E. (1999). Drugs and falls in older people: A systematic review and meta-analysis: II. Cardiac and analgesic drugs. *Journal of the American Geriatrics Society, 47*, 40–50.

Minnick, A.F., Mion, L.C., Johnson, M.E., Catrambone, C., & Leipzig, R. (2007). Prevalence and variation of physical restraint use in acute care settings in the US. *Journal of Nursing Scholarship, 39*, 30–37.

Myers, H. (2003). Hospital fall risk assessment tools: A critique of the literature. *International Journal of Nursing Practice, 9*, 223–235.

Myers, H., & Nikoletti, S. (2003). Fall risk assessment: A prospective investigation of nurses' clinical judgement and risk assessment tools in predicting patient falls. *International Journal of Nursing Practice, 9*, 158–165.

Nelson, A., Powell-Cope, G., Gavin-Dreschnack, D., Quigley, P., Bulat, T., Baptiste, A.S., et al. (2004). Technology to promote safe mobility in the elderly. *Nursing Clinics of North America, 39*, 649–671.

Neufeld, R.R., Libow, L.S., Foley, W.J., Dunbar, J.M., Cohen, C., & Breuer, B. (1999, October). Restraint reduction reduces serious injuries among nursing home residents. *Journal of the American Geriatrics Society, 47*(10), 1202–1207.

Oliver, D. (2008). Falls risk-prediction tools for hospital inpatients. Time to put them to bed? *Age and Ageing, 37*, 248–250.

Oliver, D., Hopper, A., & Seed, P. (2000, December). Do hospital fall prevention programs work? A systematic review. *Journal of the American Geriatrics Society, 48*(12), 1679–1689.

Parker, K., & Miles, S.H. (1997, July). Deaths caused by bedrails. *Journal of the American Geriatrics Society, 45*(7), 797–802.

Parker, M.J., Gillespie, L.D., & Gillespie, W.J. (2006). Effectiveness of hip protectors for preventing hip fractures in elderly people: systematic review. *British Medical Journal, 332*, 571–574.

Perell, K.L., Nelson, A., Goldman, R.L., Luther, S.L., Prieto-Lewis, N., & Rubinstein, L.Z. (2001). Fall risk assessment measures: An analytic review. *Journal of Gerontology. Series A, Biological Sciences and Medical Sciences, 56*, M761–M766.

Peterson, J.F., Kupeman, G.H., Shek, C., Pate, M., Avorn, J., & Bates, D.W. (2005). Guided prescription of psychotropic medication for geriatric in patients. *Archives of Internal Medicine, 165*, 802–807.

Ray, W.A., Taylor, J.A., Meador, K.G., Thapa, P.B., Brown, A.K., Kajihara, H.K., et al. (1997, August 20). A randomized trial of a consultation service to reduce falls in nursing homes. *JAMA, 278*(7), 557–562.

Reed, L., Blegen, M.A., & Goode, C.S. (1998). Adverse patient occurrences as a measure of nursing care quality. *Journal of Nursing Administration, 28*, 62–69.

Rohde, J.M., Myers, A.H., & Vlahov, D. (1990). Variation in risk for falls by clinical department: Implications for prevention. *Infection Control and Hospital Epidemiology, 11*, 521–524.

Rutledge, D.N., Donaldson, N.E., & Pravikoff, D.S. (2003). Update 2003: Fall risk assessment and prevention in hospitalized patients. *Online Journal of Clinical Innovation, 6*, 1–55.

Schwendimann, R., Bühler, H., De Geest, S., & Milisen, K. (2008). Characteristics of hospital inpatient falls across clinical departments. *Gerontology, 54*, 342–348.

Tinetti, M.E., Liu, W.L., & Ginter, S.F. (1992, March 1). Mechanical restraint use and fall-related injuries among residents of skilled nursing facilities. *Annals of Internal Medicine, 116*(5), 369–374.

Tzeng, H.M., & Yin, C.Y. (2006). The staff-working height and the designing-regulation height for patient beds as possible causes of patient falls. *Nursing Economics, 24*, 323–327.

Tzeng, H.M., & Yin, C.Y. (2007). Height of hospital beds and inpatient falls: A threat to patient safety. *Journal of Nursing Administration, 37*, 537–538.

Tzeng, H.M., & Yin, C.Y. (2008). The extrinsic risk factors for inpatient falls in hospital patient rooms. *Journal of Nursing Care Quality, 23*, 233–241.

Tzeng, H.M., Yin, C.Y., & Grunawalt, J. (2008). Effective assessment of use of sitters by nurses in inpatient care settings. *Journal of Advanced Nursing, 64*, 176–183.

van der Velde, N., Stricker, B.H., Pols, H.A., & van der Cammen, T.J. (2007). Withdrawal of fall-risk-increasing drugs in older persons: Effect on mobility test outcomes. *Drugs & Aging, 24*, 691–699.

Vassallo, M., Amersey, R.A., Sharma, J.C., & Allen, S.C. (2000). Falls on integrated medical wards. *Gerontology, 46*, 158–162.

Vassallo, M., Poynter, L., Sharma, J.C., Kwan, J., & Allen, S.C. (2008). Fall risk-assessment tools compared with clinical judgment: An evaluation in a rehabilitation ward. *Age and Ageing, 37*, 277–281.

von Renteln-Kruse, W., & Krause, T. (2007). Incidence of in-hospital falls in geriatric patients before and after the introduction of an interdisciplinary team-based fall-prevention intervention. *Journal of the American Geriatrics Society, 55*, 2068–2074.

Vu, M.Q., Weintraub, N., & Rubenstein, L.Z. (2006). Falls in the nursing home: Are they preventable? *Journal of the American Medical Directors Association, 7*(3 Suppl), S53–S58.

Resources

Fall Prevention Guidelines

Best Clinical Practices in Acute Care Hospitals and Nursing Facilities

PURPOSE

To provide a summary of best clinical practices to prevent patient falls in hospitals and nursing facilities, the most frequently occurring factors that increase fall risk, and the most commonly used interventions that reduce fall risk. Best clinical practices are simply ideas that work. Best practices in terms of fall prevention are strategies or interventions and practices that produce effective outcomes and decrease falls and injury. By knowing what causes falls and what strategies prevent falls, facilities can develop programs and protocols aimed at eliminating falls.

BEST PRACTICES IN ACUTE CARE HOSPITALS

The first part of this chapter deals with best clinical practices in acute care hospitals. Best practices of nursing facilities are discussed beginning on page 172.

Risk Factors

While many older patients are at some degree of risk of falling, certain factors have been consistently identified with high risk of falling. These include the intrinsic, extrinsic, and patient risk factors.

Intrinsic Risk Factors

- Age: Elderly patients older than age 75

- History of falling: Reported fall(s) during hospitalization; patients tend to repeat the circumstances of the first fall in subsequent falls

- Mental status: Impaired cognition—confusion, disorientation, poor memory, and inability to understand

- Medications: Psychotropic drugs such as sedatives and tranquilizers

- Dizziness or vertigo
- Lower extremity weakness
- Impaired mobility: Impaired transfers, gait/balance impairment
- Altered elimination: Urinary/bowel incontinence, urgency.

Extrinsic Risk Factors

- Equipment issues: Broken wheelchair locks, bed wheels not locked
- Floor surfaces/treatments that promote slips
- Raised beds
- Full-length bedside rails
- Furnishings: Unstable chairs/over-the-bed tables.

Patient Risk Factors

- Multiple risk factors (i.e., presence of more than one risk factor; risk increases as number of risk factors increases)
- Diagnoses:

  —Congestive heart failure (due to generalized weakness, nocturia)

  —Stroke (due to extremity weakness, aphasia/communication impairment)

  —Neoplasm (due to generalized weakness, side effects of anti-cancer drugs).

Most Frequent Causes/Sites of Patient Falls

- Transfers on and off beds (account for up to 50% of falls)
- Elimination (i.e., trips to bathroom)
- Types of units (unit-specific risk factors):

  —Psychiatry (depression, dementia, anxiety, antidepressants, orthostatic hypotension, wandering, aggressive behavior)

  —Rehabilitation units (incontinence, polypharmacy, stroke).

- Disability requiring assistance with activities of daily living [ADLs], and impaired wheelchair transfers.

Assessment of Risk

Fall risk assessment tools should be employed to identify risk factors. By identifying specific fall risk factors, appropriate interventions aimed at minimizing risk can be identified and implemented. Risk assessments should be completed at the time of admission (within 24 hours) and, thereafter, whenever patients experience a change of status (e.g., acute illness, change in function, a move to another hospital unit).

Facilities can either use available risk assessment tools or develop their own risk assessments and incorporate them into the admission form for initial assessment and into the daily nursing assessment form for continual risk evaluation. Although established risk assessment tools are beneficial in identifying risk, tailoring risk assessments is helpful in meeting the unique needs of patient populations in specialty units (e.g., intensive care units, rehabilitation, telemetry, psychiatry).

Fall Preventive Interventions[1]

Staff Related

- Providing education (increasing awareness of patient fall risk during hospitalization and strategies to reduce risk)

- Communicating "at-risk" status (identifying fall risk status in patient's medical/nursing chart).

Patient Related

- Providing education (increasing patient/family awareness of fall risk during hospitalization and strategies to reduce risk)

- Attempting medication reduction (regularly reviewing patient medications, eliminating high-risk drugs as appropriate)

- Moving confused patients near nurses' station (close observation)

- Using sitters to sit with confused patients

- Using bed alarms (to alert staff when at-risk patients are attempting unsafe mobility tasks)

- Using identification bracelets (to identify high-risk patients)

- Using nonskid footwear

- Meeting elimination needs (placing patients near toilets, using bedside commodes, routine toileting schedules)

- Providing ambulation programs (e.g., walking high-risk patients in hallway once per shift).

Environment Related

- Keeping bed in low position, bed wheels locked

- Using half side rails as enablers (side rails to prevent falls is not successful)

- Reducing pathway clutter around patient's bed/bedroom

- Maintaining stable furnishings (beds/chairs used to maintain balance; help with efficient transfers)

- Improving lighting (night-lights at bedside/toilet)

- Installing toilet grab rails (to support safe transfers).

BEST PRACTICES IN NURSING FACILITIES

While all nursing facility residents are at some degree of risk of falling, certain factors have been consistently identified with high risk of falling.* These include the following risk factors:

Risk Factors

Intrinsic Risk Factors

- History of falling: Reported fall(s) previous to institutionalization and/or during institutionalization

- Mental status: Impaired cognition—confusion, disorientation, poor memory, and inability to understand; dementia

- Vision impairment: Glaucoma, cataracts, macular degeneration, and functional vision loss

- Medications: Use of antidepressants and sedatives; use of more than four medications (i.e., polypharmacy)

- Post-prandial hypotension

- Lower extremity weakness

- Impaired mobility (e.g., impaired transfers, gait/balance impairment)

- Assistive devices (e.g., canes, walkers)

- Toileting needs (i.e., urinary/bowel incontinence, urgency)

- Use of restraints.

Extrinsic Risk Factors

- Equipment issues (e.g., wheelchair wheels not locked, bed wheels not locked)

- Slippery or wet floors

- Raised beds

- Inadequate assistive devices (e.g., canes, walkers)

- Lack of toilet grab rails

- Malfunctioning nurse call systems

- Use of full-length side rails.

---

*Because the population of residents is similar or the same as that represented in the hospital practices listed previously, some of these risk factors are the same or similar.

Patient Risk Factors[2]

- Presence of multiple risk factors (e.g., residents of advanced age with accompanying multiple chronic diseases, polypharmacy, cognitive impairment, and/or unsteady gait/balance)

- Diagnoses:

    —Congestive heart failure (presumably causes generalized weakness, nocturia)

    —Stroke (may cause extremity weakness, aphasia/communication impairment)

    —Parkinson's disease (may cause associated gait/balance impairment)

    —Degenerative joint disease (may cause associated lower extremity weakness).

Most Frequent Causes/Sites of Patient Falls

- Transfers on and off beds (account for up to 50% of falls)

- Elimination; trips to bathroom

- Transfers on and off chairs/wheelchairs.

Assessment of Risk

Fall risk assessment tools can be employed to identify risk factors. The Minimum Data Set (MDS) contains some—but not all—of the information relevant to assessing fall risk. By identifying specific fall-risk factors (both intrinsic and extrinsic), appropriate interventions aimed at minimizing risk can be identified and implemented. Facilities either use available risk assessment tools or develop their own risk assessments and incorporate them into the admission form for initial assessment, and into the daily nursing assessment form for continual risk evaluation.

The Resident Assessment Protocols (RAPs) provide some information about fall risk (e.g., previous falls, medications/recent medication changes, assistive devices, environmental factors, neuromuscular/functional factors, orthopedic factors, sensory factors, and cognitive/behavioral factors). This information can be used to supplement risk factors identified on the fall risk assessment.

A fall risk assessment for all residents should be completed upon admission (within 24 hours) to the nursing facility, on a regular basis (i.e., to coincide with the MDS and/or whenever residents experience a change in condition), and post-fall.

Every time a resident falls, an assessment of the details or circumstances of the fall, causes of the fall, and contributing intrinsic and extrinsic factors should occur. The information obtained can be used to develop interventions to prevent further falls.

Recognize that using assessments to predict fall risk is not an exact science (i.e., some low-risk residents will fall and some high-risk residents may not fall). An effective fall risk assessment, however, should anticipate risk accurately more often than not.

Fall Preventive Interventions[3]

Staff Related

- Providing education (increasing awareness of resident fall risk and strategies to reduce risk)

- Communicating "at-risk" status (identifying fall risk status in resident's medical/nursing chart; reporting risk status at time of shift changes)

- Examining staffing patterns and maintaining adequate staff to assist high-risk residents

- Anticipating need of high-risk residents

- Monitoring high-risk residents (frequently observe fall-risk residents during the first week of institutional stay)

- Monitoring fall-risk residents during acute illnesses (represents high-risk time for falling)

- Monitoring residents during post-fall period (risk of further falls is increased)

- Developing an interdisciplinary falls consultation team to address high-risk residents with multiple falls

- Developing fall incident reports (ones that incorporate circumstances of falls/interventions)

- Developing an "Eyes/Ears" program aimed at early detection of fall risk (see "Eyes and Ears Program," pages 203–205).

Resident Related

- Attempting medication reduction (regularly reviewing resident's medications, eliminating high-risk drugs as appropriate)

- Moving confused residents near nurses' station (close observation)

- Using sitters to sit with confused residents

- Using bed alarms (to alert staff when at-risk residents are attempting unsafe mobility tasks)

- Using identifiers such as bracelets, stickers, or special socks (to identify high-risk residents)

- Having residents use nonskid footwear

- Meeting elimination needs (placing residents near toilets, using bedside commodes, routine toileting schedules)

- Providing assistive devices (canes, walkers), as appropriate
- Providing supervised ambulation programs (walking high-risk residents in hallway once per shift)
- Providing exercise programs (chair-based exercises, stretching/flexibility programs, and targeted strengthening exercises)
- Using hip protectors/pads (to reduce risk for hip fractures)
- Using gait belts to assist residents with unsteady transfers, ambulation, and balance
- Avoiding physical and chemical restraints (e.g, including use of side rails solely to prevent falls).

Environment Related

- Keeping beds in low position or using low platform beds
- Placing mats on floor along the bedside to reduce risk for injurious falls
- Keeping bed wheels locked or replacing wheels with immobilizer legs
- Using half side rails as enablers to support bed mobility
- Reducing pathway clutter around resident's bed/bedroom
- Maintaining stable furnishings (beds/chairs used to maintain balance; help with efficient transfers)
- Improving lighting (night-lights at bedside/toilet) and access to light switches
- Installing toilet grab rails (to support safe transfers)
- Installing carpeting on floor (avoids slipping on linoleum flooring)
- Maintaining wheelchair safety (removing/fixing broken wheelchairs)
- Providing frequent rest areas along hallways and other areas where residents ambulate
- Evaluating all assistive devices to ensure that they are the appropriate types.

ENDNOTES

1. Despite considerable research addressing falls in acute care hospitals, it remains somewhat unclear as to what interventions are most effective in preventing falls. Based on fall risk assessments, designing targeted, multiple interventions is the most effective way to reduce risk, especially for high-risk patients.
2. High-risk factors may differ somewhat from institution to institution.
3. Care planning by an interdisciplinary team soon after admission to design targeted, multiple interventions is the most effective way to reduce fall risk in high-risk patients.

Fall Prevention Program: Organizational Self-Assessment

One of the critical success factors in developing effective fall prevention practice is having knowledge of one's own fall prevention program, its strengths and shortcomings with respect to process and structure, and having a strategic plan to address shortcomings. Table III-1 can be used as an organizational self-assessment of your facility's fall prevention program.

Directions

For Sections 1 and 2, check off the level of implementation for each component of your fall prevention program. Section I may also be used to evaluate a specific unit or floor within your facility/organization.

Table III-1. Section I. Care process steps and components of fall prevention

Steps	Components	Implemented?
Fall Risk Assessment	Fall risk assessments are conducted on all patients/residents?	Yes ❏ No ❏
	Baseline fall risk assessments are completed upon 2 hours of admission?	Yes ❏ No ❏
	Reassessment of fall risk is completed whenever patients/residents experience a "change of condition" (e.g., decline in health/functional status, medication change)?	Yes ❏ No ❏
	Reassessment of fall risk is completed daily/every shift for certain high-risk patients/residents (e.g., recent confusion, taking sedatives, recent fall, acute illness)?	Yes ❏ No ❏
	Assessment or reassessment of fall risk is completed immediately post-fall?	Yes ❏ No ❏
	Fall risk assessment tool(s) are readily available for front-line caregivers and are easy to locate when needed?	Yes ❏ No ❏
	Fall risk tool(s) are specific for patients/residents and populations/units (e.g., rehabilitation, psychiatric/behavioral health, geriatric, ICU, long-term care, memory care)?	Yes ❏ No ❏
	Fall risk assessment includes intrinsic risk factors, such as recent fall(s), poor vision, muscle weakness, impaired sensory function, unsteady gait/balance, use of cane/walker, elimination problems, altered cognition, medications, mobility impairment, foot disorders?	Yes ❏ No ❏
	Fall risk assessment includes extrinsic or environmental risk factors, such as toilets (lack of equipment for support [e.g., grab bars]); furnishings (inappropriate bed/chair heights); floors (loose or thick-pile carpeting, sliding rugs, highly polished or wet ground surfaces); lighting (lack of night-lights); footwear (ill-fitting shoes, slippery soles); assistive devices (improper and/or broken cane, walker, or wheelchair); use of bed rails (rather than preventing falls, bed rails can increase fall risk); clutter in rooms or hallways?	Yes ❏ No ❏
	Fall risk assessment includes situational risk factors, such as new admission/post-fall (many falls occur during the first week after admission and immediately following a fall); post-meal times (need for toileting); nighttime activity (many falls occur at night, often while traveling to the bathroom and/or transferring from bed); changes in health status; exhibiting unsafe behavior (overestimation of one's abilities to self-transfer and ambulate, poor safety awareness, desire not to "bother" staff for assistance, resistance to care, not using prescribed ambulation device)?	Yes ❏ No ❏
	Following risk assessment, multidisciplinary referral is made to evaluate the cause(s) of all risk factors identified?	Yes ❏ No ❏

(continued)

Table III-1. *(continued)*

Steps	Components	Implemented?
	Fall risk signage/colored wristbands are available and used to identify at-risk status?	Yes ❑ No ❑
	Hand-off procedures are in place to communicate risk status/plan of care between caregivers, shift changes, and unit transfers?	Yes ❑ No ❑
	Strategies/procedures for monitoring at-risk patients/residents are available (e.g., fall alarms, hourly rounding, sitters)?	Yes ❑ No ❑
Care Planning	For at-risk patients/residents, multidisciplinary strategies are considered (e.g., medical, nursing, rehabilitative, and environmental interventions)?	Yes ❑ No ❑
	Use of safety technology is considered to help prevent falls and injury (e.g., fall alarms, hip protectors, low beds, floor mats, gait belts, bedside commodes, bathroom grab rails)?	Yes ❑ No ❑
	Interventions are designed around identified risk factors?	Yes ❑ No ❑
	Procedures are in place to see that the preventive plan of care has been reliably implemented?	Yes ❑ No ❑
	All caregivers are aware of risk status of patients/residents and plans of care?	Yes ❑ No ❑
Post-Fall Assessment	Post-fall assessments are conducted on all patients/residents who fall?	Yes ❑ No ❑
	Post-fall assessment includes evaluation of injuries, identification of all intrinsic/extrinsic factors contributing to the fall as well as presence of any new or additional fall risk factors, and implementation of a root cause analysis to determine "What happened?" and "Why did it happen?"	Yes ❑ No ❑
	Patients'/residents' plan of care is reviewed and appropriate strategies to prevent further falls are implemented?	Yes ❑ No ❑
	Updated plan of care and how the fall might have been avoided/prevented is communicated to all staff caring for patients/residents?	Yes ❑ No ❑

Table III-1.   Section II. Organizational components of a fall prevention program

Steps	Components	Implemented?
Culture of Safety	A "culture of safety" is in place (i.e., an environment of "no shame, no blame" in which staff are not blamed for falls, but rather falls are looked at as an opportunity for doing things better)?	Yes ❑ No ❑
	An open atmosphere is in place wherein staff members can report falls and safety concerns without fear of punishment?	Yes ❑ No ❑
	Clinical and administrative staff voluntarily report fall and injury hazards?	Yes ❑ No ❑
	All falls and injuries are discussed with patients/residents (as appropriate) and families?	Yes ❑ No ❑
Falls Coordinator	A falls coordinator or champion is available (i.e., a specifically trained nurse who can support and follow through with your fall prevention program)?	Yes ❑ No ❑
	The fall coordinator pulls together your fall prevention program (i.e., takes responsibility to coordinate fall prevention activities and sees what needs to be changed/improved)?	Yes ❑ No ❑
	The fall coordinator oversees the analysis of fall-related injuries and their causes and coordinates improvement activities?	Yes ❑ No ❑
Education	Ongoing staff education regarding fall prevention is available?	Yes ❑ No ❑
	Staff education occurs during orientation and, subsequently, on a regular basis?	Yes ❑ No ❑
	Staff receives education aimed at increasing their knowledge, skills, and abilities in identifying patients/residents at risk of falling and selecting the appropriate interventions for the prevention of falls?	Yes ❑ No ❑
	Staff receives training on the fall prevention care process and available interventions used by your facility to prevent falls, including the appropriate use of safety technology (e.g., bed alarms, low beds, hip protectors)?	Yes ❑ No ❑
	Staff receives education on specific medications, diseases, and disorders associated with falls/fall risk within your facility?	Yes ❑ No ❑
	Staff receives regular/updated education on fall prevention policies, procedures, and protocols used in your facility?	Yes ❑ No ❑
	Your facility educates patients/residents (as appropriate) and/or their family about falls and safety awareness, individual risk factors, and interventions aimed at preventing falls?	Yes ❑ No ❑

(continued)

Table III-1. *(continued)*

Steps	Components	Implemented?
Fall Management Committee	A fall management or safety committee is in place composed of medical and nursing staff, physical and occupational therapists, and administration?	Yes ❏ No ❏
	The fall committee discusses patients/residents at risk for falls, specific cases of falls, and strategies to minimize fall risk, especially in those patients/residents with recurrent falls?	Yes ❏ No ❏
Quality Improvement Activities	Auditing the fall prevention process occurs on a regular basis (i.e., evaluating whether staff are assessing risk, implementing interventions)?	Yes ❏ No ❏
	A falls surveillance system is available for monitoring the nature/severity of falls and contributing factors?	Yes ❏ No ❏
	Reviewing incident reports, tracking and trending falls, measuring fall rates, and making recommendations for improvements takes place?	Yes ❏ No ❏
	Staff are provided with timely/routine feedback on fall/injury data, improvement results, significant events, and near misses?	Yes ❏ No ❏
Administrative Support	Falls and safety are a priority in your facility?	Yes ❏ No ❏
	Management supports staff in their efforts to prevent falls?	Yes ❏ No ❏
	All policies, procedures, and manuals are updated on a regular basis?	Yes ❏ No ❏
	Required staff and/or safety technology resources are available?	Yes ❏ No ❏
	Management facilitates periodic "walk-rounds" and unit/floor meetings to learn about problems and/or to find out firsthand how fall prevention activities/efforts are going?	Yes ❏ No ❏
	The fall prevention program is analyzed annually and evaluated for potential risk factors and opportunities for improvement?	Yes ❏ No ❏

Fall Risk Assessment

PURPOSE

- To outline the approach of managing patients/residents who are at risk for falls

- To provide staff with guidance for decisions regarding fall avoidance.

STEPS

Step 1: Problem Definition

Decide whether the patient/resident is at fall risk. Common problems placing individuals at fall risk include the following:

- History of recent fall(s)

- Polypharmacy

- Cognitive impairment

- Bladder or bowel dysfunction

- Sensory changes (vision and hearing)

- Unsteady gait/balance

- Mobility impairment.

Step 2: Assessment/Problem Analysis

Complete a fall risk assessment to identify what factors place patients/residents at fall risk. Formal risk assessments should be completed at the time of admission (within 24 hours) and thereafter whenever patients/residents experience a significant change in condition (i.e., onset of acute illness, worsening of chronic diseases, medication changes).

Fall risk assessment tools help to identify whether patients/residents are at risk for falling. In order to ensure staff compliance with risk evaluation, and the likelihood of the tool being effective in terms of falls reduction, fall risk assessment tools should

- Be quick to complete and simple to use

- Include the most common factors related to falls, including a functional and environmental assessment

- Be able to identify patients/residents "at risk" or with a "high risk" of falling

- Use prompts to initiate referrals aimed at further in-depth interdisciplinary assessments, and contain immediate actions or interventions aimed at fall avoidance.

In addition to formal risk assessments, staff should assess patients/residents

- Each day for ability to transfer/ambulate

- Each shift for change of condition/environmental hazards

- Any time that a fall risk is observed (such as acute illness and/or changes in mental status).

In those patients/residents with falls

- Assess the patient/resident for injury (e.g., pain, abrasions, bruises, fractures)

- Identify circumstances surrounding the fall. Often, identifying and correcting the cause of a fall can reduce the likelihood of subsequent falls

- Communicate high-risk fall status to all members of the patient's/resident's interdisciplinary team.

Step 3: Problem Management

Use the information gathered to decide and plan how best to manage the patient's/resident's problems (i.e., what causes or risk factors are correctable). As patients/residents may have several fall risk factors, designing a care plan aimed at preventing falls is most effective when achieved through an interdisciplinary approach.

Step 4: Monitoring

Regularly evaluate the patient's/resident's progress (i.e., effectiveness of interventions and/or the need to redesign interventions).

SAMPLE TOOL

No single fall risk assessment tool meets the needs of every facility. Health professionals will either have to choose from the wide variety of risk assessment tools already available or create their own tools. Although the effectiveness of fall risk assessment tools is somewhat controversial (i.e., some tools identify a high percentage of patients/residents at risk), the real value of a risk assessment tool is that it raises staff awareness of patients/residents who are at risk of falling, and staff awareness of risk is an important first step in preventing falls. Table III-2 on pages 184–185 includes an example of the most relevant risk factors and immediate safety interventions that should be included in a fall risk assessment tool. The goal of the form is not to determine the cause(s) of risk or impairments, which should occur during routine multidisciplinary assessment and plan of care, but to provide at-risk patients/residents with *immediate* safety. Section Three, Part C includes a Fall Risk Checklist that is also helpful.

Further information/copies of fall and fall risk guidelines can be obtained from

- American Medical Directors Association (800-876-2632; www.amda.com)

- University of Iowa Nursing Interventions Research Center, Department of Nursing-RDDC, 4118 Westlawn, Iowa City, IA 52242–1100.

Table III-2. Risk factors and recommended interventions

Risk factors	Specific types of risks	Recommended interventions
Medications	Medication changes within 24 hours Anticholinergics Antipsychotics Diuretics Sedatives	Physician evaluation (drug review) Pharmacist evaluation (drug/drug and drug/food interactions) Monitor postural blood pressure (sitting/standing)
Cognitive impairments	Disorientation/delirium Dementia Depression Anxiety Impaired communication Impaired judgment	Physician evaluation Frequent observation checks Assess need to utilize sitters Assess need for bed alarms Consider moving confused patient/resident near nurses' station
History of recent fall(s)	Injurious fall(s) Fear of falling	Physician evaluation Identify/communicate "at-risk" for falls Frequent observation checks
Bladder dysfunction	Incontinence Nocturia Frequency	Physician evaluation Evaluate toileting needs/routines Consider placing patients/residents with urgency near toilets Assess need for bedside commode Consider night-lights at bedside/toilet
Sensory changes	Impaired vision Impaired hearing	Physician evaluation Provide easy access to glasses/hearing aids Observe mobility in patients/residents environment; note any difficulties encountered and modify as needed
Postural hypotension/ dizziness	Cardiovascular diseases/ medication	Physician evaluation Orthostatic vital sign checks Assess need for assistance with transfers
Unsteady gait/balance	Stroke Parkinson's disease Musculoskeletal conditions Neuromuscular conditions Foot problems	Physician evaluation Physical therapy evaluation Assistive devices (cane, walker) Assist with ambulation as needed Evaluate footwear safety (consider nonslip socks/footwear)

Table III-2. *(continued)*

Risk factors	Specific types of risks	Recommended interventions
Mobility impairment	Transfer impairment Ambulation impairment Ambulation device (cane, walker)	Physician evaluation Physical therapy evaluation Place bed in low position Consider using side rails as enablers Assist with ambulation/transfers as needed Consider use of chair/bed alarms Keep call bell within reach Evaluate safety of ambulation devices Environmental evaluation (e.g., bedroom and furnishings, bathroom, surrounding hazardous conditions), modify as needed

Fall Prevention and Restraint Avoidance Programs

PURPOSE

A commitment to patient and resident safety requires a clearly defined, coordinated, and ongoing Fall Prevention and Restraint Avoidance (FPRA) program. The goals of any FPRA program are

- To prevent and/or reduce the risk of falls and fall-related injury

- To promote patient/resident mobility and autonomy

- To avoid the use of restraints to maintain safety.

STRUCTURE

Structure and *process* represent the basic building blocks of a successful FPRA program, whether it is housed in an acute care hospital or a nursing facility. Structure refers to the "who"—the individuals needed to accomplish a program, and the "what"—the resources needed to achieve success or positive outcomes. Process refers to the "how"—the care-planning steps needed to achieve positive outcomes. Putting the two together, structure plus process equals *outcomes*. Outcomes refer to the set of goals one hopes to accomplish by having a fall prevention program in place, including reduced falls and injurious falls, reduced use of physical restraints, and enhanced mobility. The basic components for a comprehensive fall prevention and restraint reduction program follow.

Knowledge and Expertise of Health Professionals

- Educate all staff on why it is important to assess for fall risk and restraint-use risk (e.g., on the potentially harmful effects of restraints), and provide clear guidance on how and when to assess risk (e.g., once per shift, daily, only when there is a change in condition and/or medications).

- Educate all staff on the relationship between fall risk and risk for restraint use and the contributory factors for both. Staff awareness of this relationship is crucial in order to produce effective strategies.

- Educate all staff on available facility strategies for reducing/preventing falls and restraint use. Any time new devices or equipment, such as bed alarms and/or least-restraining appliances are introduced into the facility, staff should receive education and training on their benefits and how to use them properly and safely.

- Educate all staff on the institutional definition of what counts as a fall; for instance, only witnessed falls or "near falls" such as observed episodes of an individual experiencing imbalance or of being assisted down to the floor or into a chair or bed following imbalance, and unwitnessed events such as "found down on the floor." In general, an episode where the patient or resident experienced imbalance and would have fallen were it not for staff intervention or the support of walls and furnishings should be counted. Similar to actual falls, episodes of imbalance and/or "found down" can represent the first sign or symptom of an underlying intrinsic and/or extrinsic problem requiring evaluation. By correcting the underlying cause of the problem, an actual fall may be prevented from occurring. The importance of reporting both falls and near falls is to identify and communicate problems and potential problems in order to implement interventions.

- Educate all staff on why falls occur and how to evaluate patients/residents with falls (e.g., using a process of root cause analysis that attempts to identify the intrinsic, extrinsic, and organizational or process factors causative of falls).

- Educate all staff on safety policies and procedures related to fall prevention and restraint avoidance. This education should begin at the time of a staff member's orientation and should be ongoing. It is important that aides, orderlies, and those individuals providing custodial services (e.g., housekeeping, maintenance) receive education as well because they can notice patients/residents early on who may be at fall risk; for example, they may be the first to observe the onset of an individual's confusion or unsteady balance. In addition, the roles and responsibilities of each staff member need to be spelled out in terms of what they can do to prevent falls.

Number and Type of Health Professionals

Examine the number and type of health professionals needed. The precise number of staff needed is highly dependent on the number of patients/residents at fall risk and number of staff available to provide care (i.e., patient/resident mix). The type of staff includes all multidisciplinary staff needed to accomplish the fall prevention and restraint-avoidance program.

Physical Environment and Resources

- Examine the elements of the physical environment that might be placing older individuals at risk. The physical environment includes the structure of units (e.g., beds; furniture placement; types/conditions of walking surfaces; lighting/glare; safety or grab bars in hallways, bathrooms, and common areas). Environmental hazards can contribute to falls, especially in high-risk patients/residents, and interventions or modification of identified hazards can reduce risk of falling.

- Determine resources needed. Resources include availability of equipment and devices to reduce falls and restraint use (e.g., bed alarms, ambulation devices and wheelchairs, bedside commodes, wedge pillows/cushions and other positioning cushions, nonslip socks, bed transfer bars, non-restraint alternative devices). A lack of resources can contribute to falls and restraint use, and conversely, maintaining adequate resources can assist with safe mobility and can reduce the risk of falls and restraint use.

Leadership Support

Organizational leadership support (e.g., from department heads, senior management, and administration) for the FPRA program is crucial in order to move any risk reduction or avoidance practices forward. The benefits of strong leadership include

- Providing adequate resources such as staff and equipment so that interventions can be implemented

- Providing support for staff education

- Helping to break down barriers between departments so that staff work together in a multidisciplinary manner

- Ensuring dissemination of the FPRA program throughout the facility, and supporting a systemic approach to designing, implementing, analyzing, and improving efforts to prevent falls and reduce restraints

- Fostering a "culture of safety" throughout the facility (i.e., communicating the importance of fall prevention and restraint avoidance within the facility). A culture of safety includes making it safer or non-punitive for staff to report falls.

Not all falls are reflections of poor or substandard care because patients and residents who fall may show no evidence of risk for falling (e.g., when a fall is due to an unanticipated acute illness). In turn, promoting a culture of safety will result in positive attitudes and "buy-in" by staff toward the FPRA program.

Protocols and Guidelines

Facilities should have protocols and guidelines governing the FPRA program (i.e., systematically developed statements to assist staff and patient/resident decisions about the care-planning process with respect to fall prevention and restraint reduction activities). All staff need to be regularly oriented and educated to the protocols and guidelines. The most effective protocols and guidelines:

- Are straightforward, explaining who does what and when they should do it, and easy for staff to follow

- Are readily available for staff

- Describe the most common risk factors/interventions related to falls and restraint use

- Are updated periodically.

Falls/Restraint Prevention Committee

Setting up a falls/restraint prevention committee is beneficial. The purpose of this committee, composed of multidisciplinary representatives from medicine, nursing, rehabilitation, pharmacy, and social services, is to investigate falls (i.e., research the circumstances of patients and residents with injurious falls, multiple falls, or those experiencing excessive restraint use) and make recommendations for safety. In addition, it is recommended that maintenance, custodial, or housekeeping personnel also be involved in the process because facilities' layout and maintenance (e.g., lighting levels, floor conditions, broken equipment) contribute to falls.

Within the committee, identify a falls coordinator and a team leader. The falls coordinator should be an individual with knowledge and experience in falls and restraints; one who is able to provide the committee with guidance and reference resources as needed. The team leader should be an individual who is well respected in the facility (such as the director of nursing or medical director); one who can help the committee move forward within the facility. The committee may have several functions:

- Review and analyze institutional falls/restraints (e.g., incidence of fall/injurious fall frequency and restraint use; fall/injurious fall and restraint circumstances). This information will help determine causes of falls and restraint use as well as actions that can be taken to reduce falls and restraints.

- Review and revise (as needed) the current facility fall risk/restraint reduction process (i.e., identify risk and available interventions and care planning), and fall reporting mechanisms including the effectiveness of incident reports.

- Educate staff about falls and restraints. Organize a staff orientation program on fall prevention and restraint reduction, to include precautions to take and methods for preventing falls and avoiding restraints, and education on fall- and restraint-related policies, procedures, and protocols.

- Review and disseminate current government regulations related to falls and restraints, and revise policies and procedures accordingly to ensure facility compliance with regulatory mandates.

STEPS

Step 1: Risk Identification

The most important action that hospitals and nursing facilities can take is to identify an individual's risk for falls at the time he or she is admitted. To say that all older patients and residents are at risk for falls is basically true but somewhat meaningless because some patients and residents are more at risk than others. Therefore, each patient and resident should receive a falls risk assessment that uncovers factors and combinations of factors that place him or her at fall risk.

Risk assessments should address both intrinsic factors (i.e., related to the individual) and extrinsic factors (i.e., related to the environment). When health care professionals identify and correct risk factors, the majority of falls can be prevented. Hospitals and nursing facilities may choose different methods to identify fall-risk individuals. (See pages 169–170 and 172–173 for a list of risk factors.)

Facilities should have a method for all staff to recognize patients and residents at high risk for falls. Visual reminders of patients/residents who are "at risk," such as colored identification bands, colored nonslip socks, and/or bedroom door and bed stickers indicating "at risk" are the most commonly used ways of identifying patients/residents at fall risk. Wrist identification bands and nonslip socks are the most effective because they are a portable method of identification; wherever "at-risk" patients/residents are on the unit, staff will recognize them.

Facility staff should investigate all falls and complete a written report for each. Incident or occurrence reports should include circumstances of the fall, responsible causes or contributing factors, and presence of any injury. A re-assessment of fall risk should be done post-fall, since the patient/resident may have new risk factors.

Step 2: Develop a Care Plan

After completing the risk assessment, staff should develop a care plan for patients/residents with specific, individualized interventions matched to identified fall risk factors. The care plan should identify various risk factors that increase the likelihood of falls and restraint use, interdisciplinary interventions aimed at reducing fall and restraint-use risk, intervention goals, responsible disciplines for completing the interventions, and a time frame for evaluating the effectiveness of interventions. If falls continue to occur, consider other possible reasons for fall risk besides those already identified. For those patients and residents who fall repeatedly and/or require restraints (i.e., where the cause cannot be modified or controlled), identify ways to reduce the risk of injurious falls and restraint complications.

Step 3: Follow-Up

Evaluate and re-evaluate outcomes or the effectiveness of interventions included in the care plan on a continual basis, and revise the patient's/resident's plan of care as needed. Steps of a good follow-up plan include the following:

- Complete a fall and restraint risk assessment whenever a patient/resident experiences a change of condition and/or states problems with imbalance, mobility, and so forth.

- Observe and communicate "at-risk" status (includes keeping an eye on patients/residents, particularly those individuals at risk, and communicating with physicians and ancillary providers regarding the current risk status of patients/residents).

- Document and evaluate all falls when they occur to see what other interventions can be put into place to prevent falls.

Step 4: Evaluation

Monitor and measure fall rates and restraint use rates over time. Monitoring falls and restraint use trends is of benefit from two perspectives: evaluating the effectiveness of FPRA programs, and assessing patient/resident outcomes (i.e., whether fall and restraint rates have decreased). Methods for calculating fall rates and restraint use rates are listed in Measuring Fall Rates and Restraint Use Rates (pp. 200–202).

Audit the process of care. This step is crucial, especially if no improvements in falls and/or restraint use occur. Information obtained can help to determine areas for improvement. Documentation should reflect steps in the care-planning process (e.g., consistently using fall-risk tools, identifying risk factors and appropriate interventions in the patient's/resident's care plan), the benefits of interventions, and the patient's or resident's response.

Provide staff with regular feedback on the audit results, especially if positive. Staff are more likely to be compliant with the care-planning process if they know that their efforts are improving care.

Critical steps in determining the effectiveness of a facility's care planning process include a review of the facility's policies and procedures that govern the care-planning process. Evaluating the process of care in conjunction with analysis of falls and restraint data assists facilities in creating a cycle of continuous improvement (i.e., changes or modifications continue to be made in the FPRA program in response to the audit's results).

BARRIERS TO A SUCCESSFUL FALL PREVENTION AND RESTRAINT AVOIDANCE PROGRAM

Certain situational factors or hidden disaster risks always exist to a certain extent in any facility that can hinder the care-planning process or implementation of strategies intended to prevent falls. Any breakdown in structure and process has the potential to make the difference between an organized versus an unorganized process, and whether good versus poor outcomes occur. As well, any failure in process can expose facilities to liability risk. By identifying structure and process problems, facilities can greatly improve the care-planning process and increase the likelihood of reducing the risk of falls and avoiding restraints. Some of the most important structural and process barriers interfering with successful outcomes include:

- Poorly trained staff (i.e., those with a lack of knowledge about risk assessment, procedures, and/or preventive interventions)

- Inadequate or inaccurate risk assessments

- Sub-optimal or lack of communication among staff related to patient/resident risk

- Lack of chart documentation related to patient/resident risk

- Delayed multidisciplinary referrals (i.e., further evaluation by necessary professional or trained staff of patient/resident risk and/or identification of underlying problems)

- Staff shortages

- Inadequate staff/patient and resident ratios (i.e., insufficient staff to properly care for the number of patients/residents requiring care)

- Constant staff turnover

- Delayed or insufficient medical and nursing care

- Reduced use of restraints without available non-restraint alternatives

- Malfunction of equipment (e.g., nurse call system, bed alarm systems, bed wheel locking systems, wheelchairs)

- Lack of established policies and procedures regarding falls and restraint prevention

- Staff noncompliance with protocols/procedures

- Inadequate resources (e.g., bed alarm devices, assistive devices, non-restraint alternatives).

Restraint/Non-Restraint Utilization Assessment

PURPOSE

- To outline the approach to managing patients/residents who are at risk for physical restraint use

- To provide staff with guidance for decisions regarding the use of physical restraints and non-restraint use.

STEPS

Step 1: Problem Definition

Decide whether there is a problem indicating need for physical restraint use. Common reasons for physical restraint use include

- Falls/fall risk

- Unsafe wandering

- Agitated behavior

- Interference with medical treatment (i.e., use of tubes, intravenous lines, catheters, and so forth).

Step 2: Assessment/Problem Analysis

- Identify the root cause of the problem or what is causing the patient's/resident's behavior.

- Talk to the patient/resident in order to determine circumstances surrounding the behavior.

- Review the patient's/resident's health problems and medications.

- Identify factors that place the patient/resident at risk for restraint use.

Step 3: Problem Management

- Decide how to best manage the patient's/resident's condition (i.e., which causes are correctable or modifiable and which conditions require consideration of restraints or non-restraint alternatives).

Step 4: Monitoring

- Evaluate the patient's/resident's progress in relation to the problem and effectiveness of interventions.

SAMPLE TOOL

A blank restraint assessment tool that can be used to compile the most relevant information is included in Part C of Section Three. Further information/copies of physical restraint guidelines can be obtained from

- American Medical Directors Association (800-876-2632; www.amda.com)

- University of Iowa Nursing Interventions Research Center, Department of Nursing-RDDC, 4118 Westlawn, Iowa City, IA 52242-1100.

Framework
for Reducing
Physical Restraints

PURPOSE

The purpose of this framework is to provide the basis necessary for facilities to reduce or eliminate physical restraints (Table III-3).

Definition

Patients or residents who are frail, medically complex, or cognitively impaired are at greatest risk of being placed in or considered for physical restraints.

USE OF RESTRAINTS

The most common reasons given for using restraints are for:

- Safety (i.e., preventive measure against falling)

- Management of situations that may be difficult or time-consuming for staff (e.g., altered mental status, disruptive behavior, and functional dependence)

- Prevention of treatment interference (e.g., protection of nasogastric tubes, Foley catheters, bladder catheters).

The overall prevalence of restraint use in acute and long-term care facilities ranges from 4% to 68%. This wide variation may be explained by a number of contributing factors, which include the following:

- Facility's staffing mix and workload

- Facility's leadership support

- Availability of restraint-free alternatives

- Beliefs about whether restraints provide a safer environment

Table III-3. What are physical restraints?

- Physical restraints are items used to restrict, restrain, or prevent movement of a patient or resident. According to the Omnibus Budget Reconciliation Act (OBRA)* guidelines of 1991, restraints are defined as "any method or physical or mechanical device, material or equipment attached or adjacent to the patient's body that the individual cannot remove easily which restricts freedom of movement or normal access to one's body." Examples include waist belts, geri-chairs, restraint jackets, hand mitts, and wheelchair safety bars. Bedside rails that keep a person from getting out of bed are considered a physical restraint as well. Staff practices that may be defined as physical restraint include tucking in a sheet so tightly that a patient or resident cannot move and placing a wheelchair by a wall so that the person in it is prevented from rising.

- Whether or not a particular device or item is considered a physical restraint depends on the purpose and effect of its use. If an item is used to restrict movement, it is a restraint. The same item may not be considered a restraint if it is used to enable mobility or function. For example, a bed rail could be used to keep someone from getting out of bed (restraint), or it could be used to help someone turn over in bed (enabler).

- The federal regulations do not specifically prohibit the use of restraints; rather, they set parameters that must be met for use of a restraint to be considered appropriate. First and foremost, the physical restraint must be used only to treat medical symptoms and only after a comprehensive assessment indicating that the device is the least restrictive intervention and that it promotes the patient's or resident's highest level of function. In addition, if the restraint is deemed the most appropriate intervention, its use must be monitored for adverse effects, and ongoing attempts must be made to find less restrictive alternatives. Such alternatives include personal strengthening and rehabilitation programs, use of assistive devices (e.g., transfer aids, mobility devices), efforts to design a safer physical environment, and use of fall alarms to alert staff when a resident needs assistance.

*Omnibus Budget Regulation Act (OBRA) of 1987, 1989, and 1990. Health Care Financing Administration, as published in the *Federal Register*, September 26, 1991, and March 6, 1992, and Interpretive Guideline of April 1, 1992.

- Fear of litigation

- Concern about negative state and federal survey results.

ADVERSE EFFECTS OF RESTRAINT USE

Physical restraints are associated with a number of negative health outcomes:

- Increased falls (i.e., restraints do not lower the risk of falls or fall-related injuries); removing restraints does not increase fall risk (i.e., restrained people are three times more likely to be injured during a fall than are unrestrained people)

- Premature death (i.e., as many as 200 deaths occur every year as a result of strangulation or suffocation from restraints)

- Urinary incontinence and problems with elimination

- Circulation impairment

- Orthostatic hypotension

- Skin breakdown and pressure ulcer development

- Joint contractures

- Decreased mobility

- Decreased muscle mass and strength

- Reduced sensory and perceptual input

- Symptoms of withdrawal or depression and resulting social isolation

- Increased agitation, confusion, combativeness, and delirium.

In addition to adverse health outcomes, physical restraints may affect staff resources:

- Patients or residents who are restrained consume more staff resources than do unrestrained ones.

- Documentation and care of restrained patients or residents consume staff time.

- Response to adverse restraint outcomes consumes staff time.

ACHIEVING RESTRAINT REDUCTION

The success of a restraint elimination program depends on the following (see also Table III-4):

- Staff adhering to an organized clinical practice

- Training and education

- Strong leadership and organizational commitment.

Assessment

- Screen patients or residents for fall risk, behavioral symptoms, medical treatments that increase fall risk, and any other associated care issues related to risk of restraint use.

- Empower all members of the interdisciplinary team to continually assess problems, such as fall risk, that may lead to restraint use.

- Ensure that assessment tools capture the necessary data to address risk factors related to falls, behaviors, and related care issues.

- Obtain information from the patient or resident, family, or caregivers regarding the person's life experiences, interests, and social patterns in order to provide an individualized approach to care.

Care Planning

- Incorporate assessment data into care plans.

Table III-4.   Benefits of removing restraints

- Unrestrained patients or residents tend to be less agitated, less fatigued, and more social.
- Unrestrained patients or residents experience fewer injurious falls.
- Unrestrained patients or residents exhibit greater independence with toileting, mobility, feeding, dressing, and strength, which decreases the burden of care.
- Reducing restraints increases staff morale and decreases staff turnover.

- Designate staff responsibility and accountability for care plan development, implementation, and oversight.

- Develop individualized, targeted interventions and goals related to providing the highest functional status and least restrictive environment.

- Integrate approaches for restraint elimination and prevention of complications (i.e., contractures, skin breakdown, and incontinence) in care plans.

- Implement an interdisciplinary team approach (including certified nursing assistants, nurses, and other staff who interact with patients or residents) for achieving the goals in the care plan.

- Use an interdisciplinary approach and involve the patient or resident and family (or legal decision maker) in development of an individualized care plan to meet the specific social and personal needs of the patient or resident.

Management

- Offer adequate activity and exercise for all patients or residents in an environment that provides frequent structured supervision.

- Address individual needs for staff assistance and equipment during toileting, transfer, ambulation, and all activities of daily living to promote safety.

- Modify the environment to accommodate special needs and limitations of patients or residents.

- Ensure that treatment is addressing the true root cause of the problem.

- Standardize processes for communicating treatment plans to all members of the interdisciplinary care team, patients or residents, and family members.

- Provide a supportive structure to staff, family, and patients or residents to allow feedback on care planning, environment and equipment, safety, and satisfaction.

- Consistently assign staff to the same person or unit to encourage learning of patients' or residents' routines and preferences.

Monitoring

- Standardize processes for monitoring and documenting the patient's or resident's response to the care plan and for revising care plans.

- Regularly inspect and repair environmental safety hazards (clutter, poor or insufficient lighting, unstable furniture, hard-to-reach personal items, unsafe flooring) in all bedrooms, bathrooms, hallways, and common areas.

- Regularly inspect and repair all wheelchairs, canes, walkers, and other equipment such as geri-chairs and lifts.

- Reassess and modify care plans until patients or residents are achieving the highest level of functioning in the least restrictive environment.

Training and Education

- Staff must have education, training, and demonstrated knowledge of assessment techniques to identify patient or resident behaviors, events, and environmental factors that may trigger the need to use restraint and to choose the least restrictive interventions based on individualized assessment.

- Staff must demonstrate competency related to restraint reduction (i.e., recognize underlying causes of behavior that may warrant the use of restraints and know about least restraint interventions to implement).

- Restraint reduction training and education (i.e., general and specific behavior management strategies, comprehensive fall management, and appropriate fall response techniques) must be incorporated into new staff orientation and annual training for all staff.

ORGANIZATIONAL COMMITMENT

Organizational support is an important element of a successful restraint reduction program. One of the most important factors in reducing restraint use is the commitment of administrative leadership to guide facilities in the process of restraint reduction. Administrative tasks include the following:

- Establish a facility-wide commitment to developing and maintaining an environment of restraint reduction.

- Provide effective ongoing training on physical restraint elimination for staff and family members; discuss the risks and consequences of physical restraints and the facility's commitment to a restraint-free environment.

- Identify a team of key staff to participate in interdisciplinary physical restraint elimination.

- Implement policies and protocols related to restraint reduction.

- Evaluate the effectiveness of the physical restraint elimination program.

- Indicate the staffing and other resources necessary to implement restraint reduction.

- Provide staff with rewards and incentives in recognition of physical restraint reduction or elimination.

Measuring Fall Rates and Restraint Use Rates

PURPOSE

Measuring fall rates and restraint use rates in a standardized manner helps organizations to:

- Monitor internal performance over time and trends in order to identify opportunities for improvement

- Compare rates with external organizations (e.g., organizations with "similar" populations) in order to provide target goals.

Fall rates and restraint use rates are usually expressed as percentages and calculated by month and quarter, with comparisons throughout the year to show trends and relationships to fall-preventive and restraint-reduction activities.

Rate of Falls

The rate of falls is calculated by dividing the number of falls by the number of patient/resident days[1] and multiplying the resulting quotient by 1000.

Number of Falls × 1000 ÷ Number of Patient/Resident Days = Rate of Falls

Rate of Residents with Repeated Falls

The rate of patients/residents with repeated falls is calculated by dividing the number of patients/residents with more than one fall by the number of patients/residents experiencing one or more falls during the reported period and multiplying the quotient by 100.

Number of Patients/Residents with More Than One Fall ÷ Number of Patients/Residents Experiencing One or More Falls × 100 = Rate of Patients/Residents with Repeated Falls

Rate of Injurious Falls

The rate of injurious falls is calculated by dividing the number of injurious falls by the number of falls and multiplying the resulting quotient by 100.

Number of Injurious Falls × 100 ÷ Number of Falls = Rate of Injurious Falls

OTHER WAYS TO RATE FALLS

Several other ways to further stratify fall rates to assist organizations in determining risk factors and identifying opportunities for improvement are used:

- By unit type (e.g., rehabilitation, geropsychiatry, ICUs)

- By cause of falls (e.g., medical/functional conditions, medication types, environmental hazards, time of day, length of stay, location).

Physical Restraint-Use Rates

The rate of physical restraint events (defined as the period between restraint initiation time and release time) is calculated by dividing the number of physical restraint events by the number of patient/resident days[1] and multiplying the resulting quotient by 100.

Number of Physical Restraint Events ÷ Number of Patient/Resident Days
× 100 = Rate of Physical Restraint-Use Events

Rate of Patients/Residents with Restraints

The rate of patients/residents with physical restraints is calculated by dividing the number of patients/residents with one or more physical restraint events by the number of patients/residents and multiplying the resulting quotient by 100.

Number of Patients/Residents with One or More Physical Restraints
÷ Number of Patients/Residents × 100 = Rate of Patients/Residents with Restraints

Rate of Repeated Restraint Use

The repeated restraint-use rate is calculated by dividing the number of patients/residents with more than one physical restraint event by the number of patients/residents with one or more physical restraint events and multiplying the resulting quotient by 100.

Number of Patients/Residents with More than One Physical Restraint Event
÷ Number of Patient/Residents with One or More Physical Restraint Events
= Repeated Restraint-Use Rate

Rate of Duration of Physical Restraint Events

The rates for physical restraint events by specified duration[2] are calculated by dividing the number of physical restraint events for a specified duration by the total number of physical restraint events and multiplying the resulting quotient by 100.

Number of Physical Restraint Events by Specified Duration ÷ Number of Physical Restraint Events × 100 = Rate of Physical Restraint Events by Duration

Rate of Physical Restraint Events by Reason

The rates for physical restraint events by reason are calculated by dividing the number of physical restraint events by specified reason (e.g., to prevent falls, agitation) by the total number of physical restraint events and multiplying the resulting quotient by 100.

Number of Physical Restraint Events by Specified Reason ÷ Number of Physical Restraint Events × 100 = Rate of Physical Restraint Events by Reason

ENDNOTES

1. The "number of patient/resident days" is calculated by adding the number of patient/resident days, or census, for each calendar day of the month.
2. Restraint duration is the cumulative time from restraint initiation to restraint removal for each restraint event.

Eyes and Ears Program

PURPOSE

To train staff to detect clinical change of not-yet-visible problems/illness and risk before falls occur; to prevent falls by heightening staff's awareness of patients/residents at high risk for falls. The more eyes available to watch older adults at high risk (e.g., observing warning signs such as unsteady balance or a change in condition such as agitation, confusion, weakness or tiredness, needing help with their daily activities) and the more ears available to hear the messages of high-risk older adults that indicate fall risk (e.g., listening to an individual talk about his or her symptoms, such as feeling dizzy or unwell, or problems with balance and/or functional activities), the better it is. Changes noted in an individual's behavior and functional activities can often serve as an early alerting mechanism to the clinical staff (e.g., to look for an underlying cause, disease/drug reaction) and help to prevent falls.

Who Should Watch

All facility employees who are in regular contact with patients/residents and/or their environments. This group should include nursing aides/assistants, housekeeping, dietary, laundry, clerical, maintenance, and administrative staff in addition to medical, nursing, rehabilitation, pharmacy, and social services staff who are already involved in daily care responsibilities. As well, available family members can be involved in the program.

Who Should Be Watched

Patients/residents most likely to benefit from an eyes and ears monitoring program include:

- Frequent fallers (e.g., those with two or more falls)

- Frequent wanderers

- Patients/residents with dementia and gait/balance impairments.

It is important to limit the number of patients to be monitored as part of the Eyes and Ears program because identifying too many patients/residents to monitor may desensitize staff from paying attention to those most at risk for falling.

STEPS

Step 1: Educate All Employees

Educate all employees about the program. Arrange a half-hour in-service presentation on the importance of fall prevention within the facility (i.e., for both the facility in terms of legal liability and patients/residents with regard to harmful consequences), the necessity for identifying patients/residents at fall risk, an explanation of the eyes and ears program, and what role or responsibilities employees have in the program. It's important to educate employees by sharpening their observational and listening skills while recognizing employee limitations. For example, maintenance employees can be taught to conduct weekly rounds to observe for environmental factors, such as lighting levels, floor conditions, broken or defective wheelchairs, bed brakes, and so forth.

Step 2: Formalize a Reporting System

Employees participating in the program need to have an established person with whom they can share their patient/resident and environmental observations (e.g., the head nurse).

Step 3: Determine the Patients/Residents Who Will Be Included

Identify patients and residents who should be included in the program and document their program participation in their chart.

Step 4: Visibly Identify "At-Risk" Program Participants

Identify at-risk program participants by a colorful identification wristband or sticker (e.g., a falling star or leaf). This enables employees to quickly identify patients and residents who are part of the program and at high risk for falling. A colorful identification wristband or sticker is a signal to observe the patient/resident closely and to intervene if the patient/resident displays any unsafe behaviors (getting up from bed without assistance) and/or voices any problems. This also helps alert staff who may not be familiar with patients/residents (such as agency nurses and other staff) to the individual's risk status. Affix the sticker

- By the patient's/resident's room

- Above the bed

- To his or her ambulation device (e.g., cane, walker, wheelchair).

Step 5: Identify Times of High Risk for Falls

Identify times when patients/residents may be most at risk for falls in order to anticipate their needs, such as before or right after meals; while going to the bathroom, getting out of or back into bed, or during toileting; late afternoon (because of shift changes, sundowning, or late afternoon confusion); or downtime between activities (because of boredom, patients/residents may become restless and try to get up from chairs/beds and fall). This alerts all employees in contact with the patients/residents that special care and supervision are required.

Step 6: Evaluation

Monitor outcomes of the Eyes and Ears program. This will help determine if the program and actions taken to reduce fall risk are effective.

Ambulation
Device Measurement

Cane Measurements

The measurement of cane height is the same regardless of cane type. Ask the person wearing everyday shoes to stand erect, with arms hanging loosely by his or her sides. The cane (or center of a multistem cane) is placed approximately 6 inches to the front and side of the person's shoe.

Two landmarks are used to determine proper height: the greater trochanter and the angle of the elbow. The top of the cane should come to approximately the level of the greater trochanter and the elbow should be flexed at 20°–30°. The degree of elbow flexion is the most important indicator of correct height because it allows the arm to shorten or lengthen during different phases of gait. This degree of flexion prevents the person from leaning forward or into the cane (if too short) or away, or leaning precariously backward (if too tall).

Walker Measurements

The measurement of walker height is similar to that of a cane. Place the walker 10–12 inches in front of the person's feet so that the walker partially surrounds the person. In this position, the handles should come to approximately the greater trochanter and the elbow is flexed at 20°–30°.

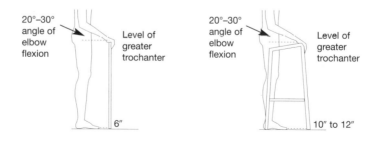

20°–30° angle of elbow flexion

Level of greater trochanter

6"

20°–30° angle of elbow flexion

Level of greater trochanter

10" to 12"

Ambulation Device Utilization

Cane Ambulation: Level Ground

For cane ambulation on level ground, the cane is held on the side of the body that is opposite to the affected limb. This position provides the greatest base of support and simulates normal gait. When the cane is held on the same side of the body as that of the affected limb, the person's center of gravity shifts from side to side. This position produces an abnormal, uncomfortable gait and leads to instability.

The cane and the involved extremity are advanced simultaneously (see figure on page 208). The cane is held relatively close to the body and should not be placed ahead of the affected limb. Placing the cane too far to the side or forward will cause lateral bending, forward bending, or both, resulting in a loss of stability.

Walker Ambulation: Level Ground

Standard Walker   Ambulation using the standard walker on level ground requires the person to have enough stability to balance on one or both feet while he or she picks up the walker and moves it forward. The "step to" and "step through" gaits are the ones used most often for stability and to protect arthritic joints. Weight is placed on the hands (i.e., hands push down on walker) and, at the same time, the other, unaffected foot is moved forward, either parallel to ("step to" gait) or past ("step through" gait) the opposite, affected foot. The person should not step too close to the front bar of the walker because this motion decreases the base of support and may cause the person to fall backward.

Sliding Walker   The use of the sliding walker is similar to that of the standard walker, except that the sliding walker is not picked up but slid along the floor. A "step to" or "step through" gait is employed.

Rolling Walker   Weight is shifted from all four walker legs to the forward (wheeled) legs. The walker is rolled forward until the hands are 10–12 inches ahead of the feet. A "step to" or "step through" gait is employed.

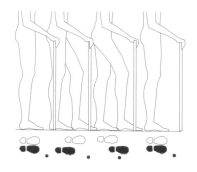

Step pattern using cane.

Cane Ambulation: Turning

Turning is accomplished by moving to the unaffected side using a gait similar to that used when walking on level ground surfaces. To start, feet are kept slightly apart in order to maintain balance. The cane and feet are moved in a small circle. The following sequence is used: First, the cane and the affected limb are moved, then the unaffected limb is moved. The unaffected limb is kept on the inside of the circle. The person should not pivot on the unaffected limb to maintain his or her balance. The process is repeated until the turn is complete (see the figure on page 209).

Walker Ambulation: Turning

Turning with a walker is similar to that of turning with a cane. A "step to" or "step through" gait is employed.

Cane Transfers: Standing

In making a cane transfer to the standing position, the person slides forward to the edge of his or her seat. The standard cane is placed against the chair armrest; the quad cane or hemi-walker cane is positioned in front of and to the unaffected side of the body. The person places his or her feet in the stride position (i.e., unaffected leg behind affected leg) with both hands on the armrests, leans forward and comes to a standing position, and then grasps the cane.

Walker Transfers: Standing

In making a walker transfer to the standing position, the person moves forward to the edge of his or her seat. The walker is positioned directly in front of the chair. The person places his or her feet in the stride position (i.e., unaffected leg behind affected leg), grasps both armrests of the chair, leans forward and comes to a standing position by pushing down on the armrests, and then reaches for the walker.

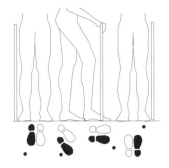

Step pattern while turning with cane.

Cane Transfers: Sitting

In making a cane transfer to the sitting position, the person approaches the chair, turns in a small circle toward the unaffected side of the body, and backs up until the chair edge is felt against the legs. The person reaches for the chair armrest with his or her free hand, releases the broad-based cane or leans the standard cane against the chair, grasps the opposite armrest, and sits down.

Walker Transfers: Sitting

In making a walker transfer to the sitting position, the person approaches the chair, turns in a small circle toward the unaffected side of the body, and backs up until the chair edge is felt against the legs. The person reaches for one chair armrest at a time, releases his or her grasp on the walker, and sits down.

Bed Safety

PURPOSE

To help care providers learn strategies for preventing falls from beds. One of the most common locations of falls in hospitals and nursing facilities is from bed, and the act of transferring in or out of bed is one of the most common causes of falls. The key to preventing falls from bed is for caregivers and patients to adhere to an organized process, which consists of the following steps.

STEPS

Step 1: Assessment

Bed mobility is best assessed by observing the patient/resident transferring from his or her bed and observing whether the individual is able to accomplish the task in a safe manner (see the "Performance-Oriented Environmental Mobility Screen" [POEMS] in Section Three, Part C). This takes only a few minutes to complete and provides more useful information than simply asking patients/ residents about whether they are able to transfer safely from bed. Some patients/residents overstate their transfer ability because they may feel embarrassed about having difficulty getting up from bed. Other patients/ residents may think that their transfers are safe, when in fact they are hazardous. Finally, patients/residents with dementia and other communication impairments will not be able to accurately describe their bed transfers.

In those patients/residents exhibiting poor bed mobility, it is important to assess for any underlying diseases and/or medications that may be interfering with safe transfers and to treat any problems found. Strategies include management of active chronic diseases and discontinuation of all offending medications.

Step 2: Intervention

- Exercise programs aimed at improving upper/lower extremity strength and joint range of motion as well as balance performance can increase transfer skills.

- Maximizing transfer tasks by choosing beds that meet functional needs can help promote safe transfers and reduce the likelihood of falling. Adaptive strategies to make beds safer for patients/residents include (1) proper bed height to allow for safe transfers, (2) firm mattress to support sitting balance, (3) application of non-slip adhesive strips on the floor along the length of the bed for stable footing during transfers, and (4) locking bed wheels or using immobilizer legs to prevent the bed from rolling away during transfers.

Step 3: Consideration of Bedside Rails

Some patients/residents will continue to remain at fall risk despite these interventions and/or bed modifications. Occasionally, side rails may be used to support safe bed activities. (See "Side Rail Utilization Assessment," page 213, which list the potential benefits of side rails.) When considering the use of a bedside rail, it is important to first assess the patient/resident and identify what, if any, factors place the individual at risk for problems related to side rail use (see "Side Rail Utilization Assessment"). The indiscriminate use of side rails can be hazardous, but side rails can be both appropriate and beneficial when evaluated and considered through a well-thought-out, individualized assessment and plan of care involving patients/residents in the decision process as appropriate. Second, determine the following:

- Does the patient/resident want side rails?

- What is the intent of side rails (i.e., what do you want to accomplish)?

- What is the effect on the patient's/resident's function (i.e., will side rails hinder or assist mobility)?

- Will side rails prevent or facilitate what the patient/resident wants to do?

- Do the benefits of side rails outweigh the risks of potential harm for this individual?

Types of Side Rails

- Full-length side rails are most useful for patients/residents who are immobile because they prevent the individuals from rolling out of bed. The use of side rail pads or protective coverings can help to prevent injuries in patients/residents at risk for thrashing about while in bed, such as those with dementia.

- Half side rails are beneficial as enablers to assist patients/residents with poor bed mobility/transfers.

- Bed alarm systems, which alert staff to individuals who are leaving their beds so that staff can check on them immediately, may be used in conjunction with both full- and half-length rails to help detect fall risk and avoid falls early on.

Alternatives to Side Rails

If side rails pose a risk of harm for an individual, some alternatives to consider include:

- Equipping the bed with a trapeze bar to increase bed mobility
- Keeping the bed in the lowest position with bed wheels locked
- Using low platform beds or beds that can be lowered close to the floor
- Placing mats on the floor next to the bed to prevent falls from bed from being injurious (Caution: Individuals with gait/balance impairments may be at risk of tripping over the mat. For these individuals, placing the mat on the floor after the person is in bed and taking up the mat before they get out of bed may be tried.).

Step 4: Monitoring

- Anticipate the reasons patients/residents get out of bed, such as to go to the bathroom. By meeting the patient's/resident's needs, the risk of falls can be averted.
- Re-evaluate mobility on a regular basis, especially following falls.
- Re-evaluate the risks and possible effects of side rails against the risks and potential beneficial effects of alternatives to side rails. As the patients/residents either improve or worsen, the indications for side rails are subject to change.
- Inspect bed frames, side rails, and mattresses regularly for potential entrapment hazards. It's important to use compatible side rails and mattresses to prevent gaps in which patients/residents could be entrapped. Beds, mattresses, and side rails are designed to fit together, but commonly, pieces are purchased separately and replaced as equipment wears out. This can leave gaps large enough to trap an individual between the mattress and side rail, putting the individual at risk of injury or suffocation.

Side Rail
Utilization Assessment

PURPOSE

To assist staff in determining the appropriate use of side rails. Side rails can be regarded as physical restraints if they restrict the movement of a patient/resident, or as "enablers" if they support the bed mobility of a patient/resident. When side rails are used or considered to enable mobility, assessment should include a review of the following factors regarding a patient/resident:

- Bed mobility (i.e., does the side rail assist the patient/resident to turn from side to side while in bed or is the patient/resident totally immobile and unable to shift without assistance?)

- Bed transfers (i.e., does the side rail help the patient/resident get up safely from bed with minimal risk of falling?).

STEPS

- *Step 1:* Gather baseline data.

- *Step 2:* Describe rationale for potential side rail use.

- *Step 3:* Determine side rail use recommendations. Describe when and why side rails are used (i.e., how long and under what circumstances).

- *Step 4:* Include any physicians' orders for side rail use.

- *Step 5:* Notify patient/resident and family of side rail use.

- *Step 6:* Obtain staff signatures and dates (include all members of the patient's/resident's interdisciplinary care team).

SAMPLE TOOL

A blank restraint assessment tool that can be used to compile this information is included in Part C of Section Three.

Using Adjustable Low Beds

PURPOSE

To provide guidance on the use of height-adjustable low beds in helping to prevent injurious falls from bed.

Definition

An important goal of fall prevention is to reduce the risk of injurious falls from bed. Low beds (i.e., beds that rest 7–13 inches above the floor) are often recommended for those at risk for falling out of bed. The reduced bed height is effective in reducing the likelihood of a fall-related serious injury. Adjustable-height low beds are preferred over fixed-height low beds.

- The low height allows patients or residents to rest comfortably at the lowest height level, eliminating the risk of serious injury caused by falls from greater heights.

- Adjustable low beds are designed to rise to a comfortable working height, which allows nursing, housekeeping, and other multidisciplinary staff greater ease and less strain in performing daily caregiver tasks.

LOW BED PROTOCOL

A best practice clinical approach to using low beds consists of the following:

Step 1: Assessing Fall Risk

The purpose of risk assessment is to identify patients or residents most likely to fall and raise staff awareness of fall risk (Table III-5). The rationale for this assessment is that if patients or residents at high risk can be identified, then appropriate interventions (including the use of low beds) can be instituted to minimize their risk of falling and injury.

Step 2: Assessing Bed Mobility

Several internal risk factors by themselves can increase susceptibility to falls. However, a true measure of bed fall risk is more accurately reflected by the

Table III-5.   Fall risk factors

Internal or Health Factors

- Recent falls (a history of falls is the best predictor of future falls)
- Poor vision (cataracts, macular degeneration, glaucoma)
- Lower extremity dysfunction (arthritis, muscle weakness, impaired sensory function)
- Unsteady gait or balance (e.g., stroke, Parkinson's disease)
- Use of a cane or walker (ambulation aids are a marker for underlying gait and balance disorders)
- Elimination problems (excessive nighttime urination, incontinence)
- Altered cognition (dementia, depression, agitation)
- Fear of falling (leads to overcaution, fear of walking, and consequently weakness, poor balance, and increased fall risk)
- Polypharmacy (four or more prescription drugs)
- Medication side effects (especially drugs that affect central nervous system, such as sedatives and tranquilizers)
- Mobility impairment (bed, toilet, and chair or wheelchair transfers)
- Foot deformities (corns, calluses, and bunions can destabilize gait)

External or Environmental Factors

- Toilets (lack of equipment for support, such as grab bars)
- Furnishings (inappropriate bed and chair heights)
- Floors (loose or thick-pile carpeting, sliding rugs, highly polished or wet ground surfaces)
- Poor lighting (lack of night-lights)
- Footwear (ill-fitting shoes, slippery soles)
- Assistive devices (improper or broken cane, walker, or wheelchair)
- Bed rails (rather then preventing falls, bed rails increase the risk of injurious falls)
- Clutter in rooms or hallways

Behavioral Factors

- Walking in stocking feet or in shoes with high heels
- Rushing to the bathroom (especially at night when not fully awake or when lighting is inadequate)
- Failing to use a cane or walker for balance support
- Exhibiting unsafe behavior (overestimation of one's abilities to self-transfer and ambulate, poor safety awareness, desire not to "bother" staff for assistance, and resistance to care)

Situational Factors

- New admission (many falls occur during the first week after admission)
- Recent fall (many falls occur immediately after a fall)
- Post-meal times (need for toileting)
- Nighttime (many falls occur at night, often while one is traveling to the bathroom or transferring from bed)
- Acute diseases or changes in condition (e.g., urinary infection, pneumonia, acute dehydration, cerebrovascular accident, transient ischemic attack, acute medication reaction, sudden hypoglycemia or hyperglycemia)

effect of internal risk factors on the patient's or resident's ability to transfer safely and independently from bed. Any observed impairment in bed transfers is a strong predictor of fall risk. This is accomplished by asking patients or residents to perform a number of simple bed mobility maneuvers and observing whether they can accomplish these activities safely and independently. (See "Performance-Oriented Bed Mobility Screen," in Section Three,

Part C.) Patients or residents who are able to complete the maneuvers normally are considered independent in bed mobility and represent a low fall risk, despite the presence of intrinsic or extrinsic risk factors. Conversely, patients or residents demonstrating one or more abnormal maneuvers have poor bed mobility and are at high risk, due to internal or external factors or a combination of both, and may be suitable candidates for a low bed.

Step 3: Assessing Injurious Fall Risk and the Need for a Low Bed

The purpose of this assessment is to identify those most likely to suffer injurious falls. The rationale for this assessment is that if patients or residents at high injury risk can be identified, then appropriate interventions, such as providing a low bed, can be instituted to minimize their risk of injury. Patients or residents at greatest risk for injurious falls and most suitable for a low bed include those with

- Unsteady balance and frequent falls from bed

- History of injurious falls from bed

- Osteoporosis

- Diseases (e.g., stroke, Parkinson's disease, diabetes, Alzheimer's disease) associated with balance loss and risk for injurious falls

- Medications associated with balance loss and injurious falls (e.g., narcotics, sedatives, or antidepressants)

- Seizure disorders

- Dementia with agitated behaviors.

Step 4: Assessing the Need for Added Injurious Fall Precautions

When using a low bed, other precautions may be needed, especially in old, frail adults. Because falling onto a hard surface can increase the risk of injury, a foam mat placed at the side of the low bed or the use of a hip protector can further reduce the impact of a fall. The use of a fall or bed exit alarm may be helpful; the alarm notifies the nurse if the patient or resident has rolled out of bed.

Step 5: Monitoring

Because fall and injury risk is a dynamic process, often subject to change, patients or residents should be monitored regularly. Also, monitoring should include evaluating the effectiveness of low beds in reducing injurious falls.

ACHIEVING SUCCESS WITH LOW BEDS

Acute hospitals can take a number of steps to achieve success with low beds.

Appoint a Low Bed Nurse Coordinator

The coordinator's tasks may include the following:

- Familiarize staff with low beds and their role in the prevention of injurious falls.

- Provide ongoing education of staff and training of new staff with respect to low beds.

- Oversee staff use of low beds.

- Collect data and evaluate outcomes with respect to low beds.

- Provide supportive feedback to staff regarding use of low beds.

- Maintain low beds and serve as the main connection with low bed vendors.

- Maintain and update low bed guidelines, policies, and protocols.

- Provide administration with feedback on low beds (e.g., low bed effectiveness, numbers of low beds needed).

Provide Education

An ongoing staff in-service regarding low beds is essential. The purpose of education is to increase staff knowledge and skills in identifying patients or residents at risk of injurious falls and the appropriate use of low beds. Education should occur during facility orientation and, subsequently, on a regular basis (i.e., audits of the care process can be used to detect any deficient practices and identify topics for in-service). Housekeeping staff also should be in-serviced with respect to low beds.

Ensure Administrative Support

Strong administrative leadership is essential for the successful use of low beds. The primary role of leadership is to make injurious fall prevention a top priority within the hospital and to support staff in their efforts to prevent injurious falls, including the use of low beds. Important tasks to consider include the following:

- Make low beds an important aspect of the hospital's planning program and budget allocation.

- Conduct regular audits of the fall prevention program (i.e., determine whether staff are assessing injury risk and implementing low beds appropriately). This helps separate what you think is happening from what is really happening.

- Ensure that an adequate number of low beds is available.

- Keep all policies, procedures, and manuals related to low beds updated.

Using Hip Protectors

PURPOSE

To provide guidance on the use of hip protectors.

Definition

Hip protectors are designed to absorb the impact of a fall on the hip bone, which helps to reduce the risk of hip fracture. In essence, hip protectors act as shock absorbers around the hip, providing a cushion between the hip bone and the impact surface.

Who Benefits from a Hip Protector?

Although all patients or residents may benefit from wearing a hip protector, the best use of a hip protector is in those who are at the greatest risk of hip fracture. These include patients or residents with

- History of injury after a fall

- History of osteoporosis and multiple falls

- Balance impairment

- Diseases (e.g., stroke, Parkinson's disease, diabetes, Alzheimer's disease) associated with balance loss and hip fracture risk

- Medications associated with balance loss and falls (e.g., narcotics, sedatives, antidepressants)

- Seizure disorders

- Frequent nocturia (i.e., nighttime toileting)

- Dementia with agitated behaviors

- Fear of falling or injury.

KEY COMPONENTS OF USING HIP PROTECTORS

To use hip protectors appropriately, nursing staff must adhere to a clinical process or practice of care that assists in identifying factors contributing to hip fracture risk and deciding on the use of hip protectors as a strategy. A best-practice approach to implementing hip protectors consists of

- Identifying patients or residents at risk of falls and hip fracture

- Assessing the need for a hip protector

- Determining hip protector use

- Communicating the patient's or resident's risk status and hip protector use to all staff

- Monitoring hip protector use and compliance.

Step 1: Assess Fall and Injury Risk

The purpose of risk assessment is to determine which patients or residents are most likely to fall and raise staff awareness of hip fracture risk. The rationale for this assessment is that if those at high risk can be identified, then appropriate interventions, such as providing a hip protector, can be instituted to minimize their risk of injury. Therefore, a fall and injury risk assessment is an important starting point in attempting to reduce hip fractures (Table III-6).

Using a formal risk assessment is important because relying on staff judgment alone is risky; some staff have better judgment than others. A basic fall and injury risk assessment is included in Table III-6. Risk assessment should take place at the time of admission, after a fall, and whenever patients or residents experience a change of condition, especially loss of balance.

Step 2: Assess Need for Hip Protectors

If the patient or resident has one or more of the risk factors included in Table III-6 plus altered mobility, he or she may be a candidate for a hip protector. The patients or residents who are most suitable for a hip protector include those who are unsteady and have frequent falls, a history of fractures from falls, osteoporosis, or limitations of activity secondary to fear of falling.

Step 3: Determine Use of Hip Protectors

Once the decision has been made to use a hip protector, the next step is to determine when the hip protector is used (e.g., every day, every night, every day and night, or during specific activities such as bathing, showering, or exercising).

Step 4: Communicate Risk

The patient's or resident's risk status and hip protector use must be communicated to all care staff involved. Communication can be achieved by the following means:

- Use of colored stickers (e.g., placing a hip protector symbol on the patient's or resident's chart, on the bedroom wall above the bed) or wristbands to identify patients or residents who should wear hip protectors

Table III-6. Fall and injury risk assessment

Inquire about
- Previous falls and injurious falls
- Drugs (especially psychotropics and sedatives)
- Altered cognitive function
- Lower or upper extremity weakness
- Osteoporosis
- Elimination problems (urinary incontinence, frequency)
- Ambulatory aid use (cane or walker)
- Altered mobility, including unsteady gait or balance and impaired transfers

Observe the patient or resident
- Get up from a chair (without use of armrests, if possible)
- Stand still momentarily
- Walk forward 10 feet
- Turn around and walk back to chair
- Turn and sit down in the chair

Factors to note:
- Ability to transfer from sitting to standing
- Stability of walking
- Ability to turn without staggering or balance loss

- Using shift reports or posting a daily list of patients or residents assigned to wear hip protectors and when.

In this way, the staff know who should be wearing a hip protector and when.

Step 5: Monitor

Hip protector use should be monitored regularly. The purposes of monitoring are as follows:

- Detect any change of condition (e.g., diseases, cognition, mobility, new medications) and reassess injury risk.

- Evaluate compliance and the effectiveness of the hip protectors in reducing hip fracture risk. Low compliance is a major obstacle in the successful use of hip protectors. Major compliance problems associated with the use of hip protectors and solutions to increase compliance are included in "Achieving Hip Protector Compliance," page 223).

- Decide what to do next if the hip protector is not effective in reducing risk.

Developing an Effective Hip Protector Program

PURPOSE

To provide guidance on developing an effective hip protector program.

Key Components

Organizations can take a number of steps to achieve a successful hip protector program.

Step 1: Appoint a Hip Protector Nurse Coordinator or Champion

Identify a nurse champion to support and follow through with the hip protector program. This person pulls together a facility's hip protector program, takes responsibility to make things happen, and sees what needs to be changed and improved. The hip protector champion's task may include the following:

- Familiarize staff with hip protectors and their role in preventing hip fractures.
- Provide ongoing education of staff and training of new staff with respect to hip protectors.
- Oversee staff compliance with hip protectors.
- Ensure that information about which patients or residents are using hip protectors is communicated between staff and shifts.
- Collect data and evaluate resident outcomes with respect to hip protectors.
- Provide supportive feedback to staff regarding hip protector use.
- Maintain hip protectors and serve as the main connection with hip protector vendors.
- Maintain and update hip protector guidelines, policies, and protocols.
- Problem solve; address compliance and other issues with hip protector use.
- Provide administration with feedback on hip protectors (e.g., hip protector effectiveness, numbers of hip protectors needed).

Step 2: Provide Education

Staff Education   Ongoing staff in-service regarding hip protector use is essential. The purpose of education is to increase staff knowledge and skills in identifying patients or residents at risk of hip fracture and the appropriate use of hip protectors. When designing in-service programs, it is important to include discussions on measuring patients or residents for proper size, types of patients or residents best suited for hip protectors, number of hip protectors each patient or resident should receive, how hip protectors should be worn, and how to overcome common hip protector compliance problems. It is important to include nursing assistants because they are the ones who will use hip protectors the most. Education should occur during facility orientation and, subsequently, on a regular basis (i.e., audits of the care process can be used to detect any deficient practices and identify topics for in-service training). Laundry and housekeeping staff should be trained in the handling and laundering of hip protectors.

Patient or Resident and Family Education   Ongoing communication and involvement with the patients or residents and their families are an important ingredient in the success of a hip protector program. Educate patients or residents, as appropriate, and their family members about hip fracture risk and hip protectors. It is important to enlist the help of families because they can assist in preventing hip fractures (i.e., if families are aware of why the person is at risk, they can communicate any potentially risky behavior or conditions to staff).

Step 3: Create a System of Administrative Support

Strong administrative or management leadership is essential for the successful use of hip protectors. The primary role of leadership is to make hip fracture prevention a top priority in the facility and to support staff in their efforts to prevent fractures, including the use of hip protectors. Important tasks to consider include the following:

- Make hip protectors an explicit and important aspect of the facility's planning program and budget allocation.

- Conduct regular audits of fall and injury prevention activities (i.e., determine whether staff are assessing hip fracture risk and implementing hip protectors appropriately). This helps separate what people think is happening from what is really happening.

- Ensure that adequate numbers of hip protectors are available.

- Keep all policies, procedures, and manuals related to hip protectors updated.

- Develop a process for recognizing and rewarding the efforts of staff for their efforts related to the successful use of hip protectors.

Achieving Hip Protector Compliance

PURPOSE

To provide guidance on the common factors or reasons responsible for non-compliance with hip protectors and solutions to increase compliance (Table III-7).

Table III-7. Compliance factors, problems, and solutions

Compliance Factors	Problems	Solutions
Patient or resident	Does not accept hip protector (HP); perception of low hip fracture risk	Education: Compliance increases with information on specific risk of hip fracture and need for HPs. Individuals who fall tend to have a more positive view of HPs than those who don't.
		Committed staff: Caregivers who understand HP need are vital in encouraging ongoing HP use.
	Uncomfortable (too tight, poor fit, pads move)	Make sure the HP fits correctly. HP must fit snugly.
	Incompatibility with urinary incontinence	Select HP specific for incontinence. HPs can be worn with incontinence garments if necessary.
	Difficult to put HP on independently	Amount of help needed putting HPs on varies depending on upper extremity strength and dexterity; using an HP that is one size larger may help (make sure pads remain aligned with and cover hips).
		Note: Because dressing and undressing can increase the risk of balance loss and falls, only staff should put on or take off HPs. If patient or resident self-dresses, observe balance while he or she puts on HP and determine whether this is a safe activity.

Table III-7. *(continued)*

Compliance Factors	Problems	Solutions
	Incompatibility with cognitive impairment and dementia (inability to comprehend reason for HPs; may see HPs as nuisance item)	In general, when patients or residents with dementia acquire the habit of wearing HPs, they continue to wear them.
Staff	Skepticism about HPs (caregiver does not perceive usefulness or efficacy)	Structured education of staff can substantially improve adherence with HPs.
		Allowing involvement and input of staff in the implementation process helps with HP buy-in.
		Attitude and motivation are crucial in achieving good staff compliance with HPs. Also, motivated staff are instrumental in convincing patients or residents to wear HPs.
		Compliance is likely to be improved when staff are educated about the likely benefits of HPs and HPs become part of everyday practice.
	Forgets to use HPs	Incorporating HPs into fall prevention guidelines or protocols helps staff with compliance.
	HPs not available	Keep HPs at bedside.
	HPs not available	Have a sufficient number of HPs available in different sizes. Number of HPs needed depends on number of patients or residents at risk. In general, each person will need 3 HPs.
		Assign one staff member to be responsible for HP program and purchase decisions.
Facility	HPs not available because of laundering practices (long turnaround period, getting lost in wash)	Each facility must formulate a policy for staff handling of soiled HPs and laundering of HPs.
		To avoid the need for daily washing, HPs can be worn over light underwear.

Using Fall Alarms

PURPOSE

To provide guidance on the appropriate clinical use of fall alarms.

Definition

Fall alarms, sometimes called exit alarms or fall prevention alarms, are tools designed to warn nursing staff via an auditory signal that patients or residents who should not leave their bed, chair, wheelchair, or toilet unassisted are doing so. Fall alarms are not designed to prevent a person from getting up, nor are they designed to prevent the person from falling. Alarms only let staff know that a hazardous situation is occurring, which can improve the timeliness of staff response. In other words, it is not the alarm but the response of staff to the alarm that can prevent falls from occurring.

Indications for Fall Alarms

Fall alarms can serve a variety of useful functions:

* Warn staff that the patient or resident has changed position and is about to leave the bed, chair, wheelchair, or toilet. This may give staff enough time to assist him or her.

* Warn staff that the patient or resident has left the bed, chair, wheelchair, or toilet. This may give staff enough time to intercept him or her before a fall.

* Promote speedy assistance to patients or residents who have already fallen in order to provide care. This can help reduce fall complications, such as the amount of time that a patient or resident lies on the floor unaided.

* In some cases, warn patients or residents themselves. When a person attempts to leave his or her bed, the alarm can activate a verbal reminder through speakers reminding the person to wait for staff. In some cases the sound of the alarm may prompt the patient or resident to sit back in the bed, chair, wheelchair, or toilet or reminds him or her to call for assistance.

* May serve as an alternative to nurse call bells for patients or residents who are noncompliant or unable to use their call bell because of cognitive or physical impairments. Alarms, which do not require active participation

to trigger, may be preferable to nurse call systems, which demand active participation to activate.

- May serve as an assessment or planning tool by monitoring the frequency of attempts to leave the bed, chair, or wheelchair, which can help identify emerging trends and interventions. Coupled with initial and ongoing risk assessments, alarms can inform staff about a patient's or resident's habits. For example, one may consistently attempt to arise at a certain hour to go to the bathroom, whereas another may get up at nonspecific times, driven by an urge to wander. As a result of such information, nurses can adjust their attention and care to each patient's or resident's habits and needs.

- Allow staff more time (avoiding constant supervision of patients or residents at risk) and, theoretically, eliminate the need to continually check on those who tend to fall. This gives staff more opportunity to work with patients or residents rather than spending time on surveillance or being frequently interrupted to observe patients or residents.

The use of alarms should be based on specific patient or resident criteria, risk factors, and clinical processes.

Criteria

- Patient or resident experiences a fall from the bed, chair, wheelchair, or toilet.

- Patient or resident experiences a fall shortly after leaving the bed, chair, wheelchair, or toilet or is found on the floor after an unwitnessed fall.

- Patient or resident has impaired mobility or demonstrates unsafe bed, chair, wheelchair, or toilet transfers.

- Patient or resident has a history of cognitive or communication problems (e.g., forgets to use call bell or ask for assistance, cannot remember or follow instructions).

- Patient or resident has a history of nocturia (i.e., excessive urination at night).

Risk Factors

History of Falls   Patient or resident has fallen at least one time in the past 30 days (or other specified time frame). A history of falling is one of the most reliable predictors of future falls. Patients or residents with recurrent falls may repeat the circumstance or characteristics of their falls, such as leaving their bed and toileting at night. Knowing the circumstances of a patient's or resident's falls can help in the design of targeted interventions and the appropriate use of alarms.

Balance or Gait Problems   Patient or resident has problems walking or standing without assistance from a walker or needs staff assistance. Common disorders such as stroke, Parkinson's disease, dementia, and arthritis can affect balance and ambulation skills.

Four or More Medications   Multiple medications can impair a patient's or resident's motor skills and personal safety awareness and increase fall risk. Common drugs include those that act on the central nervous system, such as sedatives and tranquilizers.

Muscle Weakness   Any weakness or impairment of the legs or arms (e.g., from arthritis, muscular weakness, stroke) can inhibit a patient's or resident's safe transfers, ambulation, and balance.

New Admission   Any patient or resident who is newly admitted to a facility should be watched closely until his or her condition is fully assessed. Many falls occur within the first 72 hours of stay.

Continence Problems   Patients or residents who have bladder problems will be more inclined to get up without assistance to use the bathroom. Patients or residents with nocturia or incontinence and those needing toileting assistance are especially at high fall risk.

Cognitive Problems   Altered mental status (e.g., confusion, disorientation, or impaired memory) is one of the most important risk factors for falling. Cognitive losses can cause errors in judgment (i.e., inability to recognize a difference between safe and hazardous transfers), forgetting to use the nurse call bell or not recognizing the purpose of the call bell (i.e., not making a connection between pushing a button and getting help), and not asking for assistance or not recognizing a need for assistance (i.e., overestimating the ability to transfer and walk safely or denying any mobility limitations).

Mobility Problems   Diseases directly affecting mobility (i.e., strength, flexibility, and balance) include acute and chronic conditions that affect the muscular, skeletal, or neurological systems and limit the patient's or resident's ability to move about safely and independently.

Clinical Processes

Use of Fall Alarm as a Risk Assessment Tool

Assess patterns of behavior that may increase fall risk during bed and chair transfers or toilet egress, including

- Nonadherence with nurse call bell (or cognitive or physical inability to use call bell)

- Nonadherence with asking for caregiver assistance

- Staff nonadherence with completion of risk and postfall assessments.

Use of Fall Alarm as a Care Planning Tool

By identifying times of unsafe bed or chair egress, caregivers can design appropriate fall reduction interventions (e.g., anticipated care, monitoring strategies).

Use of Fall Alarm as a Monitoring Tool

Error Reduction   Used in conjunction with monitoring strategies (e.g., observation, rounding, and sitters), a fall alarm can reduce the risk of nonadherence or errors in monitoring strategies caused by staff shortages (number of staff, nonavailability of staff during shift changes) or staff fatigue from stress and overwork. Used at the time of admission or change of condition, a fall alarm can detect risk that might result from risk assessments not being completed in a timely manner or completed accurately.

Medication Side Effects   Monitor anticipated side effects with medications that increase fall risk (e.g., by causing orthostatic hypotension or gait or balance impairment) and necessitate caregiver assistance.

Toilet Egress   Identify when patients or residents who need assisted toilet egress are getting up from the toilet, which is the most common time for toilet-related falls.

Low Bed Egress   Identify times of roll out and increased fall or injury risk that may occur if patients or residents rise after rolling out.

Injury Reduction with Hip Protectors   Identify times and patterns of mobility and fall risk in patients or residents at risk for injurious falls.

Patient Compliance and Use of Canes or Walkers   Identify which patients or residents who need a cane or walker to assist with poor balance are not using the ambulation device or not using it correctly.

Unsafe Wandering   Identify times of wandering that can be addressed by intervention in the plan of care.

Use of Fall Alarm as a Postfall Tool

A fall alarm can help staff identify circumstances of falling (i.e., location and activity) when unwitnessed falls occur.

Keys to Success

In addition to selecting the right fall alarm, the effective use of alarms depends on several factors:

- Maintaining strong organizational or management support for fall prevention programs, including the use of exit alarms.

- Educating and training staff on the use of fall alarms (i.e., what alarms are, how they work, and which patients or residents will benefit from an alarm). Ongoing staff education on fall prevention and the use of alarms as a preventive strategy is important.

- Checking fall alarms on a regular basis to ensure that they are functioning properly (i.e., to verify that they send an alarm if a patient or resident arises), that they are sufficiently audible, and that staff respond to alarms appropriately.

- Auditing the use of fall alarms to ensure that staff are using them properly and that alarms are effective in helping to reduce falls.

- Choosing a champion or coordinator. Assigning a designated staff member to provide leadership, oversight, and coordination for both fall alarms and fall prevention can help ensure the successful integration of alarms.

Selecting
Fall Alarms

PURPOSE

To provide guidance on the selection of fall alarms.

Types of Fall Alarms

Several types of fall alarms are available; all alarms function similarly (Table III-8). They allow patients or residents to maintain a free-movement zone, or an area adequate for normal activity. If the patient or resident exceeds the free-movement zone, an alarm sounds indicating that he or she is about to leave the bed, chair, wheelchair, or toilet or has already done so. The alarm may be set (via a control unit) to sound in the patient's or resident's room or at the nurses' station, in a hallway, or on a staff pager (using a nurse call system interface or a remote receiver console).

Steps

Selection of the most appropriate fall alarm for an organization should be based on the following process:

Step 1: Identify a multidisciplinary team. The decision to introduce fall alarms affects many levels of the organization; as a result, a multidisciplinary team involving all stakeholders who may be affected by the introduction of alarms should be formed. Team members should include key personnel from nursing, medicine, and rehabilitative therapy, as well as staff responsible for purchasing decisions, administrative leadership, front-line staff who will be using the technology, family representatives, insurance and legal representatives, quality improvement staff, and risk managers.

Step 2: Identify which patients or residents could benefit from alarms (see "Using Fall Alarms," pp. 225–228) or specific groups that alarms are intended to target (see Table III-9). Performing a root cause analysis of falling events (i.e., asking why the fall occurred and how future falls may be prevented) can sometimes help identify the need for alarms.

Step 3: Consider how fall alarms will affect or complement a fall prevention program. Fall alarms work best when integrated into a well-designed fall prevention program (i.e., in other words, alarms should not be considered the sole

Table III-8. Types of fall alarms

Pressure pad alarms

These consist of a thin pad (placed on top of or underneath a bed mattress or on a chair or wheel-chair seat) and a control unit (typically mounted on the bed or chair). The pad senses changes in weight and pressure; if the patient or resident gets up from a bed or chair, the alarm sounds. Pad alarms are also available for use on toilet seats to detect unsafe egress.

Pull-string alarms

These consist of an adjustable-length cord and garment clip that is attached to the patient's or resident's clothing. The end of the cord is attached to the control unit via a small magnetic disc or ball. The alarm is activated when the patient or resident exits the bed, chair, wheelchair, or toilet and the cord detaches from the control unit. Pull-string alarms equipped with a prerecorded voice message (i.e., instructing the patient or resident not to get up until help arrives) are available. These alarms activate automatically when the cord detaches from the control unit. (Some alarm companies have incorporated the prerecorded voice message design into pressure pad alarms.)

Leg band alarms

These consist of a small, lightweight control unit that attaches to the patient's or resident's thigh by means of a washable fabric band. When the patient or resident changes position (i.e., getting up from bed, chair, wheelchair, or toilet) the alarm is activated.

Postural change alarms

These are applied directly to the patient or resident (by means of an adhesive sensor patch to the thigh) and are activated by changes in position. When the patient or resident attempts to stand from bed, chair, wheelchair, or toilet (i.e., leg becomes weight-bearing) the adhesive patch sends a signal to a receiver unit, which activates an alarm.

Floor mat alarms

These consist of a pressure pad mat placed on the floor alongside the bed, chair, wheelchair, or toilet. The alarm unit is activated when foot pressure is applied to the mat.

Infrared alarms

These consist of directional infrared sensors that send a beam over the top of or alongside the bed. The alarm is activated when the beam is broken (i.e., patient or resident sits up and puts his or her legs over the side of the bed).

Built-in alarms

Some bed manufacturers have equipped their beds with fall alarms. These alarms function very similarly to pressure pad alarms.

---

solution to fall or injury prevention). This is a fact that is not always clearly understood. To be effective, alarms must be implemented with care and with a clear understanding of their benefits and limitations.

Step 4: Choose the right fall alarms for patients or residents. There are benefits and disadvantages to most alarms. To a large degree, the right alarm depends on certain patient or resident characteristics that may interfere with or defeat the use of alarms (Table III-10).

Step 5: Choose the right fall alarm for staff. Many technologies, including fall alarms, directly affect staff workload and procedures. Consideration of these issues is paramount when deciding which alarms to purchase. The best alarm is one that care staff find easy to use and that does not malfunction or result in nuisance alarms. Nursing feedback and involvement in the evaluation, purchasing, and implementation process are essential.

Once a decision has been made to purchase fall alarms, certain features will help determine which type is the most appropriate (Table III-11).

Table III-9.   Fall Alarm Criteria

Criteria for Bed Use

- Fall out of bed
- Fall shortly after leaving bed
- Fall risk from bed (i.e., impaired transfers)
- Fall risk shortly after leaving bed (i.e., impaired gait or balance)

The goal of the alarm is to prevent falls from bed or shortly after leaving bed in at-risk patients or residents.

Criteria for Chair Use

- Fall from chair or wheelchair
- Fall shortly after leaving chair
- Fall risk from chair or wheelchair (i.e., impaired transfers)
- Fall risk shortly after leaving chair (i.e., impaired gait or balance)

The goal of the alarm is to prevent falls from chairs or shortly after leaving chairs in at-risk patients or residents.

Criteria for Toilet Alarm Use

- Fall from toilet
- Fall shortly after getting up from toilet
- Fall risk from toilet (i.e., impaired transfers)
- Fall risk shortly after getting up from toilet (i.e., impaired gait or balance)

The goal of the alarm is to prevent falls from the toilet or shortly after leaving the toilet in at-risk patients or residents.

Table III-10.   Potential conditions interfering with fall alarms

- Agitation or restless behavior
- Skin irritation (at risk for pressure ulcers)
- Urinary or bowel incontinence
- Being lightweight
- Obesity
- Restless sleep
- Dementia

Table III-11.   Features to look for in fall alarms

- Alarm emits a distinctive alarm that is loud enough to be heard by staff.
- Alarm is quiet in patient's or resident's room (interface with nurse call system), if desired.
- Alarm has the ability to differentiate and prioritize calls.
- Alarm has a built-in time delay, which reduces the number of false alarms.
- Alarm is equipped with automatic reactivation if staff forgets to reset alarm.
- Alarm has different mounting options (bed, wheelchair).
- Alarm has the ability to operate on battery.
- Alarm does not interfere with daily patient or resident care.
- Alarm is easy to use and maintain by staff.
- Alarm is durable; warranty and service contract are included.
- Alarm has performed reliably (prior user satisfaction).

Maintaining Effective Fall Alarm Systems

PURPOSE

To provide guidance on troubleshooting fall alarm ineffectiveness.

Reasons for Ineffective Fall Alarms

Fall alarm ineffectiveness occurs for a variety of reasons. Common problems include the following.

Staff Error

- Staff are unaware of what fall alarms are, what alarm means, or how to set up or activate alarms.

- Staff do not list fall alarm in the care plan along with other fall prevention interventions.

- Staff do not respond to alarms in time to assist patients or residents.

- Staff apply or operate alarms incorrectly.

Organizational Error

- Staff are not properly trained in the use of alarms.

- Protocols or guidelines to assist staff with alarm operation are absent or insufficient.

- Number of alarms is insufficient to meet patient or resident needs.

- Staff cannot locate alarms when needed.

Alarm Error

- Alarm does not sound or false alarms occur; too many false alarms increase risk of true alarms being ignored or alarm being shut off.

- Staff do not hear alarm because of inappropriate volume setting (although high ambient noise levels can also interfere with detecting alarm).

Patient or Resident Error

- Patient or resident removes or defeats alarm.

Strategies for Improving the Effectiveness of Fall Alarms

- Review current alarm problems (e.g., failures, errors). Ask staff whether alarms are working and whether they can hear alarms when sounding. (If not, find out why not.) Look for patterns of failure or error.

- Review the type and design of all alarms used in the facility. Are problems associated with the specific type of alarm?

- Review staff response to and reasons for sounding alarms (e.g., getting out of bed, needing to toilet). Documenting the circumstances of sounding alarms (e.g., why person is getting out of bed) helps to determine patterns or circumstances and times of risk (e.g., nights, weekends, and holidays), patient or resident safety needs, and anticipatory interventions.

- Review incidence of nuisance alarms or alarms being defeated by the patient or resident. These problems typically can be overcome by selecting the right type of alarm for a particular person's condition (e.g., cognitive impairment, restlessness, incontinence).

- Revise or implement a formal fall alarm assessment process, including guidelines and clinical criteria specific for each type of alarm used. Include a self-check procedure for verifying alarm operation before and during use, especially for prevention of false alarms.

- Implement a regular program of maintenance and testing of alarms, as defined by the manufacturer's recommendations. Make sure that alarms are regularly tested to detect any problems and that alarms are loud enough to be heard within the unit (audibility is one of the most frequently reported alarm problems). To ensure that alarms are functioning properly, they should always be tested before and during use.

- Educate and train all staff. Understanding which patients or residents benefit from a fall alarm and when to use alarms can increase both staff compliance and effectiveness of alarms. All staff members using a fall alarm should be knowledgeable about alarms and properly trained in their use (e.g., setup of alarm, what to do if an alarm sounds). Education and training must be ongoing (e.g., repeated reinforcement due to staff changes, orientation of new staff).

- Design methods for evaluating staff understanding of the correct use of fall alarms (e.g., setting up alarms, managing alarms during use, responding to alarms).

- Review fall alarm selection and purchase process. Be sure to involve staff in the decision-making process when selecting and purchasing alarms; their positive and negative experiences with fall alarms can be invaluable. Remember that a single type or design of fall alarm does not fit all patient or resident safety needs.

Fall Risk
Monitoring Strategies

PURPOSE

To provide guidance on strategies for monitoring fall risk.

Definition

Fall risk is a dynamic, ongoing process, one that depends on acuity of illness, medication changes, and environmental conditions affecting mobility, physical status, and cognition. Having a means of monitoring patients or residents who are at risk is a central component of efficient fall prevention (Table III-12).

Monitoring Strategies

Because many falls are foreseeable and preventable, monitoring or observing patients or residents at risk of falling is based on the principle that risk can be managed (i.e., the early detection of risky activities or conditions can facilitate efforts to prevent falls). A number of strategies can be used to monitor patients or residents and reduce the risk of falls.

Safety Rounds

The purpose of safety rounds, in which caregivers conduct walking rounds every 30 minutes or so, is to visibly check on the safety of patients or residents at fall risk. Adjustment of staffing levels may be needed to increase supervision at times of day when many patients or residents are carrying out activities of daily living and therefore are at higher risk of falling. Although the ability to observe at-risk patients or residents may be limited by both the number of staff (i.e., caregivers can become overloaded by monitoring too many people simultaneously) and the design of facilities (i.e., patients' or residents' rooms are located far from the nursing station, which necessitates increased travel times for caregivers), there are several options to ease the burden:

- Target rounds to patients or residents with high-risk conditions or circumstances.

- Maintain continuity of caregivers because caregivers who already are familiar with a patient's or resident's care and routines are most likely to detect unsafe conditions and intervene in a timely fashion.

Table III-12. Fall risk conditions or circumstances suggesting the need for surveillance or observation

- New admission: Many falls occur within 72 hours of admission.
- Postfall period: A high number of repeat falls occur within 72 hours of the original fall.
- Change of condition (e.g., agitation, restlessness, poor sleep or altered sleep patterns, nocturnal wandering, postural hypotension, dizziness, onset of toileting frequency).
- Change of medication regimen (i.e., new medication or increasing dosages).
- Reduced staffing levels or staff shift changes (i.e., lack of caregivers for mobility and care assistance).
- Noncompliance with nurse call system.
- Unit or floor relocation (i.e., new environment, new staff, and new routines).
- Post-meal times (i.e., increased need for toileting activity and fall risk).
- Caregiver and family concern. Always err on the side of safety; if the caregiver or family member thinks that there is any risk whatsoever, the patient or resident should be monitored as a precaution. Monitoring is much less expensive than fixing a fall after it occurs.

- Place high-risk patients or residents in a high-traffic area such as near a nursing station or in a multipurpose day room or dining room.

- Educate families about their loved one's risk of falling and involve them in monitoring risk. Family members who have been educated about the risk of falling can tell staff if their loved one is experiencing any physical or behavioral changes that might increase the risk of falling. When involving families, it is important to formalize a reporting system for them (i.e., families need to have an established staff member with whom they can share their observations, such as the head nurse).

Eyes and Ears Program

From a risk management viewpoint, having insufficient numbers of caregivers available to watch over and anticipate the needs of residents at risk of falling can undermine the best plans to prevent falls. One solution to the problem of caregiver shortages is to involve all facility staff and employees who are in regular contact with patients or residents and their environments (e.g., nursing assistants, housekeeping, dietary, laundry, clerical, maintenance, administrative staff) in monitoring of patients or residents. The purpose of this monitoring strategy (sometimes called a "falling leaf" or "falling star" program) is to prevent falls by increasing staff and employee awareness of patients or residents at risk for falls and training them to detect changes in patients or residents that may lead to falls.

In essence, this program provides another set of eyes and ears for the nurses to help monitor fall risk. The more eyes available to watch over patients or residents at risk (e.g., observing warning signs such as unsteady balance or a change in condition such as agitation, confusion, weakness, or tiredness, needing help with daily activities) and the more ears available to listen to patients (e.g., complaints of dizziness, weakness, unsteady balance), the better it is. Any changes reported can serve as an early warning system, allowing clinical staff to evaluate patients or residents for an underlying cause, disease, or drug reaction that may result in a fall. Patients or residents likely to benefit from an eyes and ears program are frequent fallers, wanderers, and those with dementia and gait or balance impairments. It is important to limit the number of patients or residents participating in this program. Identifying too many people who need monitoring may distract staff from paying attention to those most at risk for falling.

Sitter Program

Sitters (also called companion observers, constant observation, or one-to-one care) provide intensive or constant surveillance. Sitters are generally certified nursing aides who situate themselves in the patient's or resident's bedroom or other locations and maintain a constant vigil. Sitters are especially recommended for certain groups of patients or residents, such as those who are frail or disoriented and at increased risk of falls from bed, and in certain circumstances, such as at night, when the risk of falling may be high.

The use of sitters can be an effective approach to preventing falls, but this practice can sometimes be an inefficient use of personnel. For instance, caregivers who are used as sitters are unable to care for other patients or residents, so additional caregivers may be needed. Targeting sitters to patients or residents who are most at risk for falls, such as those who experience sudden disorientation or who are intermittently confused and those who have had a recent fall or a fall from bed between the hours of 7 P.M. and 7 A.M. when many bed falls occur, can be beneficial in managing the costs of one-to-one care.

Fall Alarms

Fall alarms, safety devices used to monitor patients or residents at fall risk, are designed to warn caregivers about patients or residents who try to get up from a bed or chair without staff assistance. Common indications for a fall alarm include a record of falls from a bed or chair and poor or unsafe chair transfers. Other indications for an alarm include poor gait or balance after getting up from a bed or chair; nocturia (i.e., excessive urination at night); cognitive dysfunction (i.e., poor communication or poor judgment), which may interfere with the ability to ask for mobility assistance; and noncompliance with nurse call bell systems. The use of fall alarms may avoid the need for frequent safety rounds or one-to-one care, thus allowing caregivers to focus their attention on patients or residents and other important responsibilities.

Deciding on Monitoring Strategies

Decisions about which monitoring strategy to use should be based on the patient's or resident's needs (i.e., specific fall risk factors and the likelihood of falling; in general, those with multiple risk factors and previous falls are at greatest risk for future falls) and staffing levels. The key to an effective monitoring strategy is to identify times when patients or residents may be most at risk in order to anticipate their needs (e.g., before or right after meals, while going to the bathroom, getting out of bed) and develop an appropriate strategy.

It is important to remember that just as fall risk is a dynamic process, monitoring strategies may have to change as well. For instance, if a patient or resident continually sets off a fall alarm by constant efforts to get out of bed, a sitter may be needed. Likewise, if a sitter is provided for a patient who does not exhibit any risk behavior or falls, consider a less intensive strategy such as safety rounds or a fall alarm. In the event of a fall, focus on improving the processes used to deliver care, not on placing blame on the caregivers involved. Rather, determine what happened and whether there is a better way to monitor the patient.

Using Fall Management Technologies

PURPOSE

To provide an overview of various technologies or products available to assist with fall prevention and injury reduction efforts. The focus here is on specialized equipment or product systems that may be commercially acquired.

Definition

To support caregivers in their efforts to manage falls, a number of technologies have been designed to reduce the hazards associated with falls. Three distinct approaches to fall management are technologies aimed at (1) reducing the risk of a fall, (2) reducing the risk of injury from a fall, and (3) warning caregivers when a patient or resident is engaging in potentially risky behavior. Some of the most noteworthy fall management technologies include the following:

- *Assistive devices.* These include four-wheeled walkers or rollators designed to improve ambulation performance, bed transfer aids designed to assist with independent and safe bed egress, and automatic wheelchair locking systems designed to ensure that wheels are locked before transfers.

- *Injury protection devices.* Available products include hip protectors designed to reduce the impact of a fall, low beds designed to reduce risk of fall-related injury from bed, and cushioned floor mats designed to create a landing area and prevent an injury in the event of a fall out of bed. These products assume that patients or residents will fall, so the goal is to reduce the likelihood of an injury associated with a fall.

- *Warning devices.* Fall or exit alarms are designed to alert nurses that a person is getting up from bed, chair, wheelchair, or toilet unassisted. Wandering alarms are designed to prevent adverse events associated with unsafe wandering.

Fall management technology can play a vital role in preventing falls or minimizing the adverse effects associated with falls. However, technology that is inappropriate for patients or residents or is poorly implemented into existing delivery systems may actually increase the risk of falls and injuries.

Assistive Devices

Rollator (Four-Wheeled Walker)

Walkers are often prescribed to support patients or residents in their ambulation. A two-wheeled walker allows the patient or resident to ambulate by pushing or rolling the walker forward and is generally easier to use than the standard pick-up walker (i.e., those without wheels). The advantage of the wheels is that patients or residents do not have to lift the walker during ambulation; they simply roll the walker along the ground. A rollator is a walker with four wheels; the front two wheels typically are on swivel casters for easy maneuverability. Some rollator models are equipped with three wheels (i.e., one front wheel and two rear wheels). Rollators offer important advantages over standard wheeled walkers.

First, rollators are equipped with hand braking systems (i.e., caliper brakes, much like those of a bicycle) to prevent the walker from rolling away. The user squeezes the hand brakes to lock the wheels in place or releases them to continue walking. Patients or residents with arthritis or cognitive dysfunction sometimes find hand brakes difficult to use and the rollator may actually roll away and increase the risk of falls. For the most part, however, clinical experience has not shown this to be a problem, as those who rely on walkers tend to have a slow gait and rarely build up enough speed to cause the rollator to roll away unexpectedly. Some rollators are equipped with automatic braking systems (i.e., brakes that engage when the user leans forward excessively on the rollator). However, some people may be better off with two-wheeled walkers equipped with automatic weight-activated brakes that slow down the walker's forward movement.

Most rollators have foldable, padded seats and back rests built into them. If the user gets tired while walking, he or she can fold the seat down and rest on it. This feature is especially beneficial for those with arthritis whose legs give way after walking a distance, and for those with underlying pulmonary disease or heart disease who tire easily and need to stop frequently and rest while walking. Caution is advised, however, because some seat designs may be difficult for people with impaired sitting balance to use, resulting in the risk of falls.

Rollators are also equipped with a basket for carrying objects, which is often larger and more stable than the wire basket attachment of a standard walker. The carrying basket allows the person to keep both hands on the rollator while transporting objects (e.g., books, newspapers, eyeglasses) from place to place. The carrying basket is recommended for those who attempt to ambulate with one hand pushing the walker and the other hand carrying objects, or for those who carry an object with both hands, risking a loss of balance, and retrieve the walker later. Both tasks can be extremely hazardous. Sometimes wheelchairs are used for similar purposes; people place objects on the seat and push the chair along. Likewise, this choice is not ideal for maintaining safe balance because the chair may tip.

Rollators offer more gait and balance stability and maneuverability on thick carpets and uneven ground surfaces (e.g., door thresholds, sidewalks) than standard two-wheeled rolling walkers. The rollator's wheels are designed to turn, pivot, and maneuver in a way that walkers cannot, which makes it much easier to get around. Rollators with smaller wheels are for indoor use, and those with bigger wheels are ideal for outdoor use.

Lastly, and perhaps most important, rollators are aesthetically more appealing than conventional rolling walkers, thereby improving both acceptance and compliance. Rollators come in various sizes, shapes, styles, and colors to meet individual needs.

Bed Transfer Aids

Many falls occur in the bedroom; typically while the patient or resident attempts to get up from bed. Those with impaired transfers are at the greatest risk of falling from bed. To facilitate transferring in or out of a bed, caregivers often resort to the use of side rails for transfer support. Although various types of side rails may be used depending on a patient's or resident's medical and functional needs, side rails pose a risk of falls and entrapment injuries. An alternative to side rails is the use of a transfer bar or transfer pole that supports residents with poor sitting and transfer balance.

Transfer Bar   This is a sturdy support rail that attaches to the bed frame and is designed specifically to assist in bed exit and entry. The transfer bar is grasped by mobility-impaired patients or residents when getting in and out of bed. A transfer bar offers more support and confidence during bed transfers than standard side rails.

Transfer Pole   A transfer pole (also known as a floor-to-ceiling pole) is designed to help patients or residents with balance and transfers from bed (i.e., the patient or resident grasps onto the pole when seated and pulls himself or herself up to a standing position when getting out of bed). The transfer pole extends from the floor to the ceiling and mounts via a screw mechanism at the pole's base, without the use of tools. The pole's height adjusts from 7 feet 8¼ inches to 8 feet 2½ inches; the one drawback is that the pole may not be appropriate for facilities with dropped ceilings (i.e., dropped ceilings are not strong enough to support the ceiling mount).

The transfer pole should be positioned close enough to the exit side of the bed to be reached from a seated position and far enough away from the side of the bed to prevent entrapment injuries. Unlike the transfer bar, a transfer pole is easy to remove or relocate for use whenever extra support is needed, such as safely assisting patients or residents with chair and toilet transfers.

The use of a transfer aid should be based on the patient's or resident's assessed medical needs, and he or she should be observed using a transfer bar or pole to ensure it is being used correctly and safely. Also, the effectiveness of transfer aids should be reviewed on a regular basis.

Wheelchair Locking Systems

Wheelchairs are involved in falls. Most wheelchair falls take place during transfers; nearly two thirds occur because patients or residents do not lock wheelchair brakes before transfers, or the wheelchair brakes are not working properly. Patients or residents with dementia or stroke and those taking medications that impair cognition are particularly susceptible to injuries due to wheelchair falls (i.e., they may not remember or be able to lock their wheels before exiting the chair). Automatic wheelchair brakes and anti-rollback devices help prevent falls by wheelchair users who cannot or do not consistently lock the manual brakes on their wheelchairs.

Automatic Wheelchair Brakes   This device installs under the seat of sling-seat wheelchairs and works by sensing weight on the chair. When weight is lifted from the seat (i.e., patient or resident gets up), the brake engages, preventing backward rolling but leaving forward movement of the wheelchair unhindered. When the wheelchair is unoccupied, the brakes remain engaged and do not release until the patient or resident is safely seated or the caregiver releases the locking mechanism. When the chair is in use, the brake disengages to allow unimpeded backward or forward chair movement.

Wheelchair Anti-Rollback Device   This supplemental wheel locking device consists of a pair of stainless steel brake arms that are held just off the surface of the wheelchair's rear tires. When a patient or resident rises from the chair, the brake arms grab the tires to prevent the chair from rolling backwards (i.e., the greater the rearward force on the chair, the greater the braking power). Once the patient or resident is seated, the device releases and the wheelchair returns to standard operation.

Injury Protection Devices

Hip Protectors

The majority of hip fractures occur as a result of a fall. Hip protectors are devices designed to ease the impact of a fall on the hip bone and help to prevent hip fractures. The risk of hip fracture when falling while wearing hip protectors is significantly lower than that of a fall with no hip protector in place. The best use of hip protectors is in those at greatest hip fracture risk (e.g., highly medicated people or those with seizure disorders, balance impairment, cognitive impairment, brittle or weak bones, or multiple falls). In addition to preventing hip fractures, hip protectors offer psychological benefits: Wearers feel more confident in completing tasks safely and, as a result, become more physically active and need less assistance with activities of daily living. Also, caregivers have less fear of injury when patients or residents at fall risk are wearing hip protectors. (See "Using Hip Protectors," pages 218–220.)

Low Beds

Low beds, which sit less than 8 inches from the floor, may be used to eliminate the risk of serious injury caused by falls from beds at higher heights. These beds are typically used for patients or residents who are at risk for falling so that if they do fall out of bed they only fall a short distance, thus minimizing the injury associated with falling out of bed (see "Using Adjustable Low Beds," pages 214–217). There are two types of low beds:

- Fixed or stationary low beds rest about 3 inches from the floor. Although these beds are effective in reducing the risk of injurious falls, they may increase the risk of caregiver injury (i.e., back and other ergonomic injuries) because the beds are not height adjustable.

- Height-adjustable low beds are a good choice for both high-risk patients or residents and their caregivers. The advantage of height-adjustable over fixed-height beds is that caregivers can raise the bed to waist height or a comfortable working height while providing care (e.g., turning and lifting residents, changing linens and clothing, transferring residents to chairs and other devices). Also, height-adjustable beds are beneficial for short patients or residents who have difficulty getting up from standard height beds safely because their feet do not reach the floor.

Fall Mats

- For those with repeated falls, cushioned floor mats may be used to prevent injurious falls. High-density foam in the mat absorbs the impact if a person falls. Fall mats can be used in areas where a patient or resident could be injured from a fall on a hard floor, such as the side of a bed, by a toilet, or in front of a chair.

- Mats are available in various sizes and 1 or 2 inches thick; some mats have beveled edges to prevent tripping and allow wheelchairs to roll on and off the mat easily. Floor mats have a durable vinyl cover, which wipes clean for easy care, and a slip-resistant bottom that keeps the mat securely in place; several types fold in half for easy storage. Some floor mats are designed for use in conjunction with a fall alarm mat (i.e., when the patient or resident gets up from bed or chair and steps on the mat, his or her body weight activates an alarm).

- The downside of floor mats, especially thick ones, is that some people with poor balance can experience even more unsteadiness when walking or standing on the mat, which can increase their risk of falling. Height-adjustable low beds kept in the low height position can be used as an alternative to floor mats.

Warning Devices

Fall Alarms

Despite all fall prevention strategies, some people remain at fall risk. Fall alarms are designed to warn caregivers that patients or residents who should not be leaving the bed, chair or wheelchair, or toilet unassisted are doing so. Fall alarms are not designed to prevent patients or residents from getting up, nor are they designed to prevent them from falling. Alarms only let caregivers know that a hazardous situation is occurring, which can improve the timeliness of staff response to a fall risk situation. In other words, it is not the fall alarm but the response of staff to the alarm that can prevent falls from occurring.

There are benefits and disadvantages to most fall alarm systems. Consequently, choosing the right fall alarm is crucial. To a large degree, the right alarm depends on certain resident characteristics that may interfere with or defeat the use of fall alarms, such as dementia, restless behavior, incontinence, and light weight (see "Using Fall Alarms," pages 225–228).

Wandering Alarms

Wandering behavior, most often characterized by walking around without apparent purpose or direction, may increase a patient's or resident's risk for falls (i.e., wandering people with poor physical conditioning are at great fall risk). Technological solutions available to assist with wandering behavior include the following:

- *Door alarms.* These range from simple battery-powered devices, which monitor one door or area, to alarm systems that can monitor many doors throughout the facility.

- *Electronic tagging alarms.* The devices include a transmitter worn by the patient or resident and a monitoring device or receiver with an alert. As the person wearing a transmitter approaches or crosses the monitored area, the alarm system can take a number of actions that include sending audible and visual alerts to caregivers, activating magnetic locks on doors, and sending a silent alert to a caregiver via a paging system. Transmitters can be of several styles, including pendants, wrist and ankle bands, and watches. These alarms can vary in their sophistication, from stand-alone alarm systems with a local alarm monitoring one door to networked alarm systems that monitor many doors and areas.

- *Monitor alarms.* From pressure-sensitive mats placed in thresholds and exits that set off an alarm when a person steps on it to infrared door monitors and motion-detecting alarms. These devices can alert caregivers when patients or residents get out of bed or exit their rooms.

Selecting and Implementing Fall Management Technology

PURPOSE

To provide guidance on selection and implementation of fall management technology in hospital and nursing home settings.

Definition

Fall management technologies include the following:

- *Assistive devices:* Four-wheeled walkers or rollators designed to improve ambulation performance, bed transfer aids designed to assist with independent and safe bed egress, and automatic wheelchair locking systems designed to lock wheels before transfers.

- *Injury protection devices:* Hip protectors designed to reduce the impact of a fall, low beds designed to reduce risk of fall-related injury from bed, and cushioned floor mats designed to create a landing area and prevent an injury in the event of a fall out of bed. These products are based on the premise that patients or residents will fall, but the goal is to reduce the likelihood of an injury associated with a fall through the use of protective devices.

- *Warning devices:* Exit or fall alarms, designed to alert nurses that the patient or resident is getting up from bed, chair, wheelchair, or toilet unassisted; wandering alarms, designed to prevent adverse events associated with unsafe wandering.

SELECTING THE BEST TECHNOLOGICAL SOLUTION

Selection of fall management technological solutions for a particular organization or population should be based on a structured, systemic step-by-step approach that consists of the following steps.

Step 1: Identify a Multidisciplinary Team

The decision to introduce fall management technology or devices affects many levels of the organization; as a result, a multidisciplinary team involving all stakeholders who may be affected by the introduction of technology or devices should be formed. Team members should include key personnel from nursing, medicine, and rehabilitative therapy; staff responsible for purchasing decisions; administrative leadership; front-line staff who will be using the technology; patient or resident representatives; family representatives; insurance and legal representatives; quality improvement staff; and risk managers.

Step 2: Identify the Need for Technology

Identify how many patients or residents could benefit from fall technologies and specific groups the technology or intervention is intended to target. Performing a root cause analysis of falling events (i.e., asking why the fall occurred and how future falls may be prevented) can help identify technologies that may be beneficial. The readiness for technology is often driven by organizational needs for technological interventions. It is also important to consider how specific technology or devices will affect or complement the fall prevention program. Fall prevention technology works best when integrated into a fall prevention program (i.e., technology by itself should not be considered the sole solution to fall or injury prevention).

Step 3: Identify Appropriate Technology

Once the need for technology is identified, the next step is to list all specific devices or products that might be appropriate in reducing falls and injury and, for each product of interest, request information from manufacturers or vendors. Questions and features to ask manufacturers or vendors about their products include the following:

- Is the product appropriate for the task to be accomplished?

- Is the product safe?

- Does the product interfere with daily care in any way?

- Does the design or use of the product affect the functional independence of the patients or residents while keeping them as safe as possible?

- Is the product easy to use? Some staff have low gadget tolerance; it is frustrating and costly to purchase technology that will not be used.

- Is the product easy to maintain? Never believe or assume that technology will not need maintenance.

- Is the product durable? Is a warranty and service contract included? If the product breaks down, how easy is it to fix? Can the product be updated easily, if needed?

- Does the product have a history of dependability? Has the product performed reliably? Ask about prior user satisfaction (i.e., many questions can be answered by talking to staff at other facilities who have used the product of interest).

- What is the cost of the product? Are there any ongoing costs?

- What information or services does the manufacturer or vendor provide on proper use of the product? Do they provide staff training on how to properly use the product? Do they provide technical support if needed?

Once specific products have been identified, and before actual purchase, it is a good idea to

- Compare similar devices or products from different manufacturers. What are the features and options of each, and what are the pros and cons for each product? What does the product really do? Often a company gets carried away with excitement about their product and presents it as more than it is.

- Invite technology vendors to present their products on site to the nursing staff and other appropriate staff. Products may be set up and demonstrated at this time, facilitating side-by-side comparisons. Nurses should be encouraged to examine and use each product and to provide feedback.

- Ask about a 30-day free trial period; to help reach a purchase decision many companies offer hands-on trials.

- Consult with an expert in the field about fall management technology, specifically the products that are under consideration.

Step 4: Implementing Technology

Deciding which technologies to use in your fall prevention program is only the first step in their successful incorporation into practice. The implementation process is equally important and has multiple potential barriers, including staff and patient or resident acceptance of the technology and ongoing maintenance and availability issues.

Staff Acceptance of Technology

Many technologies directly affect staff workload and procedures, which may entail a change in how care is provided. If the benefits of technology are not apparent or the appropriate use of the products is not understood, staff will quickly abandon the technology. Consequently, staff acceptance and understanding of technology are a major barrier to overcome in implementing technology. Approaches to gaining staff buy-in to technology include the following:

- *Provide adequate staff education and training.* The amount and quality of staff education regarding a product and how it will fit into the fall prevention program can affect the success of implementation.

- *Provide readily available protocols on using the product and accessing technical support.* Having ongoing support will encourage staff to overcome difficulties and facilitate staff acceptance of technologies.

- *Provide a staff or point person.* Select a leader in the organization to champion the change, a person with administrative skills to coordinate the process of education and implementation.

Patient or Resident Acceptance of Technology

Involve the patients or residents in any decisions made about their fall safety. This information can increase acceptance and motivation to use certain products that depend on patient or resident adherence or compliance, such as walkers, hip protectors, and bed transfer aids.

Maintenance and Availability Issues

Facility administrators should establish channels and means for patients or residents and staff to report problems with a specific device. Also, resources and procedures for repairing or replacing nonfunctioning or broken products should be in place.

Fall prevention technology is an important component of any effective fall prevention program. An organized approach to the selection and implementation of fall prevention technologies helps to ensure that the products will be of benefit in reducing the risk of falls and injuries.

Fall Management Technology Audits

PURPOSE

Audits help to separate what you think is happening from what is really happening with respect to fall management technology. The objective of an audit is to

- Ensure the appropriate use of fall management technology.
- Evaluate staff and patient or resident adherence with fall management technology.
- Measure the effectiveness of fall management technology.
- Recommend further actions for improvement.

Audit Process

Consider the following items as an example of an audit:

- Ensure the appropriate use of low beds.
- Evaluate staff and patient or resident adherence with use of low beds.
- Measure the effectiveness of low beds in reducing injurious falls.

The following steps outline the audit process:

1. *Select a question to examine.* In order to determine the effectiveness of low beds, both the intervention (low beds) and the process of care related to implementing and monitoring the intervention (low beds) should be evaluated. Start by choosing a question that you want answered, such as, "Does our staff routinely assess the need for a low bed in patients or residents at fall risk?"

2. *Define inclusion criteria* (e.g., all patients or residents at risk of falling or all patients or residents at risk for injurious falls from bed).

3. *Select a sample to examine.* Select a random number of patients or residents meeting the inclusion criteria to sample. Patients or residents should be selected from all floors or units in the organization.

4. *Determine questions to ask* (e.g., is there documentation in the medical chart or nursing records that the patient or resident was evaluated for a low bed?).

5. *Collect the data.* Use a standardized collection form for consistency (Table III-13).

6. *Analyze the data.* At the end of the audit, calculate how many at-risk patients or residents received a low bed assessment and how many did not. In cases where no low bed assessment was completed or documented, staff should be questioned as to why an assessment was not done. To maintain consistency, one staff member should undertake data analysis.

7. *Discuss the results.* If all at-risk patients or residents received a low bed assessment, then your process is working. However, if clinical practice did not meet expectations (i.e., assessment of at-risk patients or residents for low beds did not happen), you need to find out why and suggest recommendations for improvement. The aim of the discussion is to identify areas where actual clinical practice did not meet expectations, discover reasons for this, and design recommendations for improvement.

8. *Implement recommendations.* It is important for all staff providing assessment to receive the recommendations for improvement. Recommendations may be disseminated through in-service education or revisions to existing low bed policies and guidelines.

9. *Re-audit.* A re-audit should follow implementation of the recommendations to see whether the process of assessments has improved. Re-audits are usually completed 3 to 6 months after the initial audit to allow the recommendations to take place. The results of the re-audit can be compared with the results from the initial audit. The re-audit results should demonstrate an improvement from the initial audit.

Table III-13. Question: Did the patient or resident receive a low bed assessment?

Patient	Yes	No (If not, why not?)
1		
2		
3		
4		
5		

Roles of Nurses and Certified Nursing Assistants in the Use of Fall Management Technology

PURPOSE

To provide guidance on the roles of nurses (RNs) and certified nursing assistants (CNAs)* in delivering fall prevention and using fall management technology.

Definition

Fall management technologies include the following:

- Assistive devices (e.g., four-wheeled walkers or rollators designed to improve ambulation performance, bed transfer aids designed to assist with independent and safe bed egress, and automatic wheelchair locking systems designed to lock wheels before transfers).

- Injury protection devices (e.g., hip protectors designed to reduce the impact of a fall, low beds designed to reduce risk of fall-related injury, and cushioned floor mats designed to create a landing area and prevent an injury in the event of a fall out of bed). These products are based on the premise that patients or residents will fall, but the goal is to reduce the likelihood of an injury associated with a fall through the use of these protective devices.

- Warning devices (e.g., exit or fall alarms designed to alert nurses that the patient or resident is getting up from a bed, chair, or wheelchair or is toileting unassisted; wandering alarms designed to prevent adverse events associated with unsafe wandering).

---

*Nursing assistants often provide a majority of direct care yet receive the least formal education about fall prevention and fall management technology. Helping nursing assistants understand their role in preventing falls and using fall management technology could improve outcomes. Nurses and nursing assistants should engage in in-service training to learn together and talk about specific patients. These sessions can also include an occasion to provide feedback about performance and suggest any changes in care needed.

RN and CNA Roles

As members of the interdisciplinary team, RNs and CNAs play a crucial role in the effective use of fall management technology. During care planning, RNs and CNAs play a distinct and collaborative role in identifying fall and injury risk, developing strategies for fall prevention, and using fall management technology that is tailored to the unique needs of each person (Table III-14).

In the event of poor outcomes with fall management technology, consider the following:

Patient or Resident Factors

- Technology is not appropriate for identified risk factors.

- Patient or resident defeats or does not use technology.

Staff or User Factors

- Technology is not listed in the plan of care.

- Staff is unfamiliar with the technology.

- Staff misuses the technology.

- Technology is not available or not found.

- Protocols and procedures are not adequate to assist with technology operation.

REFERENCES

ECRI. (2004, May). Bed-exit alarms a component (but only a component) of fall prevention. *Health Devices*, *33*(5), 157–168.

Tideiksaar R. (2006). *Fall prevention: A guide to exit alarm systems*. Baltimore: Health Professions Press.

Tideiksaar, R. (2006). *Guide to hip protectors*. Baltimore: Health Professions Press.

Table III-14. Fall prevention care process

Steps	RN Role	CNA Role
Fall risk assessment	Identify patients or residents at high risk for falling and specific fall risk factors.	Observe patients or residents for any change in condition and report to RN any changes noticed.
Interim plan of care (POC)	Based on identified fall and injury risk factors. Consider patient or resident and nursing needs and short-term use of fall management technology to support nursing strategies in care of high-risk patients or residents. Initiate referral and further assessment of patient or resident to interdisciplinary team members.	Follow procedures and care plan for high-risk patients or residents. Observe patients or residents and report to RN any deviation from plan of care. Report to RN operational and compliance problems with fall management technology.
POC	Based on feedback from interdisciplinary referrals, design interdisciplinary strategies and interventions to reduce fall/injury risk. Consider continuing or modifying fall management technology to support POC.	Follow procedures and care plan for high-risk patients or residents. Observe patients or residents and report to RN any deviation from plan of care. Report to RN operational and compliance problems with fall management technology.
Education	Provide education to patients or residents and family members about POC and specific fall management technology in use. Educate CNA on the need for and use of fall management technology. Request feedback from CNA on knowledge and understanding of fall management technology.	Reinforce education to patients or residents and family members about POC and specific fall management technology in use. Review procedures and protocols related to fall management technology in use.
Monitor	Ensure that POC and procedures for high-risk patients or residents are in place, including fall management technology. Assess outcomes and staff compliance with fall management technology.	Observe patients or residents for any change in condition and report to RN any changes noticed. Report to RN any deviation from plan of care. Report to RN operational and compliance problems with fall management technology.
Evaluate	Following fall risk assessments and postfall evaluations, consider redesign of POC and use of fall management technology.	Provide feedback to RN on benefits and problems associated with fall management technology.

Home Safety Guidelines

Home Safety Guidelines

To prevent falls after discharge, patients and caregivers must be aware of fall risk factors and interventions. Use these tips and checklists to educate yourself and improve home safety.

TAKING CHARGE: REDUCING THE RISK OF FALLS

People of all ages fall, but falls are more common for older people. In fact, losing balance and falling down is probably the most common accident that happens to older adults. Although most people are not usually harmed when they fall, the more falls a person has, the greater the chance of injury. A serious injury can harm your health, your sense of well-being, and your independence.

RISK OF FALLING

It is important to understand that falls are not a normal part of aging. In order to stop falls from happening, it will help you to understand who is at greatest risk and why. Although anyone can fall, certain conditions or situations put older adults at higher risk. They include the following:

- *Poor eyesight.* This can keep you from seeing hazards and objects in your path and lead to trips or slips.

- *Walking and balance problems.* Disorders such as stroke, arthritis, diabetes, and neurological diseases may affect your muscle strength and reaction time. As a result, your balance may not be quite the same as it was.

- *Use of medications.* Taking too much medication or the wrong combination of drugs can sometimes affect your judgment, coordination, and balance.

- *Depression or stress.* This often causes people to pay less attention and be less alert to surrounding dangers in the environment.

- *Lack of exercise.* Inactivity results in weakened muscles and lack of flexibility. This can change your balance and the way you walk and increase the chances of falling.

PREVENTING FALLS

The good news is that many falls are preventable. By taking some simple steps, you can greatly reduce your chances of falling.

Visit Your Doctor

- Get regular physical exams, even if you are feeling fine.

- Ask the doctor to review your medications for any side effects that can affect balance. Make sure the doctor knows about all the medications you are taking (both prescription and over-the-counter drugs) so that harmful combinations of drugs can be avoided.

- Tell the doctor about any falls or balance problems you have experienced. The doctor may want to check you out for any medical conditions.

Stay Active

- A regular program of physical activity is one of the best ways to decrease your chances of falling and improve your sense of well being and confidence.

- Try to include such activities as walking, dancing, gardening, and stretching exercises to improve flexibility and balance.

Make Your Home Safer

- At least half of all falls happen at home and generally take place when people are doing ordinary things such as walking on stairs, getting up from bed, or going to the bathroom. The best way to deal with any threats to safety in the home is through prevention. It is a good idea to check your home for hazards that frequently cause slips, trips, or falls and eliminate as many potential trouble spots as possible. Use the "Checklist for Spotting and Correcting Home Safety Hazards." By making your home safe now, you can avoid a fall later.

You can further decrease your chances of falling by identifying any unsafe activities leading to risk of falls and trying to eliminate any hazards or obstacles interfering with safety. The "Self-Assessment of Fall Risk in Your Home" is a helpful guide.

CHECKLIST FOR SPOTTING AND CORRECTING HOME SAFETY HAZARDS

Hazard	Solutions
Lighting	
❏ Inadequate lighting	• Keep lights on in rooms that you are walking through. The lighting in your home must be bright so you can avoid tripping over objects that are not easy to see. Consider a night-light for dark passageways.
	• During the day, open curtains and shades to let more sunlight in.
	• Install extra lighting along the pathway from bedroom to bathroom and by steps and stairways.
Floor Surfaces	
❏ Sliding throw rugs	• Check all rugs and mats to make sure they are slip-resistant. Consider buying new rugs with nonslip backing or applying nonskid matting to backs of existing rugs to make them secure.
❏ Upended or curled carpet edges	• Use carpet tape to keep carpet edges from curling up.
Pathways	
❏ Clutter	• All pathways should be clear of objects and furnishings.
Steps and Stairs	
❏ Inadequate lighting and clutter	• Make sure stairs are well lit and free of clutter.
	• Use stairway handrails for going up or down steps.

SELF-ASSESSMENT OF FALL RISK IN YOUR HOME

Do You Have Any Trouble . . . ?	Suggested Solutions
❑ Walking about your home?	• Keep traffic lanes free of clutter and obstacles; allow plenty of walking room. • Make sure all rooms have sufficient lighting. • Remove slippery scatter and throw rugs or use rubber pads to keep them in place. • Secure all carpet edges. • Wear shoes and slippers with nonslip soles that grip the floor. • Ask your doctor about a cane to help maintain balance.
❑ Walking to the bathroom at night?	• Install night-lights in the bedroom and bathroom. • Keep a light within reach of the bed. • Keep a clear path from the bedroom to the bathroom.
❑ Getting up from chairs?	• Use sturdy chairs with armrests to help get up and sit down. • Add firm foam pads to seats of chairs and sofas to help get up.
❑ Getting up from beds?	• Move beds against the wall to prevent the bed from sliding away when getting up. • Replace existing mattress with a thinner one to lower bed height or a thicker one to raise bed height.
❑ Getting up from toilets?	• Consider an elevated toilet seat and grab bars to help sit down and get up.
❑ Getting in and out of bathtubs or showers?	• Consider using a tub or shower chair and grab bars to help get in and out. Towel bars are not designed to be used as grab bars. • Place nonskid rubber mats or decals on the floor to prevent slipping.
❑ Getting objects from kitchen cabinets and closet shelves?	• Store everyday dishes and kitchen supplies within easy reach. Consider keeping items no lower than waist level or no higher than shoulder height to avoid excessive bending, stooping, or reaching.

Forms

Performance-Oriented Environmental Mobility Screen (POEMS)

Instructions: Ask the patient or resident to perform the indicated maneuvers. If the individual uses an ambulation device (e.g., cane, walker), each maneuver is tested with the device as appropriate. For each maneuver, indicate whether the person's performance is normal (independent function) or impaired (dependent function). Suggested interventions for each impairment discovered (indicated by numbers in parentheses) are indicated. The key for the numbered interventions follows the forms.

Note: Each of the POEMS maneuvers has been printed on a separate page. The purpose of this design is to allow staff members to photocopy the POEMS and arrange the sequence of maneuvers according to their individual needs and those of patients or residents. In addition, the design allows for targeted assessments of risk (e.g., bed transfers, toilet transfers).

POEMS: Performance-Oriented Environmental Mobility Screen

Ambulation

Bedroom	Observation Normal	Impaired (Intervention)
Walk in straight line from doorway to most distant wall (approx. 10–15 feet)	❑ Gait is continuous, without hesitation	❑ Gait is noncontinuous, with hesitation (1) (2)
	❑ Gait is straight, without deviation from path	❑ Gait deviates from straight path (1) (2) (5)
	❑ Both feet clear floor surface	❑ One or both feet scrape floor surface (1) (5) (6)
	❑ Does not use walls/furniture for support	❑ Walls/furniture are used for support (1) (2) (3) (4)
		❑ Unable to perform maneuver or perform it safely (10)
Turn around, walk around both sides of bed	❑ Steps are smooth, continuous	❑ Steps are discontinuous (1) (2) (5)
		❑ Staggers, loses balance (1) (2) (5)
	❑ Does not stagger or lose balance	❑ Walls/furniture are used for support (1) (2) (3) (4)
	❑ Does not use walls/furniture for support	❑ Unable to perform maneuver or perform it safely (10)
Device used to perform maneuver: ❑ Yes Type _____ ❑ No	❑ Device appropriate for space	❑ Device inappropriate for space (2) (4)
	❑ Device used correctly	❑ Device used incorrectly (2)

Ambulation

Observation

Bedroom	Normal	Impaired (Intervention)
Walk to sink, toilet, turn around and return	❏ Gait is continuous, smooth without hesitation	❏ Gait is noncontinuous, with hesitation (1) (2)
	❏ Both feet clear floor and threshold	❏ One or both feet scrape floor or threshold (4) (5) (6)
	❏ Does not lose balance	❏ Loses balance (1) (2)
	❏ Does not use walls, sink, towel bar for balance support	❏ Uses walls, sink, towel bar for balance support (3) (4)
		❏ Unable to perform maneuver or perform it safely (10)
Device used to perform maneuver: ❏ Yes Type _____ ❏ No	❏ Device appropriate for space	❏ Device inappropriate for space (3)
	❏ Device used correctly	❏ Device used incorrectly (2)

(continued)

Ambulation

	Observation	
Hallway	Normal	Impaired (Intervention)
Walk from bedroom to nurses' station, toward exit, and return to bedroom	❑ Gait is continuous, without hesitation	❑ Gait is noncontinuous, with hesitation (1) (2) (5)
	❑ Gait is straight, without deviation from path	❑ Gait deviates from straight path (1) (2) (5)
	❑ Both feet clear floor surface	❑ One or both feet scrape floor surface (1) (5) (6)
	❑ Does not use walls/furniture/handrails for support	❑ Walls/furniture/ handrails are used for support (1) (2) (3) (4)
	❑ Able to perform maneuver without excessive fatigue	❑ Unable to perform maneuver without fatigue (1) (10)
		❑ Unable to perform maneuver or perform it safely (10)
Device used to perform maneuver: ❑ Yes Type _____ ❑ No	❑ Device appropriate for space	❑ Device inappropriate for space (3)
	❑ Device used correctly	❑ Device used incorrectly (2)

Falls in Older People: Prevention and Management, Fourth Edition,
by Rein Tideiksaar. Copyright © 2010, Health Professions Press, Inc., Baltimore, MD.

POEMS: Performance-Oriented Environmental Mobility Screen

Transfers

Observation

Bed	Normal	Impaired (Intervention)
Transfer onto bed and lie down	❏ Bed transfer is completed in smooth, controlled movement (sits on bed in one attempt)	❏ Bed transfer is not smooth (requires several attempts; falls onto mattress; uses mattress edge to guide transfer) (1) (8)
	❏ Sitting balance is stable	❏ Sitting balance is unstable (2) (8)
	❏ Does not use arm support to maintain sitting balance	❏ Uses arm support to maintain sitting balance (2) (8)
	❏ Both feet rest flat on floor	❏ Feet do not rest flat on floor (8)
	❏ Feet do not slide	❏ Feet slide away (5) (6)
	❏ Bed does not slide away	❏ Bed slides away (6) (8)
	❏ Able to lie down in one smooth, controlled movement	❏ Unable to lie down in one smooth, controlled movement (several attempts required) (8)
		❏ Unable to perform maneuver or perform it safely (8) (10)
Device used to perform maneuver: ❏ Yes Type _____ ❏ No	❏ Device appropriate for space	❏ Device inappropriate for space (3)
	❏ Device used correctly	❏ Device used incorrectly (2)

(continued)

Falls in Older People: Prevention and Management, Fourth Edition,
by Rein Tideiksaar. Copyright © 2010, Health Professions Press, Inc., Baltimore, MD.

Transfers (bed—*continued*)

Bed	Normal	Impaired (Intervention)
Rise from supine position and transfer off bed	❑ Able to rise in one smooth, controlled movement to sitting position	❑ Unable to rise in one smooth, controlled movement to sitting position (several attempts required or cannot perform) (1) (8)
	❑ Sitting balance is stable	❑ Sitting balance is unstable (2) (8)
	❑ Does not use arm support to maintain sitting balance	❑ Uses arm support to maintain sitting balance (2) (8)
	❑ Both feet rest flat on floor	❑ Feet do not rest flat on floor (8)
	❑ Transfers off bed in smooth, controlled movement (rises off bed in one attempt)	❑ Transfer off bed is not completed in smooth, controlled movement (requires several attempts) (8)
	❑ Feet do not slide ❑ Bed does not slide away	❑ Feet slide away (5) (6) ❑ Bed slides away (6) (8) ❑ Unable to perform maneuver or perform it safely (8) (10)

POEMS: Performance-Oriented Environmental Mobility Screen

Transfers

	Observation	
Chair	Normal	Impaired (Intervention)
Sit down in chair(s)	❏ Sits in smooth, controlled movement (sits in one attempt)	❏ Sitting is not completed in smooth, controlled movement (requires several attempts) (1) (7)
	❏ Does not lose balance	❏ Loses balance (falls into seat) (2) (7)
	❏ Does not use arm rests for sitting	❏ Chair tips or slides away (7)
	❏ Chair does not tip or slide away	❏ Uses arm rests for sitting (7)
	❏ Seated, both feet rest flat on floor	❏ Seated, feet do not rest on floor (7)
		❏ Unable to perform maneuver or perform it safely (10)
Device used to perform maneuver: ❏ Yes Type _____ ❏ No	❏ Device appropriate for space	❏ Device inappropriate for space (2) (4)
	❏ Device used correctly	❏ Device used incorrectly (2)

(continued)

Transfers (chair—*continued*)

Chair	Normal	Impaired (Intervention)
Rises from chair	❏ Rises in smooth, controlled movement (rises in one attempt)	❏ Rising is not completed in smooth, controlled movement (requires several attempts) (1) (7)
	❏ Does not lose balance	❏ Loses balance (falls back into/off seat) (1) (7)
	❏ Does not use armrests	❏ Uses armrests or seat (7)
	❏ Chair does not tip or slide away	❏ Chair tips or slides away (7)
	❏ Feet do not slide on floor	❏ Feet slide on floor (5) (6) (7)
		❏ Unable to perform maneuver or perform it safely (10)

POEMS: Performance-Oriented Environmental Mobility Screen

Transfers

Observation

Toilet	Normal	Impaired (Intervention)
Sit down on toilet	❑ Able to sit down in one smooth, controlled movement	❑ Unable to sit down in one smooth, controlled movement (requires several attempts) (1) (9)
	❑ Does not lose balance	❑ Loses balance (1) (2) (9)
	❑ Does not use grab bars, sink edge for balance support	❑ Uses grab bars, sink edge for balance support (3) (4) (9)
	❑ Both feet rest flat on floor in seated position	❑ Feet do not rest flat on floor in seated position (9) (10)
		❑ Unable to perform maneuver or perform it safely (9) (10)
Device used to perform maneuver: ❑ Yes Type _____ ❑ No	❑ Device appropriate for space	❑ Device inappropriate for space (3)
	❑ Device used correctly	❑ Device used correctly (2)
Reach for toilet paper receptacle; simulate toilet hygiene	❑ Able to perform without excessive reach or balance loss	❑ Unable to perform without excessive reach or balance loss (9)
	❑ Does not use toilet, walls for balance support	❑ Uses toilet, walls for balance support (3) (9)
		❑ Unable to perform maneuver, or perform safely (10)

(continued)

Transfers (toilet—*continued*)

Toilet	Normal	Impaired (Intervention)
Rise from toilet	❏ Able to rise in one smooth, controlled movement	❏ Unable to rise in one smooth, controlled movement (requires several attempts) (1) (9)
	❏ Does not lose balance	❏ Loses balance (1) (3) (9)
	❏ Does not use grab bars, sink edge for balance support	❏ Uses grab bars, sink edge for balance support (3) (4) (9)
	❏ Feet do not slide away	❏ One or both feet slide away (5) (6)
		❏ Unable to perform maneuver or perform it safely (10)

POEMS: Performance-Oriented Environmental Mobility Screen

Balance

Standing/Reaching	Observation	
	Normal	Impaired (Intervention)
Stand in place (for approx. 15 seconds) with both eyes open	❏ Steady, able to stand without losing balance	❏ Unsteady, unable to maintain standing balance (1) (2)
	❏ Does not use chair to maintain balance	❏ Uses chair to maintain balance (7)
	❏ Does not use device to maintain balance	❏ Uses device to maintain balance (1) (2)
		❏ Unable to perform maneuver or perform it safely (10)
Stand in place with both eyes closed	❏ Steady, able to stand without losing balance	❏ Unsteady, unable to maintain standing balance (1) (2) (4)
	❏ Does not use chair to maintain balance	❏ Uses chair to maintain balance (7)
Stand in place (both eyes open); lightly nudge person's sternum 3 times	❏ Steady, able to maintain balance	❏ Unsteady, unable to maintain balance (1) (2)
	❏ Does not use furniture or walls to maintain balance	❏ Uses furniture or walls to maintain balance (7)
		❏ Unable to perform maneuver or perform it safely (10)
Bend down and pick up object from floor	❏ Steady, able to bend down without losing balance	❏ Unsteady, unable to bend down and maintain balance (1)
	❏ Does not use device to maintain balance	❏ Uses device to maintain balance (1) (2)
		❏ Unable to perform maneuver or perform it safely (10)

Falls in Older People: Prevention and Management, Fourth Edition,
by Rein Tideiksaar. Copyright © 2010, Health Professions Press, Inc., Baltimore, MD. POEMS-11

POEMS: Performance-Oriented Environmental Mobility Screen

Key to Interventions

1. Medical evaluation

2. Rehabilitative evaluation
   - ❑ Nonslip strips
   - ❑ Gait assessment
   - ❑ Balance assessment
   - ❑ Exercise program
   - ❑ Hip-padding system
   - ❑ Other: _____

3. Walking space/pathways
   - ❑ Unobstructed walking areas
   - ❑ Stable furnishings for support
   - ❑ Nonslip grasp surfaces (furnishings, walls, sink, hallways)
   - ❑ Other: _____

4. Visual walking space/pathways
   - ❑ Accessible lighting
   - ❑ Adequate lighting
   - ❑ Glare reduction
   - ❑ Color contrast (furnishings, handrails, grab bars)
   - ❑ Other: _____

5. Footwear
   - ❑ Podiatrist evaluation
   - ❑ Proper fit
   - ❑ Nonslip soles/socks
   - ❑ Nontraction soles
   - ❑ Other: _____

6. Floor space
   - ❑ Nonslip finishes
   - ❑ Nonslip strips
   - ❑ Eliminate uneven surface elevations
   - ❑ Color contrast uneven surface elevations
   - ❑ Other: _____

7. Chair
   - ❑ Seat height adjustment
   - ❑ Seat depth adjustment
   - ❑ Supportive armrests
   - ❑ Stable (nonmovable) chair
   - ❑ Seat cushions/wedge cushion
   - ❑ Other: _____

8. Bed
   - ❑ Height adjustment (low/high)
   - ❑ Firm mattress support
   - ❑ Bed half side rail
   - ❑ Transfer bar
   - ❑ Bed wheel locks
   - ❑ Immobilizer legs
   - ❑ Bed alarm device
   - ❑ Accessible nurse call system
   - ❑ Other: _____

9. Toilet
   - ❑ Grab bar (wall/toilet attached)
   - ❑ Raised toilet seat
   - ❑ Accessible nurse call system
   - ❑ Bedside commode
   - ❑ Other: _____

10. Human assistance
    - ❑ One person
    - ❑ Two people
    - ❑ Other: _____

POEMS: Performance-Oriented Environmental Mobility Screen

POEMS Summary

Location	Maneuver	Normal	Impaired
Bedroom	Ambulation		
	Straight line	❑	❑
	Turning	❑	❑
	Chair transfer		
	Onto	❑	❑
	Off	❑	❑
	Standing balance		
	Eyes open	❑	❑
	Eyes closed	❑	❑
	Sternal nudge	❑	❑
	Bending down	❑	❑
	Bed transfer		
	Onto	❑	❑
	Off	❑	❑
Bathroom	Ambulation		
	Straight line	❑	❑
	Turning	❑	❑
	Toilet transfer		
	Onto	❑	❑
	Off	❑	❑
	Toilet hygiene	❑	❑
Hallway	Ambulation		
	Straight line	❑	❑
	Turning	❑	❑
	Distance	❑	❑

Falls in Older People: Prevention and Management, Fourth Edition,
by Rein Ticeiksaar. Copyright © 2010, Health Professions Press, Inc., Baltimore, MD. POEMS-13

Performance-Oriented Bed Mobility Screen

Maneuver	Observation		
Ask the patient or resident to . . .		Independent	Impaired
Rise from supine to seated position	❑	Able to rise and sit up in smooth, controlled movement	❑ Unable to rise and sit up in smooth, controlled movement
	❑	Sitting balance is stable	❑ Sitting balance is unstable
	❑	Feet rest flat on floor	❑ Feet do not rest flat on floor
	❑	Assistive device used to perform maneuver	
	❑	Assistive device used properly	
Transfer from bed	❑	Able to rise from seated position in smooth, controlled movement	❑ Unstable rising from seated position (needs several attempts to get up; falls back onto mattress)
	❑	Bed stable, does not slide or roll away	❑ Bed slides or rolls away
	❑	Feet do not slide away on floor	❑ Feet slide away on floor
	❑	Side rail or transfer bar used to perform maneuver	
	❑	Side rail or transfer bar used properly	
Stand in place	❑	Steady, able to stand without balance loss	❑ Unsteady standing balance
	❑	Side rail or transfer bar used to perform maneuver	
	❑	Side rail or transfer bar used properly	
Transfer back onto bed	❑	Able to sit down on bed in smooth, controlled movement	❑ Unstable when sitting down on bed
	❑	Feet do not slide away on floor	❑ Feet slide away on floor
	❑	Bed stable, does not slide or roll away	❑ Bed slides or rolls away
	❑	Side rail or transfer bar used to perform maneuver	
	❑	Side rail or transfer bar used properly	
Operate nurse call system	❑	Able to operate	❑ Unable to operate

Injury and Acute Medical Problems Checklist

Summon for medical assistance if patient/resident complains of

	Yes	No
Difficulty moving arms or legs?	❏	❏
Pain/injury in arms, legs, or lower back?	❏	❏
Headache/head injury?	❏	❏
Confusion/lethargy?	❏	❏
Dizziness/lightheadedness?	❏	❏
Loss of consciousness?	❏	❏
Convulsions?	❏	❏
Chest pain/difficulty breathing?	❏	❏
Fast, slow, or irregular pulse rate?	❏	❏

If you suspect a hip or pelvic fracture (e.g., pain in hip, lower back, or groin area; extremity pain that worsens with movement), do not try to move the person.

Falls in Older People: Prevention and Management, Fourth Edition,
by Rein Tideiksaar. Copyright © 2010, Health Professions Press, Inc., Baltimore, MD.

Fall Risk Checklist

Risk factors

- ❏ Previous falls
- ❏ Visual impairment
- ❏ Postural hypotension
- ❏ Balance disorder
- ❏ Cognitive impairment (depression, dementia, poor judgment)
- ❏ Gait disorder

- ❏ Lower extremity weakness
- ❏ Arthritis (knee, hips)
- ❏ Medications (psychotropics, sedatives, hypnotics, antihypertensives)
- ❏ Bladder and/or bowe dysfunction (frequency, urgency, nocturia, incontinence)

Describe circumstances of falls

Symptoms:

Location:

Time of day:

Activity:

Trauma:

_____

(continued)

Fall Risk Checklist *(continued)*

Mobility

Location	Maneuver	Independent	Impaired
Bedroom	Chair transfers		
	Sitting	❏	❏
	Rising	❏	❏
	Standing balance	❏	❏
	Immediate	❏	❏
	Romberg test	❏	❏
	Sternal push test	❏	❏
	Bending-down balance	❏	❏
	Bed transfers		
	Sitting	❏	❏
	Rising	❏	❏
	Ambulation		
	Straight path	❏	❏
	Turning	❏	❏
Bathroom	Toilet transfers		
	Sitting	❏	❏
	Rising	❏	❏
	Ambulation		
	Straight path	❏	❏
	Turning	❏	❏
	Other	❏	❏

_____

_____

High–Fall Risk Room Setup

A majority of hospital and nursing home falls are associated at least in part with extrinsic or unsafe environmental factors in the bedrooms. Consequently, creating a safe room environment for people at high fall risk is an important component of fall prevention. The following checklist can be used by hospitals and nursing homes to ensure maximum bedroom safety for at-risk patients or residents.

High–Fall Risk Room Setup and Checklist

Recommendations	Rationale
❏ Place person in a bedroom close to the nursing station.	Allows closer observation by a greater number of staff.
❏ Place high-risk signage (falling star) in the bedroom and on the outside of the room door.	Alerts all staff that the person is at fall risk.
❏ Place fall prevention storyboard (identified risk factors and interventions) on the wall in front of the bed.	Used to increase staff awareness of the care plan. Used as a teaching aid for patients or residents and families in ways to prevent falls.
❏ Place bed in a low position so that knees are at a 90-degree angle.	Bed position provides maximum safe egress.
❏ Place side rails down on the exit side of the bed and two split rails up on the nonexit side of the bed.	Protects and directs patient or resident to exit on the safe side of the bed.
❏ If patient or resident exhibits impaired transfers, place head split rail up on the exit side of the bed and two split rails up on the nonexit side of the bed.	Side rail used as an enabler (hand-hold) for safe transfers.
❏ Place nonslip strips on the floor where the patient or resident exits the bed.	Prevents the patient or resident from slipping on spilled liquids (e.g., urine, feces, blood, water).
❏ Place over-the-bed table on the nonexit side of the bed.	Prevents the patient or resident from using table for hand support during transfers.
❏ Place sturdy chairs with armrests and seats no higher or lower than 18 inches. Avoid chairs with wheels.	Provides maximum support for safe chair egress.
❏ Place a commode chair next to the bed, on the exit side of bed for people with urinary impairment (e.g., incontinence, nocturia).	Provides a safe option to meet toileting needs.
❏ Keep room illuminated during the day.	Provides greater visibility.
❏ Place motion-activated night-light by the bed and in the bathroom.	Provides a safe pathway to the bathroom at night.
❏ Place a call bell and personal items within reach.	Patient or resident does not have to stretch or exit the bed to reach items.
❏ Place IV pole on the exit side of the bed (tubes or lines not across the bed).	Prevents lines from being pulled out and patient or resident getting tangled in lines.
❏ Use bed or chair alarm.	Alarm provides an audible alert when the patient or resident attempts to stand. It can be used as an assessment tool to help identify a pattern of bed or chair exits and supervision needs.

Falls in Older People: Prevention and Management, Fourth Edition,
by Rein Tideiksaar. Copyright © 2010, Health Professions Press, Inc., Baltimore, MD.

Process Steps in Reducing Bedside Falls

A majority of institutional falls occur in the patient's or resident's room; up to half of all falls take place from or near the bed. The ability to decrease the risk of bedside falls depends on a multifaceted approach (see forms "Strategies to Reduce Bedside Falls" and "Strategies to Ensure Bed Safety").

Strategies to Reduce Bedside Falls

Intervention Strategies	Description
Assessment	Assess patient or resident • Each day for ability to transfer from bed and ambulate after leaving bed. • Each shift for hazard-free environment. • Any time medical and functional status changes. • After a fall.
Multidisciplinary referrals	• Refer and discuss with physician and multidisciplinary team identified risk factors and any changes in status (e.g., medical conditions, medications, and function) that suggest the need for further assessment of the cause or targeted interventions.
Nursing care	• Use colored wristband and decal above bed to identify patients or residents at high risk of falling. • Assist with ambulation and transfers. • Offer assistance with toileting every 2 hours while patient or resident is awake. • Provide appropriate shoes or socks with nonskid soles. • Ensure that wheels on beds are locked before transferring patients or residents. • Ensure that call light, urinal, bedpan, and drinking water are within easy reach. • Reduce clutter around bed. • Institute protective measures and additional interventions after fall (e.g., increasing surveillance, more frequent observations, bed alarms).
Technology and equipment	Consider • Nonslip bedside mats or low beds that go to within 8 inches of floor to reduce injurious fall risk. • Bed alarms that identify when patients or residents are moving out of bed. • Bed poles or transfer handles to help patients or residents transfer safely and independently. • Night sensor light to reduce nighttime falls. • Nonslip flooring or change of floor cleaning processes to reduce slippery finish.
Family and patient or resident education	Instruct patient or resident and caregiver • What factors contribute to fall risk. • What safety measures patients or residents and family members can take to reduce fall risk. Consider having a family member stay with the patient or resident when a personal nursing assistant is not available.

Falls in Older People: Prevention and Management, Fourth Edition,
by Rein Tideiksaar. Copyright © 2010, Health Professions Press, Inc., Baltimore, MD.

Strategies to Ensure Bed Safety

Intervention	Explanation
Maintain bed at appropriate height.	Bed height is appropriate when the person's knees are at 90 degrees and the feet touch the floor. This height supports the person's ability to exit a bed safely. If bed height is raised for nursing care, return the bed to a low position when care is completed.
Ensure that bed brakes are on at all times.	Prevents the bed from rolling away during bed transfers.
Always leave a nurse call bell within reach when the patient or resident is in bed.	The patient or resident should be able to operate the call bell appropriately. Demonstrate the use of the call bell and ask the patient or resident for a return demonstration. Consider the use of a fall alarm for any patient or resident who is at fall risk and is unable to use the call bell.
Ensure that frequently used items are left within reach.	Reaching for items that are out of reach may cause the patient or resident to lose balance.
Place antislip strips on the floor where the patient or resident exits the bed.	Protects the patient or resident from slipping on any spilled food or water.
Position over-bed table on the nonexit side of the bed.	Discourages the patient or resident from using the over-bed table, which can easily roll away, as a handhold when trying to exit from the bed.
If in use, place the bedside commode next to the bed, on the exit side.	Placing the commode on the exit side makes access easier for the patient or resident.
If in use, position canes and walkers next to the bed, on the exit side.	Placing the cane or walker on the exit side makes access easier for the resident or patient.
Keep the bedroom night-light illuminated at all times.	Provides greater visibility when natural light is low.
Use height-adjustable low beds to support safe transfers and prevent injurious falls.	A height-adjustable low bed (6 to 32 inches high) provides a proper bed height for safe transfers by short patients or residents and, when kept in the low position, helps prevent injurious falls (should a fall occur, distance of falling is less). Consider the use of a fall alarm (to detect rollouts from bed) or floor mat (to avoid injury from rolling onto floor) in conjunction with a bed in low position.

Restraint/Non-Restraint Assessment and Care Planning Tool

Date: _____

Patient's/resident's name: _____

PART I: Baseline Patient/Resident Information

Does the patient/resident:	Yes	No
Have poor judgment or impaired communication?	❑	❑
Have a history of recent falls?	❑	❑
Have contractures or limited range of motion?	❑	❑
Have difficulty with postural hypotension?	❑	❑
Have a diagnosis of or signs and symptoms of depression?	❑	❑
Have difficulty with standing/sitting balance?	❑	❑
Have a history of wandering?	❑	❑

Is the patient/resident:		
Able to toilet independently?	❑	❑
On any medications requiring safety precautions?	❑	❑
Able to use the call light?	❑	❑
Continent?	❑	❑
Agitated?	❑	❑
Interfering with his or her medical treatment?	❑	❑

Falls in Older People: Prevention and Management, Fourth Edition,
by Rein Tideiksaar. Copyright © 2010, Health Professions Press, Inc., Baltimore, MD.

PART II: Concern(s). Describe the patient's/resident's medical, psychological, and functional problems indicating potential need for restraint use.

PART III: Non-restraint justification. Describe the care plan (including non-restraint alternatives) provided to patient/resident and why non-restraint is being considered at this time.

Consider:

Low beds

Mats on floor

Half-side rails as enablers

Bed alarms

Wedge cushions/other positioning devices

Moving patient/resident nearer to nurses' station

Fall prevention program

(continued)

PART IV: Restraint use justification. Describe the care plan (including least-restraint/ restraint-alternative efforts to date) provided to the patient/resident and why restraint is being considered at this time.

PART V: Recommendations. Describe the restraint recommendations (including restraint-monitoring schedule).

PART VI: Physician's order for restraint.

Does the order include the following:	Yes	No
Specific type of restraint used?	❑	❑
The circumstances or conditions under which the restraint should be used?	❑	❑
Restraint release/reduction times?	❑	❑

PART VII: Notification. Inform patient/resident and family of restraint/nonrestraint recommendations.

I understand why the interdisciplinary team has recommended restraints/non-restraints as

part of care plan for _____ .
                                                        patient/resident name

I am aware certain negative outcomes such as falls are associated with [restraint/non-restraint] use.

❑ Approve

❑ Disapprove

Signature: _____ Date: _____
                    Family representative or legal guardian

Signature: _____ Date: _____
                            Patient/resident

_____

PART VIII: Staff signatures and dates. Include all members of the patient's/resident's inter-disciplinary care team.

Side Rail Assessment and Care Planning Tool

Date: _____

Patient's/resident's name: _____

PART I: Baseline Assessment Information

Is the patient/resident:	Yes	No
Ambulatory (including assistive devices)?	❏	❏
Comatose, semi-comatose, or having fluctuations in mental status?	❏	❏
Able to toilet independently?	❏	❏
Able to transfer from bed independently?	❏	❏
Able to ambulate to the bathroom (toilet) independently?	❏	❏
Continent?	❏	❏
On any medications that would require increased safety precautions?	❏	❏

Does the patient/resident:		
Have poor judgment or impaired communication?	❏	❏
Have a diagnosis or symptoms of depression?	❏	❏
Have falls from bed?	❏	❏
Have falls on the way to bathroom (toilet)?	❏	❏
Have postural hypotension?	❏	❏
Have contractures or limited range of motion?	❏	❏

(continued)

Falls in Older People: Prevention and Management, Fourth Edition,
by Rein Tideiksaar. Copyright © 2010, Health Professions Press, Inc., Baltimore, MD.

Side Rail Assessment and Care Planning Tool *(continued)*

PART II: Concern(s). Describe rationale for potential side rail use.

Include the following:

	Yes	No
Patient/resident has requested to have side rail raised while in bed.	❏	❏
Side rails serve as:		
An enabler to promote mobility while in bed	❏	❏
An enabler to promote safe bed transfers	❏	❏
Side rails are indicated to provide safety or prevent falls at this time. (If yes, explain why.)	❏	❏

_____

PART III: Recommendations. Describe when and why side rails are used (i.e., how long and under what circumstances).

PART IV: Physician's order for side rail use.

Does the order include the following:	Yes	No
Specific type of side rail?	❏	❏
Under what circumstances or conditions side rails are used?	❏	❏
Side rail monitoring times?	❏	❏

PART V: Notifications. Inform patient/resident and family of side rail recommendations.

I understand why the interdisciplinary team has recommended side rails as part of

care plan for _____.
(patient/resident name)

I am aware that certain negative outcomes are associated with side rail use.

❏ Approve

❏ Disapprove

Signature: _____   Date: _____
Family representative or legal guardian

Signature: _____   Date: _____
Patient/resident

PART VI: Staff signatures and dates. Include all members of the patient's/resident's interdisciplinary care team.

Wheelchair Problems and Modifications Checklist

Observe patient's or resident's wheelchair mobility. Ask the individual to transfer from the chair and observe whether he or she accomplishes the task safely.

	Yes	No
Did the person engage the brakes?	❏	❏
If no, consider wedge cushion to prevent independent transfers.		
Can the person reach the hand brakes?	❏	❏
If no, replace with long brake handles.		
Did the brakes lock in place?	❏	❏
If no, replace the chair or fix the problem.		
Did the person remember to move the footrests away?	❏	❏
If no, consider removing footrests (if appropriate) or consider adding a wedge cushion to prevent independent transfers.		
Did the chair tip over forward?	❏	❏
If yes, consider attaching antitip device to footplates or weights to the back of the chair.		
Does the seat interfere with transfers?	❏	❏
If yes, consider retrofitting sling seat with plywood or solid inserts.		
Does the seat interfere with sitting balance?	❏	❏
If yes, consider lateral supports to correct lean.		
Does individual slide out of chair seat?	❏	❏
If yes, consider use of Dycem mat (placed on seat to prevent sliding) or position footrests to maintain proper seating.		

Discharge Teaching Sheets

Home Fall Prevention

An injury from falling can limit a person's ability to lead an active, independent life. This is especially true for older people. Each year, thousands of older men and women are injured, sometimes permanently, by falls that result in broken bones. Yet many of these injuries can be prevented by making simple changes in the home.

As people age, changes in their vision, hearing, muscle strength, coordination, and reflexes may make them susceptible to falls. Older adults likely have treatable disorders that may affect their balance (e.g., diabetes; conditions of the heart, nervous system, and thyroid). In addition, as compared with younger adults, older people often take medications that may cause dizziness or lightheadedness.

Preventing falls is especially important for people with osteoporosis, a condition in which bone mass decreases so that bones are more fragile and break easily. Osteoporosis is a major cause of bone fractures in women after menopause and older adults in general. For people with severe osteoporosis, even a minor fall may cause one or more bones to break.

STEPS TO TAKE

Falls and accidents seldom "just happen," and many can be prevented. Each of us can take steps to make our homes safer and reduce the likelihood of falling. Here are some guidelines to help prevent falls and fractures:

- Vision and hearing should be tested regularly and properly corrected.
- The person should talk with the doctor or pharmacist about the side effects of the medicines he or she is taking and whether they affect coordination or balance. The person should ask for suggestions to reduce the possibility of falling.
- The person should limit his or her alcohol intake. Even a small amount of alcohol can disturb already-impaired balance and reflexes.

- The person should use caution in getting up too quickly after eating, lying down, or resting. Low blood pressure may cause dizziness at these times.
- The nighttime temperature in the person's home should be at least 65°F. Prolonged exposure to cold temperatures may cause a drop in body temperature, which in turn may lead to dizziness and falling. Many older adults cannot tolerate cold as well as younger people can.
- A cane, a walking stick, or a walker should be used to help the person maintain balance on uneven or unfamiliar ground or if the person sometimes feels dizzy. Special caution should be taken in walking outdoors on wet or icy pavement.
- The person should wear supportive rubber-soled or low-heeled shoes and avoid wearing smooth-soled slippers or socks without shoes on stairs and waxed floors. These surfaces make it easy to slip.
- The person should maintain a regular program of exercise to improve strength and muscle tone, and joints, tendons, and ligaments should be kept flexible. Many older people enjoy walking and swimming. Mild weight-bearing activities, such as walking or climbing stairs, may even reduce bone loss due to osteoporosis. The person should check with his or her doctor or physical therapist to plan a suitable exercise program.

MAKE HOME A SAFE PLACE

Many older people fall because of hazardous conditions at home. This checklist can be used to help safeguard the person against some likely hazards.

Stairways, hallways, and pathways should have

- ❏ Good lighting. Provide extra lighting along path from bedroom to bathroom, by one- and two-step elevations, and by top and bottom of stairway landings; use night-light, 100- to 200-watt bulbs, and 3-way lightbulbs to increase lighting levels
- ❏ A lack of glare. Eliminate glare from exposed lightbulbs by using translucent light shades or frosted lightbulbs.
- ❏ Firmly attached carpet, rough-texture or abrasive strips to secure footing, nonskid rugs and carpet runners on slippery floors, a coating of nonskid floor wax, carpeting over threshold to create a smooth transition between rooms
- ❏ No clutter, including obtrusive furnishings
- ❏ Tightly fastened cylindrical handrails running the whole length and along both sides of all stairs, with light switches at the top and bottom

Bathrooms should have

- ❏ Elevated toilet seat or toilet safety frame
- ❏ Wall-mounted or tub-attached grab bar or shower chair/tub transfer bench
- ❏ Nonskid mats, abrasive strips, or carpet on all surfaces that may get wet
- ❏ Night-lights

Bedrooms should have

❑ Night-lights or light switches within reach of bed(s)
❑ Telephones that are easy to reach near the bed(s)

Living areas should have

❑ Electrical cords and telephone wires placed away from walking paths
❑ Rugs well secured to the floor
❑ Furniture, especially low coffee tables, and other objects arranged so that they are not obstacles
❑ Couches and chairs that are of a proper height so that patients or residents get into and out of them easily (add a seat cushion to raise seat height; replace existing mattress with one that is thinner to lower bed height, or thicker to raise bed height); chairs with armrest support
❑ Frequently used objects sited at waist level
❑ A reacher device available for person to obtain objects from shelves
❑ Shelves and cupboards at accessible height

Checklist to Assess Components of a Successful Fall Prevention Program

Effective fall prevention programs are based on having an organized and structured clinical process of care as well as organizational components that are enabling or supportive. The following checklists, "Clinical Process of Care" and "Organizational Components," can be used as a quick assessment of an organization's fall prevention program.

Successful Fall Prevention Program Checklist

Clinical Process of Care

Fall Risk Assessment
- ❑ A system for identifying fall and injury risk upon admission, after a fall, and with a change of condition?
- ❑ A fall risk tool that consists of identifying diseases, drugs, cognitive factors, elimination or urinary factors, ambulatory aids, and mobility factors associated with fall risk?

Care Plan
- ❑ A process of care planning or implementing targeted interventions aimed at reducing identified risk factors?
- ❑ A process of care planning that consists of multidisciplinary strategies targeted at identified risk factors?
- ❑ A mechanism for communicating when patients or residents are at fall risk to all staff?

Postfall Assessment
- ❑ A formal postfall process for investigating falls (to identify why a fall occurred and to prevent further falls)?
- ❑ A postfall assessment that includes circumstances of the fall (symptoms, location, activity), presence of environmental hazards, reassessment of fall risk factors, and root cause analysis (cause of fall)?

Monitoring
- ❑ A process of monitoring risk or change of condition on a daily basis?
- ❑ A follow-up process to determine whether interventions are working to reduce fall risk?

Organizational Components

- ❑ Fall prevention policies, procedures, and guidelines for staff?
- ❑ Process for promoting a culture of safety throughout the facility that fall prevention is important and that many falls can be prevented?
- ❑ Comprehensive fall prevention education program to increase awareness for all staff and family members?
- ❑ Fall coordinator who can support and follow through with the fall prevention initiatives?
- ❑ Process for evaluating the effectiveness of specific strategies and overall approaches to fall prevention?
- ❑ Process for monitoring facility-wide fall and injury patterns and contributing factors as well as for implementing appropriate preventions?
- ❑ System for recognizing and rewarding the staff for their fall prevention efforts?
- ❑ Budget to support the fall and injury prevention program?

Falls in Older People: Prevention and Management, Fourth Edition,
by Rein Tideiksaar. Copyright © 2010, Health Professions Press, Inc., Baltimore, MD.

Checklist to Audit Care Plans

The steps in the fall prevention process of care include assessment of risk, multidisciplinary evaluation of identified risk factors, design of interventions based on identified risk factors, communication of risk to all caregivers, patient or resident and family education on specific risk factors and interventions, and outcome monitoring of the plan of care. This checklist can be used to determine whether staff are adhering to the fall prevention process of care.

Audit Checklist

	Yes	No
Presence of an individualized plan of care within 8 hours of admission, with a change of condition, and after a fall based on a risk assessment?	❏	❏
Plan of care reflects input from all disciplines as appropriate?	❏	❏
Staff members have integrated information from various assessments (disciplines) to identify care needs?	❏	❏
Plan of care has been communicated with staff?	❏	❏
Plan of care has been discussed with patient or resident and family?	❏	❏
Outcomes have been reviewed and updated?	❏	❏

Administrator's Safety Walk Rounds Checklist

Aside from relying on front-line staff to provide feedback regarding potential safety issues within the facility, administrators need to be involved in the milieu, and one important way to achieve this is through rounds (i.e., walking around the facility, spotting any potential safety issues, and addressing these concerns to staff). The "Safety Walk Rounds Checklist" helps focus attention on important aspects of the environment and can be used during rounds to look for the following:

- Safety trouble spots or hazardous conditions that staff may have missed

- Opportunities for improvement related to environmental safety and fall avoidance.

It is important to address any unsafe situations immediately by notifying the appropriate staff and ensuring that remedial actions are taken.

Safety Walk Rounds Checklist

	Yes	No
Are hallways and living areas well lit?	❏	❏
Are hallways and living areas uncluttered and free of spills?	❏	❏
Are hallway handrails secure and unobstructed?	❏	❏
Are furnishings (e.g., tables, chairs) sturdy, especially when leaned on?	❏	❏
Are bed wheels in good repair, and do they lock properly?	❏	❏
Are wheelchair brakes in good repair, and do they lock properly?	❏	❏
Are handrails in toilet area present and secure?	❏	❏
Are nurse call bells in working order?	❏	❏

Falls in Older People: Prevention and Management, Fourth Edition,
by Rein Tideiksaar. Copyright © 2010, Health Professions Press, Inc., Baltimore, MD.

Safety Culture Checklist

Organizations with a positive safety culture set the tone for a successful fall prevention program. Safety culture generally includes such areas as safety perception, teamwork within and between departments, communication openness, feedback and communication about error, nonpunitive response to error, organizational learning, management expectations, and actions promoting safety, staffing, and management support for safety. The "Safety Culture Checklist" can be used to identify characteristics associated with a positive safety culture within an organization.

Safety Culture Checklist

To what extent are the following items characteristic of the facility?

- ❏ Staff work together as a team.
- ❏ Team members deal constructively with disagreements.
- ❏ Staff remain focused on goals of care plan.
- ❏ Different staff perspectives are incorporated into care plan.
- ❏ Staff are not blamed when a patient or resident falls.
- ❏ Staff feel safe reporting their mistakes.
- ❏ Staff talk about ways to keep falls from happening again.
- ❏ Staff report hazardous situations or conditions that might lead to a fall.
- ❏ Management asks staff how safety can be improved.
- ❏ Changes to improve safety are easy to implement.
- ❏ Changes to improve safety are checked to see whether they worked.
- ❏ Improving quality of care and reducing falls are a high priority.
- ❏ Staff treat each other with respect and support one another.
- ❏ Sufficient staff are available for the care workload.
- ❏ Staff ideas and suggestions are valued.
- ❏ Staff engage in problem solving on challenging patients or residents.
- ❏ Team meetings are productive.
- ❏ Staff feel like part of a team.
- ❏ Staff get the training they need on fall prevention.
- ❏ Staff understand the training they get.
- ❏ Staff are told what they need to know before taking care of patients or residents for the first time.
- ❏ Ways to keep patients or residents safe from harm and falls are discussed.
- ❏ Management listens to staff ideas and suggestions about safety.
- ❏ Management pays attention to safety problems.

Appendix

Appendix A
Case Study Exercises

CASE 1

E.L. is an 80-year-old hospital patient who experienced two falls. She stated that both falls occurred shortly after she got up from bed at night to go to the bathroom. She was hurrying to the toilet in order to avoid urinating on the floor and lost her balance. Her medical problems consist of Parkinson's disease and arthritis in both knees. She takes no medication. E.L.'s ambulation is poor and she does not use a walker. Her cognitive abilities are unaffected.

Questions

1. With the information you have about this patient, what specific interventions would you include in her care plan in order to reduce fall risk?

2. Based on your care plan, for which outcomes would you monitor this patient?

CASE 2

G.B. is a 76-year-old nursing facility resident who experienced several falls from bed. He complained of unsteadiness after getting up from bed. G.B.'s medical problems include a history of hypertension, which was treated with a diuretic. The results of the medical evaluation revealed that G.B. was dehydrated and had orthostatic hypotension (i.e., dizziness on rising from a seated or lying position).

Questions

1. With the information you have about this resident, what specific interventions would you include in his care plan in order to reduce fall risk?

2. Based on your care plan, for which outcomes would you monitor this resident?

CASE 3

M.P. is an 89-year-old nursing facility resident who experienced several falls, all of which occurred while she was walking either in the bedroom or hallway in the late afternoon. M.P.'s medical problem consists of severe dementia. She exhibits poor gait and balance. M.P. has a walker but forgets to use it. Since her original diagnosis, M.P.'s cognition has deteriorated further, resulting in agitation. M.P. does not take medication.

Questions

1. With the information you have about this resident, what specific interventions would you include in her care plan in order to reduce fall risk?
2. Based on your care plan, for which outcomes would you monitor this resident?

CASE 4

J.S. is an 82-year-old hospital patient who was admitted for pneumonia. He remained in bed for 3 days. After treatment of the illness, the patient demonstrated poor bed and toilet transfers, which was the result of lower-leg weakness developed after being confined to bed.

Questions

1. With the information you have about this patient, what specific interventions would you include in his care plan in order to improve mobility and reduce fall risk?
2. Based on your care plan, for which outcomes would you monitor this patient?

CASE 5

L.R. is a 73-year-old hospital patient admitted for falls. After her most recent fall, she lay on the floor unattended for 6 hours (she lives alone). L.R.'s falls are associated with a loss of balance—which she experiences when she reaches up to retrieve objects from her kitchen and closet shelves and when she gets into and out of her bathtub. L.R. has experienced a stroke and, as a result, has mild left-side leg weakness. She expresses a fear of falling.

Questions

1. With the information you have about this patient, what specific interventions would you include in her care plan in order to improve mobility and reduce her fear of falls while she is in the hospital?
2. What specific interventions would you include in her postdischarge care plan?

CASE 6

A.C. is a 91-year-old nursing facility resident who has experienced several falls from his wheelchair. His falls occur as he attempts to transfer onto his bed and toilet. In a few instances he has slid out of his wheelchair and onto the floor; on one occasion his wheelchair tipped over during a transfer. A C.'s medical history includes a stroke with associated leg weakness and depression for which he takes an antidepressant. Occasionally, he feels dizzy when transferring from his wheelchair.

Questions

1. With the information you have about this resident, what specific interventions would you include in his care plan in order to decrease the risk of falls from his wheelchair?

2. Based on your care plan, for which outcomes would you monitor this resident?

CASE 7

R.E. is an 89-year-old nursing facility resident with moderate dementia, arthritis of the knees, and polymyalgia rneumatica (i.e., a syndrome affecting older people characterized by proximal joint or muscle pain) for which he takes steroid medication. He demonstrates poor bed transfers and ambulation. R.E. uses a walker, but the device is unsafe.

Questions

1. With the information you have about this resident, what specific interventions would you include in his care plan in order to reduce fall risk?

2. Based on your care plan, for which outcomes would you monitor this resident?

CASE 8

M.S. is an 82-year-old hospital patient admitted for falls. She demonstrates poor bed, toilet, and chair transfers, which are the result of lower limb weakness. M.S.'s cognition is mildly impaired. She has hypothyroidism and is on replacement therapy.

Questions

1. With the information you have about this patient, what specific interventions would you include in her care plan in order to improve mobility and reduce fall risk?

2. Based on your care plan, for which outcomes would you monitor this patient?

CASE 9

W.M. is a 79-year-old hospital patient. On the day she was admitted, she slipped in her urine while attempting to toilet. W.M. is now afraid to go to the bathroom by herself and has developed a fear of falling. As a result of this fear, she has developed urinary incontinence. She is able to transfer independently and her cognitive abilities are unaffected.

Questions

1. With the information you have about this patient, what specific intervention would you include in her care plan in order to reduce incontinence and her fear of falling?
2. Based on your care plan, for which outcomes would you monitor this patient?

CASE 10

M.M. is an 82-year-old nursing facility resident who has experienced several falls from bed. M.M.'s medical problems consist of Parkinson's disease and osteoporosis. She takes no medication. Recently, her nurses found M.M. sprawled on the floor by her bed. To prevent further bed falls she was placed in mechanical restraints.

Questions

1. With the information you have about this resident, what specific interventions would you include in her care plan to reduce the risk of falls and eliminate the need for mechanical restraints?
2. Based on your care plan, for which outcomes would you monitor this resident?

CASE 11

L.B. is a 76-year-old woman admitted to the hospital emergency room following a left-sided cerebrovascular accident (CVA) with aphasia. After 2 days, she was transferred to the rehabilitation unit for treatment.

Questions

1. With the information you have about this patient, what specific interventions would you include in her care plan in order to reduce fall risk?
2. Based on your care plan, for which outcomes would you monitor this patient?

CASE 12

T.S. is a 95-year-old man with Parkinson's disease. His nursing aide notices that T.S. has difficulty getting up from his bed. Until now, the patient's bed transfers have been normal.

Questions

1. With the information you have about this patient, what specific interventions would you include in his care plan in order to reduce fall risk?
2. Based on your care plan, for which outcomes would you monitor this patient?

CASE 13

S.O. is a 72-year-old nursing facility resident with confusion. She experienced a fall while walking to the bathroom.

Questions

1. With the information you have about this patient, what specific interventions would you include in her care plan in order to reduce fall risk?
2. Based on your care plan, for which outcomes would you monitor this resident?

CASE 14

A.S. is an 84-year-old hospital patient with diabetes and arthritis. He experiences gait and balance impairment but doesn't use his walker.

Questions

1. With the information you have about this patient, what specific interventions would you include in his care plan in order to reduce fall risk?
2. Based on your care plan, for which outcomes would you monitor this patient?

CASE 15

P.P. is an 88-year-old nursing facility resident. She has experienced two falls while getting up from an easy chair located in her bedroom. Now she has a fear of falling.

Questions

1. With the information you have about this resident, what specific interventions would you include in her care plan in order to reduce fall risk?

2. Based on your care plan, for which outcomes would you monitor this resident?

CASE 16

I.S. is a 71-year-old man admitted to the hospital for elective total knee arthroplasty for severe degenerative joint disease that has led to a decline in function and increasing pain. On the evening of the second hospital day, I.S. began to exhibit some confusion.

Questions

1. With the information you have about this patient, what specific interventions would you include in his care plan in order to reduce fall risk?

2. Based on your care plan, for which outcomes would you monitor this patient?

CASE 17

L.P. is a 76-year-old hospital patient who was just admitted as an emergency following a series of falls at home. L.P.'s falls were associated with a "loss of balance" and her doctor felt that she could benefit from an inpatient evaluation. L.P. has a history of osteoporosis and mild dementia. On the day of admission, L.P. exhibited poor balance and a lack of safety awareness.

Questions

1. With the information you have about this patient, what are her risk factors for suffering an injurious fall?

2. What specific interventions would you include in her care plan to reduce her risk of falls and injurious falls?

CASE 18

T.M. is an 82-year-old nursing home resident who has had a stroke (has right-sided weakness of his arm and leg) and has bladder impairment (frequent urination).

Questions

1. With this limited information, what are T.M.'s fall risk factors?

2. What interventions should be considered to decrease his risk of falling?

CASE 19

D.S. is a nursing home resident with dementia. Recently, D.S. exhibited bouts of agitation and her physician prescribed a low-dose antipsychotic to control her behavioral disturbances. The facility pharmacist advised nursing staff that antipsychotics are associated with a range of common side effects and that they should observe for: Parkinsonism (rigidity and tremor); tardive dyskinesia (jerky, abnormal, or delayed movements in the facial area, the entire head, or the trunk and extremities); tachycardia (rapid heartbeat); akathisia (a persistent feeling of restlessness in the body and muscles and the need to constantly move about); sedation and drowsiness; and hypotension (low blood pressure).

Questions

1. Which of the antipsychotic side effects place D.S. at fall risk?
2. What interventions should be considered to reduce the risk of falls?

CASE 20

G.S. is an 84-year-old hospital patient who has fallen three times in the past 2 days. All of G.S.'s falls have taken place in the late afternoon and are associated with symptoms of "dizziness and lethargy." Her medical history is notable for diabetes, which is treated with a morning dose of long-acting insulin.

Questions

1. What is the most likely cause of G.S.'s falls?
2. What interventions should be considered to reduce G.S.'s risk of falls?

CASE 21

P.S. is a 71-year-old nursing home resident with Parkinson's disease who needs frequent toileting. Upon a mobility evaluation, P.S. exhibits difficulty arising from her bed and chair without armrest support.

Questions

1. What "extrinsic" interventions are available to assist P.S. with safe bed and chair egress?
2. Based on her medical history and mobility evaluation, what is another mobility problem that P.S. is likely to exhibit and what "extrinsic" interventions can be used to modify the problem?

CASE 22

R.E. is an 83-year-old hospital patient with unsteady gait and balance and urinary incontinence. She fell while "rushing" from her bed to the bathroom.

Questions

1. What potential factors could have contributed to R.E.'s fall?
2. What interventions are available to reduce R.E.'s risk of future falls?

CASE 23

B.C. is a 90-year-old nursing home resident with severe arthrits and impaired mobility (i.e., transfer anc ambulation impairment). B.C. was found on her bedroom floor after an apparent fall.

Questions

1. To understand what caused the fall, what questions would you ask B.C.?
2. How can the information help in designing B.C.'s care plan interventions?

CASE 24

P.O. is a 78-year-old patient admitted to the hospital with a history of diabetes, arthritis, mild stroke, and urinary incontinence.

Questions

1. Based on P.O.'s medical problems, what "functional" fall risk factors might be anticipated?
2. What interventions can be put in place on the day of admission to reduce P.O.'s fall risk?

CASE 25

D.H. is a 76-year-old hospital patient who has just experienced a fall. He was found by a nursing assistant on the floor next to his bed. D.H. was reported to be confused and unable to state what happened. He has a history of heart disease and hypertension, and is currently being treated with digoxin and a diuretic. The patient was mentally intact previous to his fall and had not experienced any prior falls.

Questions

1. Awaiting a formal post-fall evaluation, what immediate preventive strategies can be put in place by the nursing staff to protect D.H. from another fall?

2. What immediate protective strategies are available to guard against an injurious fall?

Answers for Case 1

Question 1

- Primary care provider to evaluate patient's nocturia (i.e., getting up at night to urinate) for reversible causes.

- Primary care provider to evaluate patient's Parkinson's disease and arthritis and her need for Parkinson's and analgesic medications in order to improve ambulation.

- Nursing to provide a night-light in patient's bedroom in order to provide safe ambulation to the bathroom.

- Physical Therapy to evaluate patient for a walker in order to improve ambulation.

- Physical Therapy to evaluate patient and provide an exercise program in order to improve ambulation.

Question 2

- Monitor patient for further falls. If falls occur under similar circumstances, consider a bed alarm system to alert staff when E.L. gets out of bed and so that they can offer assistance with ambulation, or provide a bedside commode to eliminate E.L.'s need to travel to the bathroom.

- Monitor symptoms of nocturia.

- Monitor patient's ability to ambulate and for safe use of her walker.

Answers for Case 2

Question 1

- Primary care provider to evaluate the dose of diuretic in order to reduce risk of dehydration and orthostatic hypotension.

- Nursing to provide resident with sufficient fluid intake in order to treat dehydration.

- Nursing to request that resident ask for assistance when getting up from bed; nursing needs to provide assistance with rising from bed in order to reduce risk of falls.

- Nursing to check whether resident also experiences orthostatic hypotension with other transfer activities, such as chair and toilet transfers, and provide appropriate modifications as needed in order to support safe transfer activities.

Question 2

- Monitor G.B. for further falls. If falls occur, refer to primary care provider for another evaluation. If falls occur with rising from bed or resident fails to ask for assistance, or both, consider the use of a bed alarm system.

- Monitor G.B.'s blood pressure to ensure that it is controlled, particularly if the dose of diuretics is reduced.

- Monitor fluid intake to avoid the risk of dehydration.

Answers for Case 3

Question 1

- Primary care provider to evaluate resident's worsening cognition and agitation for reversible causes. Consider short-term medication to control agitation, but only if behavior results in harm to self or others.

- Physical Therapy to evaluate resident and provide a walker and an ambulation program in order to support safe ambulation.

- Nursing to provide resident with structured activities in the late afternoon in order to avoid agitation and eliminate need for medication to control agitation.

Question 2

- Monitor for further falls. If falls occur under similar circumstances, consider hip-padding system in order to decrease risk of hip fractures.

- Monitor cognition and agitation.

- Monitor for effectiveness and side effects of medication, if given for agitation.

- Monitor ambulation and for safe use of walker. If resident fails to use her walker, consider a Merry Walker to allow independent ambulation.

- Monitor for sundowning (i.e., late afternoon or early evening confusion).

Answers for Case 4

Question 1

- Primary care provider to evaluate patient's leg weakness for treatable causes.

- Physical Therapy to evaluate patient and provide rehabilitative exercise program to improve his leg strength.

- Nursing to evaluate patient's bed and provide modifications such as low height, half-bedside rail for transfer assistance, and nonslip floor surfaces in order to support safe transfers.

- Physical Therapy to evaluate patient's toilet and provide modifications such as grab bars, toilet riser, and nonslip floor surface in order to support safe transfers.

- Nursing to request that patient ask for help with transfers; nursing needs to provide assistance in order to support safe transfers.

Question 2

- Monitor patient for further falls. If patient falls from bed, fails to ask for assistance, or both, consider bed alarm system to alert staff when patient gets out of bed.

- Monitor for effectiveness of bed and toilet modifications.

- Monitor for effectiveness of rehabilitative exercise program.

Answers for Case 5

Question 1

- Primary care provider to evaluate the causes of the patient's falls and risk factors for further falls (i.e., to examine for treatable causes and modifiable risk factors).

- Physical Therapy to evaluate patient and provide an exercise program in order to improve L.P.'s balance and reduce her fear of falling.

- Nursing to provide assistance with patient's transfers and ambulation in order to support safe activities and reduce her fear of falling.

Question 2

- Home Care to provide patient with a personal emergency response system in order to reduce the risk of extensive lie times.

- Home Care Physical Therapy to continue exercise program, if needed.

- Home Care Occupational Therapy to evaluate the safety of L.P.'s home environment; modify kitchen/closet shelves in order to reduce risk of balance loss and provide bathtub equipment in order to support safe tub transfers.

Answers for Case 6

Question 1

- Primary care provider to evaluate resident's depression and antidepressant dosage for medication side effects and possible decreased medication dose or selection of an alternative drug.

- Physical Therapy to teach resident safe wheelchair transfer techniques, provide an exercise program to strengthen his legs, modify resident's wheelchair (e.g., brakes, seat height, and anti-tipping device to support safe transfers), and provide toilet grab bars and half-bedside rail to support safe toilet and bed transfers.

- Nursing to provide resident with a nonslip wheelchair seat cushion in order to prevent him from sliding out of his wheelchair.

Question 2

- Monitor for further falls from the wheelchair. If falls occur, reevaluate wheelchair interventions.

- Monitor depression and effectiveness/side effects of medication.

- Monitor for effectiveness of Physical Therapy and Nursing interventions.

Answers for Case 7

Question 1

- Primary care provider to evaluate resident's steroid medication for necessity or for tapering off the dosage.

- Nursing to evaluate resident's bed and provide modifications, such as lower height and half-bedside rails, for transfer assistance to support safe transfers.

- Physical Therapy to evaluate resident's walker and the need for an exercise program in order to improve leg strength and ambulation.

Question 2

- Monitor for further falls from bed.

- Monitor bed transfers and for effectiveness of bed modifications.

- Monitor ambulation and for safe use of the walker.

Answers for Case 8

Question 1

- Primary care provider to evaluate patient's leg weakness and altered cognition for treatable causes.

- Nursing to evaluate patient's bed and provide modifications in order to support safe transfers.

- Physical Therapy to evaluate patient and provide an exercise program in order to improve transfers. PT to evaluate and provide chair and toilet modifications in order to support safe transfers.

Question 2

- Monitor for further falls.

- Monitor thyroid status and for effectiveness of replacement therapy.

- Monitor cognition.

- Monitor transfers.

- Monitor for effectiveness of chair and toilet modifications.

Answers for Case 9

Question 1

- Nursing to provide patient with a bedside commode to eliminate the need for traveling to the bathroom and to reduce incontinence.

- Nursing to provide assistance with toileting, as needed.

- Nonslip strips of a noncontrasting color to be applied to patient's bathroom floor in the event that patient resumes bathroom activity.

Question 2

- Monitor for incontinence.

- Monitor for fear of falling.

- Monitor for effectiveness of bedside commode.

Answers for Case 10

Question 1

- Primary care provider to evaluate resident's Parkinson's disease for the need for medication.

- Nursing to evaluate resident's bed and provide modifications in order to support safe bed transfers. Mechanical restraints to be removed from the resident. If the resident continues to fall, consider the use of a bed alarm system.

- Nursing to evaluate resident's need for low-height bed to reduce the risk of injurious falls from bed. Provide bed, if necessary.

Question 2

- Monitor for further falls from bed.

- Monitor Parkinson's disease and for effectiveness of medications, if given.

- Monitor for effectiveness of bed alarm system, if used.

- Monitor for effectiveness of low-height bed, if used.

Answers for Case 11

Question 1

- Physical Therapy to evaluate patient's mobility and transfers, and an ambulation device (e.g., walker).

- Nursing to evaluate patient's risk of falling.

- Nursing to evaluate patient's communication (e.g., ability to use nurse call bell and request assistance).

Question 2

- Monitor mobility and bed transfers.

- Monitor ambulation and safe use of walker.

- Monitor use of call bell and consider a bed alarm system if patient is noncompliant.

- Monitor risk of falling and reassess risk as patient's condition improves.

Answers to Case 12

Question 1

- Nursing to evaluate patient's immediate risk for bed falls.

- Nursing to consider lowering bed height and/or using siderail as enabling device to support safe bed transfers.

- Physical Therapy to evaluate patient's mobility and transfers.

- Primary care provider to evaluate patient's change of condition.

- Nursing aide to observe patient's bed transfers every shift.

Question 2

- Monitor bed transfers and safety interventions established. If patient continues to experience impaired bed transfers, consider using side rail as enabling device to support bed transfers.

Answers to Case 13

Question 1

- Nursing to review circumstances of resident's fall.
- Nursing to reassess resident's risk for falls.
- Nursing to communicate resident's risk status to other staff members.
- Primary care provider to evaluate resident's cognitive status and cause of confusion.
- Physical Therapy to evaluate resident's gait and balance.
- Nursing to provide resident with daily ambulation assistance, as needed.

Question 2

- Monitor resident's ambulation status.
- Monitor resident's cognitive status.
- Monitor resident's risk for falls.
- Monitor resident for change of condition.

Answers to Case 14

Question 1

- Primary care provider to evaluate patient's medical conditions and need for disease management.
- Physical Therapy to evaluate patient's mobility and appropriateness of walker.
- Physical Therapy to evaluate patient for exercises to improve gait and balance.
- Nursing to evaluate patient for assistance with ambulation needs.

Question 2

- Monitor patient's diabetes and arthritis.
- Monitor patient's gait and balance.
- Monitor patient's compliance with walker.

Answers to Case 15

Question 1

- Nursing to provide safety with resident's chair transfers (e.g., determine level of assistance needed with transfers or replace chair with one that the resident is able to transfer safely from).

- Nursing to evaluate resident's fear of falling (i.e., has her concern about falling restricted her mobility?).

- Primary care provider to evaluate resident for change of condition.

- Physical Therapy to evaluate resident's chair transfers and need for chair modifications.

Question 2

- Monitor resident's chair transfers.

- Monitor resident's risk for further falls.

- Monitor resident's fear of falling and provide assistance with mobility until resident regains confidence.

Answers to Case 16

Question 1

- Primary care provider to evaluate for causes of patient's confusion and pain.

- Nursing to evaluate patient's risk for falls with condition change and safety interventions as needed.

- Physical Therapy to evaluate patient's functional status and needs.

Question 2

- Monitor patient's mental status.

- Monitor patient's pain.

- Monitor patient's functional status.

- Monitor patient's risk for falls.

Answers for Case 17

Question 1

- Osteoporosis, loss of balance, and lack of safety awareness (i.e., it's likely that the patient will not use her nurse call bell or ask the nurses for assistance with her balance) are factors contributing to patient's fall risk.

Question 2

- To prevent falls consider a fall alarm. To guard against injurious falls consider using a low bed, cushioned floor mat, and/or hip protector.

Answers for Case 18

Question 1

- Risk factors include poor balance, frequent urination, and, most likely due to his stroke and extremity weakness, poor bed and toilet transfers.

Question 2

- Nursing to assist with bed and toilet transfers and ambulation.
- Physical Therapy to assess for an ambulation device and implement exercise program to maintain or increase function.
- Primary care provider to evaluate bladder status.
- Nursing to consider use of a bedside commode or a half-bedside rail, which could serve as an enabler to support bed mobility.

Answers for Case 19

Question 1

- The following side effects put this resident at risk for falls: Parkinsonism, tardive dyskinesia, tachycardia, akathisia, sedation and drowsiness, and hypotension.

Question 2

- Nursing to monitor resident for medication side effects and offer mobility assistance in the event of side effects.
- Nursing to provide frequent supervision and implement use of a fall alarm to supplement monitoring, especially at night.
- Nursing to evaluate resident's need for a low bed or floor mat.
- Monitor blood pressure.

Answers for Case 20

Question 1

- The resident is most likely falling due to low blood sugar caused by long-acting insulin, which taken in the morning peaks in the late afternoon.

Question 2

- Primary care provider to evaluate insulin dosage and adjust if needed.
- Nursing to observe and monitor the patient's status in the afternoon during his readjustment of insulin dosage.
- Monitor G.S.'s diet and blood sugar.

Answers to Case 21

Question 1

- Nursing to evaluate resident's bed and provide modifications such as low bed height and half-bedside rail to enable safe bed transfers.
- Provide a chair with armrest support.

Question 2

- Physical Therapy to evaluate toilet transfers and consider the use of toilet grab rails and a toilet riser to support safe toilet transfers.

Answers to Case 22

Question 1

- Any of the following risk factors could have contributed to the patient's fall: unsteady gait and balance, rushing to bathroom (exceeding safe mobility limits), slipping on leaking urine, and distance from her bed to bathroom, which might be considerable for someone with an urge to urinate.

Question 2

- Nursing to evaluate patient for use of a bedside commode or a program of scheduled or assisted toileting.

Answers for Case 23

Question 1

- The patient needs to be asked what symptoms he experienced prior to or at the time of falling and what activity he was doing at the time of the fall.

Question 2

- Ascertaining the circumstances of a fall facilitates the design of "targeted" interventions intended to reduce the risk of further falls.

Answers for Case 24

Question 1

- The patient should be evaluated for unsteady gait and balance caused by his diabetes, arthritis, and stroke. He should be observed for impairment in bed, chair, and toilet transfers because of his history of arthritis and stroke. He may also experience visual impairment from his diabetes.

Question 2

- Physical Therapy to evaluate patient's transfers and determine the need for modifications to bed, chair, and toilet to support safe transfers.
- Physical Therapy to provide cane or walker if needed to support safe ambulation.
- Nursing to remove bedroom clutter, especially in pathway between bed and bathroom, to support safe walking (lessen visual impairment) and toileting activity (urinary incontinence).

Answers for Case 25

Question 1

- Consider implementing use of a fall alarm to detect unsafe mobility or a program of close observation (e.g., use of a "sitter").

Question 2

- Placing the patient in a low bed with a cushioned floor mat are immediate safety measures to take. He may also be a candidate for wearing a hip protector.

Appendix B
Problem Solving:
Questions and Answers

Over the years, I have received hundreds of e-mail inquiries from nurses who have asked me questions about fall prevention. It occurred to me that for every inquiry received, there were probably hundreds of nurses who had the same question in mind but did not ask and would benefit from my responses. The following represents the most frequently asked questions and my responses.

RISK ASSESSMENT

Q: Are there any fall risk assessment tools for psychiatric units or facilities? When we use the standard assessments, all of our patients become fall risks, and there is not much differentiation between degrees of risk.

A: Fall risk assessment tools are designed to predict which people are likely to fall but, perhaps more importantly, to identify individual risk factors. Identifying specific risk factors helps health care professionals design targeted interventions aimed at reducing fall risk. To my knowledge, there are no fall risk assessment tools specific for psychiatric units. Important risk factors in this population include a history of falling, dizziness, low blood pressure, confusion or disorientation (e.g., unable to follow instructions, poor safety awareness, unaware of own ability, restless or impulsive behavior), impaired mobility (assistance with transfers, and unsteady gait or balance), altered elimination (frequency, urgency, nocturia, and incontinence), and medications (e.g., polypharmacy, sedatives, psychotropics).

NURSING EDUCATION

Q: We want to improve our hospital's fall prevention education program for nursing staff. What are the important components of an effective educational program?

A: The goal of nursing education for fall prevention is to

- Increase staff awareness and knowledge of falls (both the extent and consequences within your organization), internal and external fall risk factors, and multidisciplinary strategies aimed at reducing risk.

- Increase staff awareness and knowledge of the care process aimed at re-ducing risk (e.g., risk assessment, selection of interventions based on iden-tified risk factors, monitoring risk, and postfall assessment).

- Increase staff awareness and knowledge of policies, protocols, guide-lines, assessment and evaluation tools, and equipment and devices for fall prevention.

Organizations should also perform regular audits of the care process in order to identify staffing education needs related to fall prevention (i.e., knowledge and skill deficits). Lastly, fall prevention education should be ongoing. A va-riety of innovative strategies for learning (e.g., electronic presentations and applications, case studies, reflective practice discussions, and postfall huddles) can be used to support nursing staff.

NURSING STAFF EFFECTIVENESS

Q: I was wondering whether you have any information on staffing effectiveness as it relates to falls. We were trying to look at hours per patient day related to the number of patients at risk for falls, but we are not seeing too much correlation.

A: The relationship between nursing staff and falls is complex (i.e., involving in-tensity, skill level, and consistency of nursing staff), and the relationship may be dissimilar for units of different types and for hospitals of different sizes. From my experience, knowing when falls occur (time of day or night) is cru-cial with respect to appropriate staffing levels. I was recently involved with one institution that implemented staffing changes to increase staff at the prime time for falls, which was determined from postfall analysis to be be-tween the hours of 2 and 4 P.M. This rather simple intervention contributed to a reduction in falls. In another institution, I reviewed the nurse staffing pat-terns and the characteristics of people at fall risk. Although management be-lieved that their staffing levels were adequate, several potential contributing patient factors for falls (e.g., recent changes in mobility and continence, com-plex medication regimens, communication difficulties) actually showed that their nursing levels were inadequate. When staffing levels were changed to re-flect skill mix and patient needs, the institution's fall rates began to decline.

FALL CHAMPION

Q: Can you tell me about fall champions and what their functions are?

A: A component of many successful fall prevention programs is a fall champion (often a nursing assistant, staff nurse, staff development coordinator, or di-rector of nursing who receives additional education and mentoring on fall prevention strategies and leadership skills). This person may be charged with training new staff, overseeing documentation and communication, and con-tinuing to raise awareness about the importance of preventing falls. Other possible roles include providing ongoing quality assurance audits and out-come studies, budgeting for the future, promoting fall prevention activities, and solving problems (i.e., eliminating roadblocks and communication problems between team members). In essence, the fall champion pulls it all together, sees what needs to be changed and improved, and takes responsibility to make things happen. It is crucial that the person selected as the fall champion is motivated, has leadership qualities, and is willing to take on this new role.

DEMENTIA AND FALL RISK

Q: What is your recommendation for the use of canes or walkers for people who are diagnosed with dementia? It would seem that these people have a higher possibility of getting confused and falling than those without the diagnosis of dementia.

A: Although it is correct that people with dementia can be at greater fall risk while using canes or walkers, it is a mistake to generalize. Some people experience no difficulties with their canes or walkers, whereas others do not use their walking devices correctly, forget to use it, or do not really understand what it is for. Staff should always make sure that the patient or resident receives the proper cane or walker for his or her particular gait or balance impairment, and on a regular basis staff should assess and monitor whether he or she is properly using the walking device. Some people use walls and furnishings, rather than walking aids, for balance support. In this instance, it is important to make sure that all pathways are clear of clutter and that furnishings used to support balance (e.g., chairs, tabletops) are stable enough to actually support balance. Lastly, for demented people who are noncompliant or refuse to use their walking devices and experience poor balance, nursing staff should provide assistance with ambulation.

Q: Why do some people with an unsafe gait fall and others not?

A: Fallers with unsafe gait are more likely to be confused and to use tranquilizers. Patients or residents having both factors are more likely to fall than those with none or only one factor present. Safe mobility requires an appreciation of one's limitations and of the environmental hazards. Confused people often lack insight into these matters and tend not to take safety precautions. Tranquilizers contribute to fall risk by causing drowsiness, muscle weakness, and impaired postural reflexes; their use should be reviewed critically in patients or residents with confusion and unsafe gaits.

Q: I work on a hospital psychiatric unit and we are experiencing a high number of falls. I have two questions. What are the reasons for falls in our population? Also, we have tried to use fall alarms and hip protectors to prevent falls and injuries, but many of our demented patients remove the devices; any suggestions?

A: Fall risk in hospital psychiatric units includes the usual suspects: recent history of falls, mobility impairment, elimination problems, and altered mental status. In addition, fall risk factors on psychiatric units include age (above 75 years), behavioral problems associated with overactivity, recent receipt of electroconvulsive therapy, lack of safety awareness, acute confusional states, medications (especially antipsychotics), Parkinson's disease, recent medication or mental status changes, and psychosis (mainly schizophrenia). Many falls occur during meal, bath, or toileting times.

One of the main reasons that demented or cognitively impaired people remove or defeat fall alarms and hip protectors is that they do not understand the purpose or importance of the device. Also, alarms and hip protectors sometimes can cause agitation, necessitating their removal. It has been my experience that pad fall alarms that are out of the person's sight and mind are a better choice for cognitively impaired people than pull string alarms. With respect to hip protectors, once demented people acquire the habit of wearing the hip protector, they usually continue to wear it. It is important to make sure that the hip protector is the right size (i.e., comfortable and not too tight).

POSTFALL

Q: Would you have a definition of a frequent faller? We have started a fall committee in our facility, and I am looking for a standard.

A: There is no standard definition of a frequent faller. My preference is to define frequent or recurrent fallers (in all settings) as those with two or more falls in a 30-day period. Identifying risk factors for recurrent fallers is important. Compared with one-time fallers, recurrent fallers are more likely to have a history of preadmission falls, confusion, unsafe gait, or use of tranquilizers and antidepressants.

Q: What is a fall huddle?

A: After a patient or resident falls, there are two basic questions to answer:

- Why did he or she fall?
- How can we prevent another fall?

Consequently, the ideal response to a fall is to perform an immediate postfall assessment; its purpose is to determine the causes of the fall. The postfall assessment should include the following:

- Determining the circumstances of the fall: What symptoms did the person experience at the time? What was the person doing just before falling?

- Performing a fall risk assessment (i.e., to determine the presence of new or additional risk factors).

- Conducting an environmental assessment (i.e., a quick review of the person's environment to determine possible external reasons for the fall).

A fall huddle is a team meeting by the caregivers in which information obtained from the postfall assessment is analyzed (i.e., what happened? why did it happen?), and appropriate strategies to prevent further falls are discussed. The fall huddle is very similar in function to a root cause analysis.

Q: If a fall occurs, what is the process for the multidisciplinary team to reevaluate the plan of care for additional interventions?

A: Falls are complex events caused by multiple internal factors (e.g., acute medical conditions, chronic diseases, behavioral symptoms or unsafe behaviors, and adverse medication effects) and external factors (e.g., hazardous environmental conditions such as slippery or wet floor surfaces, poor lighting, unstable furnishings, and unsafe equipment). The goal of a postfall assessment, which should occur immediately after a fall, is to identify the internal and external factors that caused the fall and to discover the presence of any new or additional risk factors. Collecting this information can help staff determine what happened and why it happened and design appropriate multidisciplinary team interventions to prevent further falls. Shortly after the fall, the multidisciplinary team members should meet and review the care plan and implement appropriate fall and injury prevention strategies as needed. Because falls are often caused by multiple factors, it is crucial that the entire multidisciplinary team (e.g., physicians, nurses, therapists) be involved in the process. Sometimes, depending on whether external factors contributed to the fall, housekeeping and maintenance staff may be involved also.

Q: Despite assessing fall risk and developing individualized strategies to reduce falls, many of our acute hospital rehabilitation patients fall. Can you offer any suggestions?

A: It has been my experience that many falls occur in the rehabilitation setting because patients are attempting to practice their newly learned skills without waiting for appropriate supervision by the staff. The patients wrongly assume that because the physical therapist had them up walking in a one-on-one therapy session, they are now able to go to the bathroom by themselves.

  What the patients forget is that it took two people to get them up and that after only 3 feet; they were ready to go back to their bed. In addition to providing these at-risk patients with adequate supervision and anticipatory care (e.g., asking patients regularly whether they need to toilet or exercise), a fall alarm can be used to monitor patients who are attempting unanticipated and unsafe activities. Aside from regular fall risk assessments, the best way to prevent falls is to have in place a postfall assessment that identifies the causes of falls in your rehabilitation patients.

Q: Do you have any evidence-based practices for monitoring a patient after a fall?

A: As a general rule, a physician should examine any indication of injury as soon as possible, and a physician should immediately evaluate any head trauma. Other injuries, such as suspected or obvious fractures, also warrant rapid treatment, as do symptoms of cardiac or neurological crisis.

  Nurses must be especially alert to possible injuries for several days after a fall. Delayed discovery of a hip or other fracture is a common occurrence. Slow internal bleeding into the brain from trauma to the head may not cause symptoms for days, and the outcome of such slow bleeds can be fatal. Watch for the following indications that anything is different about the patient:

- Altered gait or limp

- Unusual hesitation or slowness when moving

- Verbal complaints of pain

- Nonverbal indications of pain, such as facial grimaces

- Loss of appetite

- Serious bruising of any part of the body
- Redness or warmth on any part of the body
- Favoring of an appendage, such as not using an arm or hand
- Unusual sleepiness or lethargy
- Changes in behavior or cognition.

Nurses should never assume a patient's complaint of pain or signs of injury are simply the minor effects of taking a tumble and do not indicate anything serious. Just because a physician evaluates someone and declares him or her uninjured does not rule out an undetected insult to some part of the body with symptoms that may surface later.

A plan of care after a fall should include additional checks or monitoring of the patient's status for several days. The frequency of those checks depends on the individual patient and the circumstances, but in many cases, twice a shift for three or four days is sufficient.

FALL RISK WRISTBANDS

Q: Our hospital is considering colored armbands for fall risk alerts. What are some of the things we should consider to make sure that our colored armband system is effective?

A: The purpose of colored armbands or wristbands is to make staff aware of a patient's fall risk status. The effective use of armbands to communicate fall risk includes the following:

- Standardize a color to represent fall risk so that all staff knows that the color yellow, for example, signifies fall risk (i.e., the color yellow is the national standard for fall risk wristbands).

- Apply a text to the wristband, such as "fall precaution" (i.e., adding text avoids the problem of relying solely on color to communicate its meaning).

- Develop a policy and process defining wristband usage (i.e., who is responsible for applying, maintaining, and removing armbands).

- Educate all staff about the purpose and use of wristbands.

Lastly, fall risk signs and stickers that correspond with the colors used on wristbands can be used to reinforce staff awareness of fall risk.

LOW BEDS

Q: Are low beds an effective fall prevention strategy?

A: Low beds are used primarily to prevent injurious falls. The problem with fixed low beds is that they can actually increase the risk of falls in some instances (i.e., falls may occur because the patient is trying to get up from the floor and may not have the strength to do so safely). Also, nursing staff attempting to assist patients in fixed low beds are at risk of back injuries. Fixed low beds were introduced several years ago as an alternative to placing the patient's mattress on the floor, which many families objected to. A more effective method of preventing falls and staff injuries is to use a height-adjustable low bed that can be raised from the floor level to approximately the waist height of the staff; the correct height of the bed is based on the patient's safe transfers from bed. However, there is still a need for more research to examine the effectiveness of height-adjustable beds in preventing falls.

BEDSIDE FLOOR MATS

Q: I am interested in the use of bedside fall mats to prevent injuries in repeat fallers. Are you aware of any current research that would support the use of bedside fall mats?

A: In those with repeated falls from bed, floor mats (i.e., cushioned mats of various sizes 1 or 2 inches thick, with or without beveled edges) are often used to prevent injurious falls. Some floor mats are designed for use in conjunction with a fall alarm (the alarm is embedded in the mat). Floor mats may be better than current conventional carpet underlays regardless of the composition and construction of the carpet to prevent injurious falls (i.e., impact testing suggests that carpets offer poor energy absorption and injury protection in the event of a fall). Unfortunately, aside from anecdotal reports, there is no solid research supporting the effectiveness of floor mats. The downside of floor mats, especially those that are thick, is that some people with poor balance can experience even more unsteadiness when standing on the mat, which can increase their risk of falling. Also, floor mats can be a potential source of tripping for both patients or residents and staff.

Sometimes low beds that can be lowered to within 8 inches of the floor are used, either in conjunction with a floor mat or as an alternative to using floor mats. In comparison to floor mats, low beds may be more useful in reducing injuries related to inappropriate transfers from beds. Lastly, it is important to remember that a multisystem approach, rather than single interventions (such as floor mats or low beds), is needed to achieve a significant reduction in fall-related injury.

BEDSIDE RAILS

Q: Our hospital uses four rails: two upper and two lower. For patients who are identified as at high risk for falls, we would like to encourage the use of all four side rails. However, literature indicates that the use of four side rails for some patients causes worse injuries when they attempt to climb over the rails. How do you advise us to approach this?

A: Research clearly shows that bedside rails do not prevent falls, and, as you suggest, bed rails can actually lead to falls. In particular, using four side rails (two upper and two lower) is associated with increased risk of injury. For example, patients can become easily trapped between the upper and lower rail during bed exits. Using a side rail cushion to block the exit works, but patients are still at fall risk because they tend to climb over the rail or footboard of the bed. On the other hand, bedrail down polices can also lead to increased falls from bed. Although serious injuries usually do not occur, any increase in falls raises medicolegal issues, threatens patient or resident and family confidence, and may decrease staff morale.

I use side rails for two purposes: full-length side rails to prevent immobile patients from rolling out of bed (they must be incapable of self-initiated transfers) and secure half side rails (two uppers) or a bed transfer bar to enable safe transfers. For all other patients at risk, I use a wide variety of alternatives, such as bed modifications to support safe transfers, low platform beds, floor cushions or mattresses, bed or fall alarms, mattresses that curve up around the edges or swimming noodles to prevent rolling out of bed, frequent staff monitoring, and the use of family members as sitters. I also explain to patients or residents and involved family members why side rails are not being used. These strategies work in most instances, but they require a dedicated nursing staff that fully appreciates the potential dangers of side rails.

FALL ALARMS

Q: I was wondering whether you have any criteria for the use of personal safety alarms to prevent falls (bed and chair). I am specifically looking to see whether there is anything out there on when to use them, when they can be removed—really any information on their use as an intervention to prevent falls.

A: Patient safety alarms (also known as fall alarms and exit alarms) are designed to serve as an early warning system; they assist staff in detecting unsafe bed or chair egress.

Like all other fall prevention strategies, alarms that are targeted to patient or resident risk factors have the greatest chance of success. The alarm criteria I suggest are as follows: Patient or resident experiences a fall from a bed, chair, wheelchair, or toilet; patient or resident experiences a fall shortly after leaving the bed, chair, wheelchair, or toilet or is found on the floor after an unwitnessed fall; patient or resident has impaired mobility or demonstrates unsafe bed, chair, wheelchair, or toilet transfers; patient or resident has a history of cognitive or communicative problems (e.g., forgets to use call bell or ask for assistance, cannot remember or follow instructions); and patient or resident has a history of nocturia. In addition, alarms serve a variety of useful functions:

- Alarms promote speedy assistance to those who have already fallen. This can help reduce fall complications, such as the amount of time that the person lies unaided.

- Alarms may serve as an alternative to nurse call bells for those who are noncompliant or unable to use their call bell because of cognitive or physical impairments. Alarms, which do not require active participation by patients or residents to trigger, may be preferable to nurse call systems, which demand active participation.

- Alarms may serve as an assessment or planning tool by monitoring the frequency of attempts to leave the bed, chair, or wheelchair, which can help identify emerging trends and interventions. Coupled with initial and ongoing risk assessments, alarms can inform staff about a patient's or resident's habits. For example, one may consistently attempt to arise at a certain hour to go to the bathroom, whereas another may get up at nonspecific times, driven by an urge to wander. As a result of such a history, nurses can adjust their attention and care to each person's habits and needs.

- Alarms allow staff more time (avoiding constant supervision of patients or residents at risk) and theoretically eliminate the need to continually check on patients who tend to fall. This gives nurses more opportunity to work with patients or residents as opposed to spending time on surveillance or being frequently interrupted to observe patients or residents.

Lastly, alarms used in conjunction with other strategies, such as providing anticipatory care or scheduled toileting, have the greatest likelihood of preventing falls.

Q: Do you have or know of any criteria that have been used to decide who should get a bed alarm or chair alarm?

A: The use of bed or chair alarms should be based on specific criteria. Important indications following fall risk assessment include impaired mobility or unsafe bed or chair transfers, history of cognitive or communicative problems (e.g., forgets to use call bell or ask for assistance, cannot remember or follow instructions) and transfer impairment, and history of nocturia (i.e., excessive urination at night) or urge incontinence and toileting difficulties. Also, you might consider the use of bed alarms for all cognitively impaired patients or residents, even without mobility impairment, at time of admission (i.e., many bedroom- and bathroom-related falls in cognitively compromised people occur in the first 24–48 hours of stay, mainly because of unfamiliarity with environments and routines), with certain interventions such as low beds (to alert staff that the person has rolled out of bed), and with certain transient risk factors, such as dizziness or low blood pressure. Important indications following postfall assessment include a fall from a bed or chair and a fall while ambulating in the bedroom or bathroom shortly after leaving the bed or chair.

Q: The supervision requirements in Centers for Medicare and Medicaid Services Issuance of Revised Guidance for Accidents and Supervision (F323) state that "fall alarms should not be used in lieu of staff supervision." As a result, my nursing director is wondering about how to use fall alarms in our facility. What's your opinion?

A: According to the F323 guidelines, facilities are obligated to provide adequate supervision to prevent falls. Adequacy of supervision is defined by the type and frequency, based on the individual patient's or resident's assessed needs, and identified hazards in the environment. Although fall alarms do not eliminate the need for adequate supervision, fall alarms have several benefits. Fall alarms can be used to supplement staff supervision (i.e., they are beneficial in helping to monitor a patient's or resident's unsafe activities). Also, fall alarms can be used as an assessment tool to help identify a patient's or resident's supervision needs.

Q: In the past, we have used bed alarms. However, the alarm did not go off until the patient was already out of bed. This was very frustrating for the nursing staff. What do you suggest?

A: Bed alarms depend on the ability of staff to reach patients in a timely manner. One of the reported drawbacks of using alarms is that the staff believes that they do not have enough time to get to the patient to prevent a fall after the alarm is activated. This problem can be reduced by using pressure sensor pad alarms and adjusting the sensitivity of the sensor pads by way of a delay function and by positioning the sensor pads underneath the patient's or resident's upper body or shoulder level (i.e., placing the pad in this position will provide the staff with more lead time in responding to activated alarms). When alarms are activated, staff should try to determine why the patient attempted to exit the bed (e.g., hunger or thirst, boredom, toileting) and provide anticipatory care in response. When patients or residents are located far from staff, bed alarms may be inadequate, and other fall prevention measures may be needed.

Bibliography

An asterisk following a reference indicates a reference covering fall-risk assessment tools.

HOSPITAL

Aisen, P.S., Deluca, T., & Lawlor, B.A. (1992). Falls among geropsychiatry inpatients are associated with PRN medications for agitation. *International Journal of Geriatric Psychiatry, 7*, 709–712.

Ashton, J., Gilbert, D., Hayward, G., et al. (1989). Predicting patient falls in an acute care setting. *Kansas Nurse, 64*(10), 3–5.

Baker, L. (1992). Developing a safety plan that works for patients and nurses. *Rehabilitation Nursing, 17*, 264–266.

Bates, D.W., Pruess, K., Souney, P., & Platt, R. (1995). Serious falls in hospitalized patients: Correlates and resource utilization. *American Journal of Medicine, 99*, 137–143.

Berryman, E., Gaskin, D., Jones, A., et al. (1989, July/August). Point by point: Predicting elders' falls. *Geriatric Nursing*, 199–201.*

Blair, E., & Gruman, C. (2005). Falls in an inpatient geriatric psychiatric population. *Journal of the American Psychiatric Nurses Association, 11*, 351–354.

Blegen, M.A. (2006). Patient safety in hospital acute care units. *Annual Review of Nursing Research, 24*, 103–125.

Brady, R., Cheater, F.R., Pierce, L.L., et al. (1993). Geriatric falls: Prevention strategies for the staff. *Journal of Gerontological Nursing 19*, 26–32.

Brians, L.K., Alexander, K., Grota, P., et al. (1991). The development of the RISK tool for fall prevention. *Rehabilitation Nursing, 16*(2), 67–69.*

Burden, B., & Kishi, D. (1989). Patient falls: lowering the risk. *Nursing, 16*(2), 79.*

Byers, V., Arrington, M.E., & Finstuen, K. (1990). Predictive risk factors associated with stroke patient falls in acute care settings. *Journal of Neuroscience Nursing, 22*(3), 147–154.

Caley, L.M., & Pinchoff, D.M. (1994). A comparison study of patient falls in a psychiatric setting. *Hospital and Community Psychiatry, 45*, 823–825.

Chu, L.W., Pei, C.K., Chiu, A., Liu K., Chu, M.M., Wong, S., & Wong, A. (1999). Risk factors for falls in hospitalized older medical patients. *Journal of Gerontology, 54*, M38–M43.

Cohen, L., & Guin, P. (1991). Implementation of a patient fall prevention program. *Journal of Neuroscience Nursing, 23*(5), 315–319.

Commodore, D.I. (1995). Falls in the elderly population: A look at incidence, risks, healthcare costs, and preventive strategies. *Rehabilitation Nursing, 20*(2), 84–89.

Corbett, C., & Pennypacker, B. (1992). Using a quality improvement team to reduce patient falls. *Journal of Hospital Quality, 14*, 38–54 *

Coussement, J., De Paepe, L., Schwendimann, R., Denhaerynck, D., Dejaeger, E., & Milisen, K. (2008). Interventions for preventing falls in acute- and chronic-care hospitals: A systematic review and meta-analysis. *Journal of the Amercian Geriatrics Society, 56*, 29–36.

Dallaire, L.B., & Burke, E.V. (1989). Reducing patient falls. *Nursing, 19*(1), 65.

de Carle, A.J., & Kohn, R. (2001). Risk factors for falling in a psychogeriatric unit. *International Journal of Geriatric Psychiatry, 16,* 762–767.

Dunton, N., Gajewski, B., Taunton, R.L., & Moore, J. (2004). Nurse staffing and patient falls on acute care hospital units. *Nursing Outlook, 52*(1), 53–59.

Easterling, M.L. (1990). Which of your patients is headed for a fall? *RN, 53* (1), 56–59.

Evans, D., Hodgkinson, B., Lambert, L., & Wood, J. (2001). Fall risk factors in the hospital setting: A systematic review. *International Journal of Nursing Practice, 7,* 38–45.

Fischer, I.D., Krauss, M.J., Dunagan, W.C., Birge, S., Hitcho, E., Johnson, S., Costantinou, E., & Fraser, V.J. (2005). Patterns and predictors of inpatient falls and fall-related injuries in a large academic hospital. *Infection Control and Hospital Epidemiology, 26,* 822–827.

Fleck, M.M., & Forrester, D.A. (2001). The efficacy of an education program to improve direct caregiver knowledge regarding fall prevention. *Journal for Nurses in Staff Development, 17,* 27–33.

Gaebler, S. (1993). Predicting which patient will fall again . . . and again. *Journal of Advanced Nursing, 18,* 1895–1902.

Goodwin, M.B., & Westbrook, J.I. (1993). An analysis of patient accidents in hospital. *Australian Clinical Review, 13,* 141–149.

Greene, E., Cunningham, C.J., Eustace, A., Kidd, N., Clare, A.W., & Lawlor, B.A. (2001). Recurrent falls are associated with increased length of stay in elderly psychiatric inpatients. *International Journal of Geriatric Psychiatry, 16,* 965–968.

Grenier-Sennelier, C., Lombard, I., Jeny-Loeper, C., Maillet-Gouret, M., & Minvielle, E. (2002). Designing adverse event prevention programs using quality management methods: The case of falls in hospitals. *International Journal of Quality Health Care, 14,* 419–426.

Haines, T.P., Bennell, K.L., Osborne, R.H., & Hill, K.D. (2004). Effectiveness of targeted falls prevention programme in subacute hospital setting: Randomised controlled trial. *British Medical Journal, 328*(7441), 676–679.

Healey, F., Monro, A., Cockram, A., Adams, V., & Heseltine, D. (2004). Using targeted risk factor reduction to prevent falls in older inpatients: A randomised controlled trial. *Age and Ageing, 33*(4), 390–395.

Hendrich, A.L. (1988). An effective unit based fall prevention plan. *Journal of Nursing Quality Assurance, 3*(1), 28–36.*

Hendrich, A.L. (1988). Unit based fall prevention. *Journal of Quality Assurance, 10*(1), 15–17.

Hendrich, A., Nyhuuis, A., Kippenbrock, A., & Soja, M.E. (1995). Hospital falls: Development of predictive model for clinical practice. *Applied Nursing Research, 8,* 129–139.

Hill, B.A., Johnson, R., & Garrett, B.J. (1988). Reducing the incidence of falls in high-risk patients. *Journal of Nursing Administration, 18* (7/8), 24–28.*

Jones, W., & Smith, A. (1989). Preventing hospital incidence. What can we do? *Nursing Management, 20* (9), 58–60.

Kerzman, H., Chetrit, A., Brin, L., & Toren, O. (2004). Characteristics of falls in hospitalized patients. *Journal of Advanced Nursing, 47,* 223–229.

Kilpack, V., Boehm, J., Smith, N., & Mudge, B. (1991). Using research-based interventions to decrease patient falls. *Applied Nursing Research, 4* (2), 50–56.

Kim, E.A., Mordiffi, S.Z., Bee, W.H., Devi, K., & Evans, D. (2007). Evaluation of three fall-risk assessment tools in an acute care setting. *Journal of Advanced Nursing, 60,* 427–435.

Lawerence, J.I., & Maher, P.L. (1992). An interdisciplinary falls consult team: A collaborative approach to patient falls. *Journal of Nursing Care Quality, 6*(3), 21–29.

Lee, J.E., & Stokic, D.S. (2008). Risk factors for falls during inpatient rehabilitation. *American Journal of Physical Medicine and Rehabilitation, 87,* 341–350.

Lim, K.D., Ng, K.C., Ng, S.K., & Ng, L.L. (2001). Falls amongst institutionalized psycho-geriatric patients. *Singapore Medical Journal, 42,* 466–472.

Llewellyn, J., Martin, B., Shekleton, M., & Firlit, S. (1988). Analysis of falls in the acute surgical and cardiovascular surgical patients. *Applied Nursing Research, 1*(3), 116–121.

Maciorowski, L.F., Munro, B.H., Dietrick-Gallagher, M., et al. (1988). A review of the patient fall literature. *Journal of Nursing Quality Assurance, 3*(1), 18–27.

Mayo, N.E., Korner-Bitensky, N., Becker, R., & Georges, P.C. (1989). Preventing falls among patients in a rehabilitation setting. *Canadian Journal of Rehabilitation, 2*(4), 235–240.

McCollam, M.E. (1995). Evaluation and implementation of a research-based falls assessment program. *Nursing Clinics of North America, 30*(3), 507–514.*

McFarlane, M.A., & Melora, P. (1993). Decreasing falls by the application of standards of care, practice, and governance. *Journal of Nursing Care Quality, 8*(1), 43–50.

Mion, L.C., Gregor, S., Buettner, M., et al. (1989). Falls in the rehabilitation setting: Incidence and characteristics. *Rehabilitation Nursing, 14*(1), 17–22.

Morse, J.M. (2002). Enhancing the safety of hospitalization by reducing patient falls. *American Journal of Infection Control, 30*, 376–80.

Morse, J.M., Black, C., Oberle, K., & Donahue P. (1989). A prospective study to identify the fall-prone patient. *Social Science Medicine, 28*(1), 81–86.*

Morse, J.M., Morse, R.M., & Tylko, S. (1989). Development of a scale to identify the fall-prone patient. *Canadian Journal on Aging, 8* 366–377.*

Morton, D. (1989). Five years of fewer falls. *American Journal of Nursing, 89*(2), 204–205.

Myers, H. (2003). Hospital fall risk assessment tools: A critique of the literature. *International Journal of Nursing Practice, 9*, 223–235.

Myers, H., & Nikoletti, S. (2003). Fall risk assessment: A prospective investigation of nurses' clinical judgement and risk assessment tools in predicting patient falls. *International Journal of Nursing Practice, 9*, 158–165.

Oliver, D., Britton, M., Seed, P., Martin, F.C., & Hopper, A.H. (1997). Development and evaluation of evidence based risk assessment tool (STRATIFY) to predict which elderly inpatients will fall: Case-controlled and cohort studies. *British Medical Journal, 315*, 1049–1053.

Oliver, D., Daly, F., Martin, F.C., & McMurdo, M.E. (2004). Risk factors and risk assessment tools for falls in hospital in-patients: A systematic review. *Age and Ageing, 33*, 122–130.

Oliver D., Hopper, A., & Seed, P. (2000). Do hospital fall prevention programs work? A systematic review. *Journal of the American Geriatrics Society, 48*, 1679–1689.

Quinlan, W.C. (1994). The liability risk of patients who fall. *Journal of Healthcare Risk Management, 14*, 29–33.

Roberts, B.L. (1993). Is stay in an intensive care unit a risk for falls? *Applied Nursing Research, 6*, 135–136.

Rohde, J.M., Myers, A.H., & Vlahov, D. (1990). Variation in risk for falls by clinical department: Implications for prevention. *Infection Control and Hospital Epidemiology, 11*, 521–524.

Ross, J.E.R. (1991). Iatrogenesis in the elderly: Contributors to falls. *Journal of Gerontological Nursing, 17*(9), 19–23.

Ruckstuhl, M.C., Marchionda, E.E., Salmons, J., & Larrabee, J.H. (1988). Patient falls: An outcome indicator. *Journal of Gerontological Nursing, 6*(1), 25–29.*

Rutledge, D.N., Donaldson, N.E., & Pravikoff, D.S. (2003). Update 2003: Fall risk assessment and prevention in hospitalized patients. *Journal of Clinical Innovation, 6*(5), 1–55.

Salgado, R.I., Lord, S.R., Ehrlich, F., Janji, N., & Rahman, A. Predictors of falling in elderly hospital patients. (2004). *Archives of Gerontology and Geriatrics, 38*, 213–219.

Savage, T., Matheis-Kraft, C. (2001). Fall occurrence in a geriatric psychiatry setting before and after a fall prevention program. *Journal of Gerontological Nursing, 27*, 49–53.

Schmid, N.A. (1990). Reducing patient falls: A research-based comprehensive fall prevention program. *Military Medicine, 155*, 202–207.

Schwendimann, R., Bühler, H., De Geest, S., & Milisen, K. (2003). Characteristics of hospital inpatient falls across clinical departments. *Gerontology, 54*, 342–348.

Schwendimann, R., Bühler, H., De Geest, S., & Milisen, K. (2006). Fall prevention in an acute care setting reducing multiple falls. *Journal of Gerontological Nursing, 32*(3), 13–22.

Spellbring, A.M. (1992). Assessing elderly patients at high risk for falls: A reliability study. *Journal of Nursing Care Quality, 6*(3), 30–35.*

Spellbring, A.M., Gannon, M.E., Kleckner, T., & Conway, K. (1988). Improving safety for hospitalized elderly. *Journal of Gerontological Nursing, 14,* 31–36.*

Stevenson, B., Mills, E.M., Welin, L., & Beal, K.G. (1998). Falls risk factors in an acute-care setting: A retrospective study. *Canadian Journal of Nursing Research, 30,* 97–111.

Tingle, J. (2007). Preventing patient falls in hospital. *British Journal of Nursing, 16*(9), 510.

Tutuarima, J.A., de Haan, R.J., & Limburg, M. (1993). Number of nursing staff and falls: A case-control study by stroke patients in acute-care settings. *Journal of Advanced Nursing, 18,* 1101–1105.

Tzeng, H.M., & Yin, C.Y. (2007). Height of hospital beds and inpatient falls: A threat to patient safety. *Journal of Nursing Administration, 37,* 537–538.

Uden, G., Ehnfors, M., & Sjostrom, K. (1999). Use of initial risk assessment and recording as the main nursing intervention in identifying risks of falls, *Journal of Advanced Nursing, 29,* 145–152.

Vassallo, M., Amersey, R.A., Sharma, J.C., & Allen, S.C. (2000). Falls on integrated medical wards. *Gerontology, 46,* 158–162.

Vassallo, M., Poynter, L., Sharma, J.C., Kwan, J., & Allen, S.C. (2008). Fall risk-assessment tools compared with clinical judgment: An evaluation in a rehabilitation ward. *Age and Ageing, 37,* 277–281.

Vassallo, M., Stockdale, R., Sharma, J.C., Briggs, R., & Allen, S. (2005). Comparative study of the use of four fall risk assessment tools on acute medical wards. *Journal of the American Geriatrics Society, 53,* 1034–1038.

Vlahov, D., Myers, A.H., & Al-Ibrahim, M.S. (1990). Epidemiology of falls among patients in a rehabilitation hospital. *Archives of Physical Medicine and Rehabilitation, 71,* 8–12.

Way, B.B. (1992). The relationship between staff–patient ratio and reported patient incidents. *Hospital and Community Psychiatry, 43,* 361–365.

Whedon, M.B., & Shedd, P. (1989). Prediction and prevention of patient falls. *Image: Journal of Nursing Scholarship, 21*(2), 108–114.*

Zepp, S. (1991). Ban "a" fall: A nursing innovation to reducing patient falls. *Kansas Nurse, 66*(7), 13.

NURSING FACILITY

Becker, C., Kron, M., Lindemann, U., Sturm, E., Eichner, B., Walter-Jung, B., & Nikolaus, T. (2003). Effectiveness of a multifaceted intervention on falls in nursing home patients. *Journal of the American Geriatrics Society, 51,* 306–313.

Eakman, A.M., Havens, M.D., Ager, S.J., Buchanan, R.L., Fee, N.J., Gollick, S.G., Michels, M.J., Olson, L.L., Satterfield, K.M., Stevenson, K.A. (2002). Fall prevention in long-term care: An in-house interdisciplinary team approach. *Topics of Geriatric Rehabilitation, 17,* 29–39.

Franzoni, S., Rozzini, R., Boffelli, S., et al. (1994). Fear of falling in nursing home residents. *Gerontology, 40,* 38–44.

Friedman, S.M., Williamson, J.D., Lee, B.H., et al. (1995). Increased fall rates in nursing home residents after relocation to a new facility. *Journal of the American Geriatrics Society, 43,* 1237–1242.

Ginter, S.G., & Mion, L.C. (1992). Falls in the nursing home: Preventable or inevitable? *Journal of Gerontological Nursing, 18,* 43–48.

Gray-Miceli, D.G., Strumpf, N.E., Reinhard, S.C., Zanna, M.T., & Fritz, E. (2004). Current approaches to postfall assessment in nursing homes. *Journal of the American Medical Directors Association, 5,* 387–394.

Greubel, D.L., Stokesberry, C., & Jelley, M.J. (2002). Preventing costly falls in long-term care. *The Nurse Practitioner, 27*(3), 83–85.

Gross, Y.T., Shimamoto, Y., Rose, C.L., et al. (1990). Why do they fall? Monitoring risk factors in nursing homes. *Journal of Gerontological Nursing, 16*(6), 20–25.

Harris, P.B. (1989). Organizational and staff attitudinal determinants of falls in nursing home residents. *Medical Care, 27,* 737–749.

Harrison, B., Booth, D., & Algase, D. (2001). Studying fall risk factors among nursing home residents who fell. *Journal of Gerontological Nursing, 27,* 26–34.

Hill-Westmoreland, E.E., & Gruber-Baldini, A.L. (2005). Falls documentation in nursing homes: Agreement between the Minimum Data Set and chart abstractions of medical and nursing documentation. *Journal of the American Geriatric Society, 53,* 268–273.

Janitti, P.O., Pyykko, I., & Laippala, P. (1995). Prognosis of falls among elderly nursing home residents. *Aging: Clinical and Experimental Research, 7,* 23–27.

Jensen, J., Lundin-Olsson, L., Nyberg, L., & Gustafson, Y. (2002). Fall and injury prevention in older people living in residential care facilities. *Annals of Internal Medicine, 136,* 733–740.

Jonsson, P.V., Lipsitz, L.A., Kelley, M., et al. (1990). Hypotensive responses to common daily activities in institutional elderly: A potential risk for recurrent falls. *Archives of Internal Medicine, 150,* 1518–1524.

Kerman, M., & Mulvihill, M. (1990). The role of medication in falls among the elderly in a long-term care facility. *Mount Sinai Journal of Medicine, 57,* 343–347.

Krueger, P.D., Brazil, K., & Lohfeld, L.H. (2001). Risk factors for falls and injuries in a long-term care facility in Ontario. *Canadian Journal of Public Health, 92,* 117–120.

Kuehn, A.F., & Sendelweck, S. (1995). Acute health status and its relationship to falls in the nursing home. *Journal of Gerontological Nursing, 21*(7), 41–49.

Lipsitz, L.A., Jonsson, P.V., Kelley, M.M., et al. (1991). Causes and correlates of recurrent falls in ambulatory frail elderly. *Journal of Gerontology, 46,* M114–M122.

Luukinen, H., Koski, K., Laippala, P., & Kivela, S.L. (1995). Risk factors for recurrent falls in the elderly in long-term institutional care. *Public Health, 109*(1), 57–65.

Micelli, D.L.G., Wasman, H., Cavalieri, T., & Lage, S. (1994). Prodromal falls among older nursing home residents. *Applied Nursing Research, 7*(1), 18–27.

Myers, A.H., Baker, S.P., Robinson, E.G., et al. (1989). Falls in the institutionalized elderly. *Journal of Long-Term Care Administration, 17*(4), 12–15.

Myers, A.H., Baker, S.P., Van Natta, M.L., et al. (1991). Risk factors associated with falls and injuries among elderly institutionalized persons. *American Journal of Epidemiology, 133,* 1179–1190.

Myers, A.H., Van Natta, M.L., Robinson, E.G., & Baker, S.P. (1994). Can injurious falls be prevented? *Journal of Long-Term Care Administration, 22*(2), 26–29, 32.

Neufeld, R.R., Tideiksaar, R., Yew, E., et al. (1991). A multidisciplinary falls consultation service in a nursing home. *Gerontologist, 31,* 120–123.

Nowalk, P.M., Prendergast, J.M., Bayles, C.M., D'Amico, F.J., & Colvin, G.C. (2001). A randomized trial of exercise programs among older individuals living in two long-term care facilities: The FallsFREE program. *Journal of American Geriatrics Society, 49,* 859–865.

Rask, K., Parmelee, P.A., Taylor, J.A., Green, D., Brown, H., Hawley, J., Schild, L., Strothers, H.S. III, & Ouslander, J.G. (2007). Implementation and evaluation of a nursing home fall management program. *Journal of the American Geriatrics Society, 55*(3), 342–349.

Ray, W.A., Meador, J.A., Thapa, P.B., Brown, A.K., Kajihara, H.K., Davis, C., Gideon, D.G., & Griffin, M.R. (1997). A randomized trial of a consultation service to reduce falls in nursing homes. *Journal of the American Medical Association, 278,* 557–562.

Ray, W.A., Thapa, P.B., & Gideon, P. (2000). Benzodiazepines and the risk of falls in nursing home residents. *Journal of the American Geriatrics Society, 48,* 682–685.

Robbins, A.S., Rubenstein, L.Z., Josephson, K.R., et al. (1989). Predictors of falls among elderly people: Results of two population-based studies. *Archives of Internal Medicine, 149,* 1628–1633.*

Ross, J.E.R. (1991). Contributors to falls. *Journal of Gerontological Nursing, 17,* 19–23.

Rubenstein, L.Z., Josephson, K.R., & Osterweil, D. (1996). Falls and fall prevention in the nursing home. *Clinics of Geriatric Medicine, 12*(4), 881–902.

Rubenstein, L.Z., Josephson, K.R., & Robbins, A.S. (1994). Falls in the nursing home. *Annals of Internal Medicine, 121,* 442–451.

Rubenstein, L.Z., Robbins, A.S., Josephson, K.R., et al. (1990). The value of assessing falls in an elderly population. A randomized clinical trial. *Annals of Internal Medicine, 113,* 308–316.

Ruthazer, R., & Lipsitz, L.A. (1993). Antidepressants and falls among elderly people in long-term care. *American Journal of Public Health, 83,* 746–749.

Svensson, M.L., Rundgren, A., Larsson, M., et al. (1991). Accidents in the institutionalized elderly: A risk analysis. *Aging, 3,* 181–192.

Taylor, J. (2002). The Vanderbilt Fall Prevention Program for Long-Term Care: Eight years of field experience with nursing home staff. *Journal of the Medical Directors Association, 3*(3), 180–185.

Thappa, P.B., Brockman, K.G., Gideon, P., et al. (1996). Injurious falls in non-ambulatory nursing home residents: A comparative study of circumstances, incidence, and risk factors. *Journal of the American Geriatrics Society, 44,* 273–278.

Thappa, P.B., Gideon, P., Brockman, K.G., et al. (1996). Clinical and biomechanical measures of balance as fall predictors in ambulatory nursing home residents. *Journal of Gerontology, 51A,* M239–M246.

Thappa, P.B., Gideon, P., Fought, R.L., & Ray, W.A. (1995). Psychotropic drugs and the risk of recurrent falls in ambulatory nursing home residents. *American Journal of Epidemiology, 142,* 202–211.

Theodos, P. (2004). Fall prevention in frail elderly nursing home residents: A challenge to case management, Part II. *Lippincott's Case Management, 9*(1), 32–44.

Theodos, P. (2003). Fall prevention in frail elderly nursing home residents: A challenge to case management, Part I. *Lippincott's Case Management, 8*(6), 246–251.

van Dijk, P.T.M., Meulenberg, O.G.R.M., van de Sande, H.J., & Habbema, J.D.F. (1993). Falls in demented patients. *Gerontologist, 33,* 200–204.

Wagner, L.M., Capezuti, E., Ouslander, J.G. (2006). Reporting near-miss events in nursing homes. *Nursing Outlook, 54*(2), 85–93.

Wright, B.A., Aizenstein, S., Vogler, G., et al. (1990). Frequent fallers: Leading groups to identify psychological factors. *Journal of Gerontological Nursing, 16*(4), 15–19.

Young, S.W., Abedzadeh, C.B., & White, M.W. (1989). A fall-prevention program for nursing homes. *Nursing Management, 20*(11), 80Y, 80Z, 80AA, 80DD, 80FF.

RESTRAINTS

Blakeslee, J.A., Goldman, B.D., Papougenis, D., & Torell, C.A. (1991). Making the transition to restraint-free care. *Journal of Gerontological Nursing, 17*(2), 4–8.

Bower, F., & McCullough, C. (2000). Restraint in acute care settings: Can it be reduced? *Journal of Nursing Administration, 30,* 592–597.

Bradley, L., & Dufton, B. (1995). Breaking free. *Canadian Nurse, 91*(1), 36–40.

Bradley, L., Siddique, C.M., & Dufton, B. (1995). Reducing the use of physical restraints in long-term care facilities. *Journal of Gerontological Nursing, 21*(9), 21–34.

Braun, J.A., & Capezuti, E. (2000). The legal and medical aspects of physical restraints and bedside rails and their relationship to falls and fall-related injuries in nursing homes. *DePaul Journal Health Care Law, 3,* 1–72.

Brower, H.T. (1991). The alternative to restraints. *Journal of Gerontological Nursing, 17,* 18–22.

Brungardt, G.S. (1994). New guidelines for a less restrictive approach. *Geriatrics, 49,* 43–50.

Bruno, R. (1994). Policy for the people: One facility's introduction to restraint reduction. *Journal of Gerontological Social Work, 22*(3/4), 129–142.

Bryant, H., & Fernald, L. (1997). Nursing knowledge and use of restraint alternatives: Acute and chronic care. *Geriatric Nursing, 18*(2), 57–60.

Burton, L.C., German, P.S., Rovner, B.W., & Brandt, L.J. (1992). Physical restraint use and cognitive decline among nursing home residents. *Journal of the American Geriatrics Society, 40,* 811–816.

Calabrese, S., Paulic, T., Callicott, D., et al. (1992). Restraint review committee: A working model. *Perspectives, 16*, 2–6.

Capezuti, E., Evans, L., Strumpf, N., & Maislin, G. (1996). Physical restraint use and falls in nursing home residents. *Journal of the American Geriatrics Society, 44*, 627–633.

Chambers, J. (1993). Eliminating physical restraint use: Implications for practice. *Journal of Nursing Administration, 23*, 5.

Clavon, A.M. (1991). Implementation of a restraint policy: A case study. *Military Medicine, 156*, 499–501.

Conely, L., & Campbell, L. (1991). The use of restraints in caring for the elderly: Realities, consequences, and alternatives. *Nurse Practitioner, 16*(12), 48–52.

Cutchins, C.H. (1991). Blueprint for restraint-free care. *American Journal of Nursing, 91*(7), 36–42.

DeSantis, J., Engberg, S., & Rodgers, J. (1998). Geropsychiatric restraint use. *Journal of the American Geriatrics Society, 12*, 1515–1518.

Dimant, J. (2003). Avoiding physical restraints in long-term care facilities. *Journal of the American Medical Directors Association, 4*(4), 207–215.

Dodds, S. (1996). Exercising restraint: Autonomy, welfare and elderly patients. *Journal of Medical Ethics, 22*(3), 160–163.

Dunbar, J.M., Neufeld, R.R., White, H.C., & Libow, L.S. (1996). Retrain, don't restrain: The educational intervention of the National Nursing Home Restraint Removal Project. *Gerontologist, 36*(4), 539–542.

Dunn, K.S. (2001). The effect of physical restraints on fall rates in older adults who are institutionalized. *Journal of Gerontological Nursing, 27*, 41–48.

Eigsti, D.G., & Vrooman, N. (1992). Releasing restraints in the nursing home: It can be done. *Journal of Gerontological Nursing, 18*(1), 21–23.

Ejaz, F.K., Flomar, S.J., Kaufmann, M., et al. (1994). Restraint reduction: Can it be achieved? *Gerontology, 34*, 694–699.

Ejaz, F.K., Jones, J.A., & Rose, M.S. (1994). Falls among nursing home residents: An examination of incident reports before and after restraint reduction programs. *Journal of the American Geriatrics Society, 42*, 960–964.

Elk, S., & Ferchau, L. (2000). Physical restraints: Are they necessary? *American Journal of Nursing*, (Suppl), 24–27.

Evans, D., Wood, J., & Lambert, L. (2002). A review of physical restraint minimization in the acute and residential care settings. *Journal of Advanced Nursing, 40*, 616–625.

Evans, L.K., & Strumpf, N. (1989). Tying down the elderly: A review of the literature on physical restraints. *Journal of the American Geriatrics Society, 36*, 65–74.

Evans, L.K., & Strumpf, N. (1990). Myths about elder restraint. *Image: Journal of Nursing Scholarship, 22*, 124–128.

Evans, L.K., & Strumpf, N.E. (1992). Alternatives to physical restraints. *Journal of Gerontological Nursing, 18*, 5–11.

Evans, L.K., Strumpf, N.E., Allen-Taylor, S.L., et al. (1997). A clinical trial to reduce restraints in nursing homes. *Journal of the American Geriatrics Society, 45*, 675–681.

Flaherty, J.H. (2004). Zero tolerance for physical restraints: Difficult but not impossible. *Journal of Gerontology: Medical Sciences, 59A*, 919–920.

Fletcher, K.R. (1990). Restraints should be a last resort. *RN, 53*, 52–55.

Frank, C., Hodgetts, G., & Puxty, J. (1996). Safety and efficacy of physical restraint for the elderly: Review of the evidence. *Canadian Family Physician, 42*, 2402–2409.

Gilbert, M., & Counsell, C. (1999). Planned change to implement a restraint reduction program. *Journal of Nursing Care Quality, 13*, 57–64.

Guttman, R., Altman, R.D., & Karlan, M.S. (1999). Report of the council on scientific affairs: Use of restraints for patients in nursing homes. *Archives of Family Medicine, 8*, 101–105.

Hall, M., & Marr, J. (1993). Patient restraint: A new philosophy. *Leadership in Health Services, 2*(4), 22–26, 42.

Hamers, J.P.H., Gulpers, M.J.M., & Strik, W. (2004). Use of physical restraints with cognitively impaired nursing home residents *Journal of Advanced Nursing, 45*, 246–251.

Hardin, S.B., Magee, R., Stratman, D., et al. (1994). Extended care and nursing home attitudes toward restraints. *Journal of Gerontological Nursing, 20*(3), 23–31.

Helmuth, A.M. (1995). Nurses' attitudes toward older persons on the use of physical restraints. *Orthopedic Nursing, 14*(2), 43–51.

Hennessy, C.H., McNelly, E.A., Whittington, F.J., et al. (1997). Perceptions of physical restraint use and barriers to restraint reduction in a long-term care facility. *Journal of Aging Studies, 11*(1), 49–62.

Hughes, R. (2008). Chemical restraint in nursing older people. *Nursing Older People, 20*, 33–38.

Janelli, L.M. (1995). Physical restraint use in acute care settings. *Journal of Nursing Care Quality, 9*(3), 86–92.

Janelli, L.M., Dickerson, S.S., & Ventura, M.R. (1995). Nursing staff's experiences using restraints. *Clinical Nursing Research, 4*(4), 425–441.

Janelli, L.M., Kanski, G.W., & Neary, M.A. (1994). Physical restraints: Has OBRA made a difference? *Journal of Gerontological Nursing, 20*, 17–21.

Janelli, L.M., Scherer, Y.K., Kanski, G.W., & Neary, M.A. (1991). What nursing staff members really know about physical restraints. *Rehabilitation Nursing, 16*, 345–349.

Janelli, L.M., Scherer, Y.K., Kuhn, M.M., et al. (1994). Acute/critical care nurses' knowledge of physical restraints. *Journal of Nursing Staff Development, 10*, 6–11.

Johnson, S.H. (1990). The fear of liability and the use of restraints in nursing homes. *Law, Medicine and Health Care, 18*, 263–273.

Johnson, S.H. (1991). Nursing home restraints: The legal issues. *Health Progress, 23*, 18–19.

Karlsson, S., Bucht, G., Eriksson, S., & Sandman, P. (2001). Factors relating to the use of physical restraints in geriatric care settings. *Journal of the American Geriatrics Society, 49*, 1722–1728.

Kallmann, S.L. (1992). Comfort, safety, and independence: Restraint release and its challenges. *Geriatric Nursing, 13*(3), 143–148.

Kane, R.L., Williams, C.C., Williams, T.F., et al. (1993). Restraining restraints: Changes in a standard of care. *Annual Review of Public Health, 14*, 545–584.

Kapp, M.B. (1992). Nursing home restraints and legal liability. *Journal of Legal Medicine, 13*, 1–32.

Kow, J., & Hogan, D. (2000). Use of physical restraints in medical teaching units. *Canadian Medical Association Journal, 162*, 1–3.

Leger-Krall, S. (1994). When restraints become abusive. *Nurse, 24*, 55–56.

Levine, J.M., Marchello, V., & Totolos, E. (1995). Progress toward a restraint-free environment in a large academic nursing facility. *Journal of the American Geriatrics Society, 43*, 914–918.

Lofgren, R.P., MacPherson, D.S., Granieri, R., et al. (1989). Mechanical restraints on the medical wards: Are protective devices safe? *American Journal of Public Health, 79*, 735–738.

Lusis, S. (2000). Update on restraint use in acute care settings. *Plastic Surgical Nursing, 20*, 145–150.

MacPherson, D.S., Lofgren, R.P., Granier, R., et al. (1990). Deciding to restrain medical patients. *Journal of the American Geriatrics Society, 38*, 516–520.

Magee, R., Hyatt, E.C., Hardin, S.B., et al. (1993). Institutional policy: Use of restraints in extended care and nursing homes. *Journal of Gerontological Nursing, 19*(4), 31–39.

Martin, L.S., & Huges, S.R. (1993). Using the mission statement to craft a least-restraint policy. *Nursing Management, 24*(3), 65–66.

Master, R., & Marks, S.F. (1990). The use of restraints. *Rehabilitation Nursing, 15*, 22–25.

Mayhew, P.A., Christy, K., Berkebile, J., Miller, C., & Farrish, A. (1999). Restraint reduction: Research utilization and case study with cognitive impairment. *Geriatric Nursing, 20*, 305–308.

Mercurio, A.T., & Mion, L.C. (1992). Methods to reduce restraints: Process, outcomes, and future directions. *Journal of Gerontological Nursing, 18*, 5–11.

Miles, S.H., & Irvine, P. (1992). Deaths caused by physical restraint. *Gerontologist, 32*, 762–766.

Minnick, A.F., Mion, L.C., Johnson, M.E., Catrambone, C., & Leipzig, R. (2007). Prevalence and variation of physical restraint use in acute care settings in the U.S. *Journal of Nursing Scholarship, 39,* 30–37.

Minnick, A., Mion, L.C., Leipzig, R., Lamb, K., & Palmer, R.M. (1998). Prevalence and patterns of physical restraint use in the acute care setting. *Journal of Nursing Administration, 28,* 19–24.

Mion, L.C., Fogel, J., Sandhu, S., Palmer, R.M., Minnick, A.F., Cranston, T., Bethoux, F., Merkel, C., Berkman, C.S., & Leipzig, R. (2001). Outcomes following physical restraint reduction programs in two acute care hospitals. *Journal on Quality Improvement, 27,* 605–618.

Mion, L.C., Frengley, J.D., Jakovicie, C.A., et al. (1989). A further exploration of the use of physical restraints in hospitalized patients. *Journal of the American Geriatrics Society, 37,* 949–956.

Mion, L.C., Strump, N., & Fulmer, T. (1994). Use of physical restraints in the hospital setting: Implications for the nurse. *Geriatric Nursing, 15*(3), 127–134.

Mohr, W.K., Petti, R.A., & Mohr, B.D. (2003). Adverse effects associated with physical restraint. *Canadian Journal of Psychiatry, 48,* 330–337.

Morse, J.M., & McHutchion, E. (1991). The behavioral effects of releasing restraints. *Research in Nursing and Health, 14* 187–196.

Mott, S., Poole, J., & Kerrick, M. (2005). Physical and chemical restraints in acute care: Their potential impact on rehabilitation of older people. *International Journal of Nursing Practice, 11,* 95–101.

Neufeld, R.R., Libow, L.S., Foley, W., & White, H. (1995). Can physically restrained nursing-home residents be untied safely? Intervention and evaluation design. *Journal of the American Geriatrics Society, 43,* 1264–1268.

Newbern, V.B., & Lindsey, I.H. (1994). Attitudes of wives toward having their elderly husbands restrained. *Geriatric Nursing, 15,* 135–138.

Patterson, J.E., Stumpf, N.E., & Evans, L.K. (1995). Nursing consultation to reduce restraints in a nursing home. *Clinical Nurse Specialist, 9*(4), 231–235.

Phillips, C., Hawes, C., & Fries, B. (1993). Reducing the use of restraints in nursing homes: Will it increase costs? *American Journal of Public Health, 83*(3), 342–348.

Quinn, C.A. (1993). Nurses' perceptions about physical restraints. *Western Journal of Nursing Research, 15,* 148–162.

Rader, J. (1991). Modifying the environment to decrease the use of restraints. *Journal of Gerontological Nursing, 17,* 9–13

Rader, J., Semradek, J., McKenzie, D., & McMahon, M. (1992). Restraint strategies: Reducing restraints in Oregon's long-term care facilities. *Journal of Gerontological Nursing, 18*(11), 49–56.

Registered Nurses' Association of Nova Scotia. (1995). Position statement on the use of physical restraints . . . approved by the RNANS Board of Directors, April 12, 1995. *Nurse to Nurse, 6*(3), 19.

Rodgers, S. (1994). Reducing restraints in a rehabilitation setting: A safer environment through team effort. *Rehabilitation Nursing, 19,* 274–276.

Scherer, Y.K., Janelli, L.M., Wu, Y.B., & Kuhn, M.M. (1993). Restrained patients: An important issue for critical care nursing. *Heart and Lung, 22,* 77–83.

Schirm, V., Gray, M., & Peoples, M. (1993). Nursing personnel's perceptions of physical restraint in long-term care. *Clinical Nursing Research, 2,* 98–110.

Schnelle, J.F., MacRae, P.G., Simmons, S.F., et al. (1994). Safety assessment for the frail elderly: A comparison of restrained and unrestrained nursing home residents. *Journal of the American Geriatrics Society, 42,* 586–592.

Schnelle, J.F., Newman, D.R., White, M., et al. (1992). Reducing and managing restraints in long term facilities. *Journal of the American Geriatrics Society, 40,* 381–385.

Shugrue, D.T., & Larocque, K.L. (1996). Reducing restraint use in the acute care setting. *Nursing Management, 27*(10), 32H, 32J, 32L, 32O.

Simmons, S.A., Schnelle, J.F., MacRaie, P.G., et al. (1995). Wheelchairs as mobility restraints: Predictors of wheelchair activity in nonambulatory nursing home residents. *Journal of the American Geriatrics Society, 43,* 384–388.

Sloane, P.D., Papougenis, D., & Blakeslee, J.A. (1992). Alternatives to physical and pharmacologic restraints in long-term care. *American Family Physician, 45,* 763–769.

Stolley, J.M. (1995). Freeing your patients from restraints. *American Journal of Nursing, 95*(2), 26–31.

Stolley, S.M., King, J., Clarke, M., et al. (1993). Developing a restraint use policy for acute care. *Journal of Nursing Administration, 23*, 49–54.

Strumpf, N.E., Evans, L.K., Wagner, J., et al. (1992). Reducing physical restraints: Developing an educational program. *Journal of Gerontological Nursing, 18*, 21–27.

Sullivan-Marx, E.M. (1994). Delirium and physical restraints in hospitalized elderly. *Image: Journal of Nursing Scholarship, 26*, 295–300.

Sullivan-Marx, E.M. (1995). Psychological responses to physical restraint use in older adults. *Psychosocial Nursing, 33*(6), 20–25.

Sullivan-Marx, E.M. (1996). Restraint-free care: How does a nurse decide? *Journal of Gerontological Nursing, 22*(9), 7–14.

Sundel, M., Garrett, R.M., & Horn, R.D. (1994). Restraint reduction in a nursing home and its impact on employee attitudes. *Journal of the American Geriatrics Society, 42*, 381–387.

Tan, K.M., Austin, B., Shaughnassy, M., Higgins, C., McDonald, M., Mulkerrin, E.C., & O'Keeffe, S.T. (2005). Falls in an acute hospital and their relationship to restraint use. *Irish Journal of Medical Sciences, 174*, 28–31.

Thomas, A., Redfern, L., & John, R. (1995). Perceptions of acute care nurses in the use of restraints. *Journal of Gerontological Nursing, 21*(6), 32–38.

Tinetti, M.E., Liu, W., & Ginter, S.F. (1992). Mechanical restraint use and fall-related injuries among residents of skilled nursing homes. *Annals of Internal Medicine, 116*, 369–374.

Tinetti, M.E., Liu, W., Marottolil, R.A., et al. (1991). Mechanical restraint use among skilled nursing facilities: Prevalence, patterns and predictors. *Journal of the American Medical Association, 265*, 460–471.

Wells, C.F., Brown, D., & McClymount, A.A. (1994). Development of a least restraint program—one hospital's experience. *Perspectives, 18*, 10–13.

Werner, P., Cohen-Mansfield, J., Braun, J., et al. (1989). Physical restraint and agitation in nursing home residents. *Journal of the American Geriatrics Society, 37*, 1122–1126.

Werner, P., Cohen-Mansfield, J., Koroknay, V., & Braun, J. (1994). Reducing restraint: Impact on staff attitudes. *Journal of Gerontological Nursing, 20*(12), 19–24.

Werner, P., Koroknay, V., Braun, J., & Cohen-Mansfield, J. (1994). Individualized care alternatives used in the process of removing physical restraints in the nursing home. *Journal of the American Geriatrics Society, 42*, 321–325.

Wilson, E.B. (1996). Physical restraint of elderly patients in critical care: Historical perspectives and new directions. *Critical Care Nursing Clinics of North America, 8*(1), 61–70.

SIDE RAILS

Braun, J.A., & Capezuti, E. (2000). Siderail use and legal liability issues in nursing homes. *Illinois Bar Journal, 88*, 34–6, 8–9, 32, 34.

Capezuti, E., Maislin, G., Strumpf, N., & Evans, L. (2002). Side rail use and bed-related fall outcomes among nursing home residents. *Journal of the American Geriatrics Society, 50*, 90–96.

Capezuti, E., Talerico, K.A., Strumpf, N., & Evans L. (1998). Individualized assessment and intervention in bilateral siderail use. *Geriatric Nursing, 19*, 322–330.

Feinsod, F.M., Moore, M., & Levenson, S.A. (1997). Eliminating full-length bedside rails from long-term care facilities. *Nursing Home Medicine, 5*, 257–263.

Gallinagh, R., Slevin, E., & McCormack, B. (2002). Side rails as physical restraints in the care of older people: A management issue. *Journal of Nursing Management, 10*, 299–306.

Gallinagh, R., Slevin, E., & McCormack, B. (2001). Side rails as physical restraints: The need for appropriate assessment. *Nursing Older People, 13*, 22–27.

Hager, H.C. (1999). An analysis of falls in the hospital: Can we do without bedrails? *Journal of the American Geriatrics Society, 47,* 529–531.

Hammond, M., & Levine, J.M. (1999). Bedrails: Choosing the best alternative. *Geriatric Nursing, 20,* 297–300.

Healey, F., Oliver, D., Milne, A., Connelly, J.B. (2008). The effect of bedrails on falls and injury: A systematic review of clinical studies. *Age and Ageing, 37,* 368–378.

Hignett, S., & Griffiths, P. (2005). Do split-side rails present an increased risk to patient safety? *Quality and Safety in Health Care, 14,* 113–116.

Jehan, W. (1999). Restraint or protection? The use of bedside rails. *Nursing Management, 6,* 9–13.

Parker, K., & Miles, S. (1997). Deaths caused by side rails. *Journal of the American Geriatric Society, 45,* 797–802.

Si, M., Neufeld, R., & Dunbar, J. (1999). Removal of bed rails on a short-term nursing home rehabilitation unit. *The Gerontologist, 39,* 611–615.

Talerico, K., & Capezuti, E. (2001). Myths and facts about side rails. *American Journal of Nursing, 101,* 43–48.

van Leeuwen, M., Bennett, L., West, S., Wiles, V., & Grasso, J. (2001). Patient falls from bed and the role of bedrails in the acute care setting. *Australian Journal of Advanced Nursing, 19,* 8–13.

SAFETY TECHNOLOGY

Nelson, A., Powell-Cope, G., Gavin-Dreschnack, D., Quigley, P., Bulat, T., Baptiste, A.S., Applegarth, S., & Friedman, Y. (2004). Technology to promote safe mobility in the elderly. *Nursing Clinics of North America, 39,* 649–671.

Index

Note: *t* indicates table, *f* figure, *b* box, and *n* note.